# Methods in Cell Biology

**VOLUME 38**
Cell Biological Applications of Confocal Microscopy

Leslie Wilson
Department of Biological Sciences
University of California
Santa Barbara, California

Paul Matsudaira
Whitehead Institute for Biomedical Research and
Department of Biology
Massachusetts Institute of Technology
Cambridge, Massachusetts

# Methods in Cell Biology

Prepared under the Auspices of the American Society for Cell Biology

## VOLUME 38
Cell Biological Applications of Confocal Microscopy

Edited by

**Brian Matsumoto**

Microscopy Facility
Neuroscience Research Institute
University of California
Santa Barbara, California

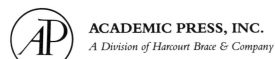

**ACADEMIC PRESS, INC.**

*A Division of Harcourt Brace & Company*

San Diego    New York    Boston    London    Sydney    Tokyo    Toronto

*Cover photograph:* From chapter 4 by T. Clark Brelje. For details see Color Plate 8.

Academic Press, Inc.
1250 Sixth Avenue, San Diego, California 92101-4311

*United Kingdom Edition published by*
Academic Press Limited
24–28 Oval Road, London NW1 7DX

International Standard Serial Number: 0091-679X

International Standard Book Number: 0-12-564138-9 (Hardcover)
International Standard Book Number: 0-12-480430-6 (Paperback)

PRINTED IN THE UNITED STATES OF AMERICA
93  94  95  96  97  98    EB    9  8  7  6  5  4  3  2  1

# CONTENTS

**13.** Three-Dimensional Confocal Light Microscopy of Neurons:
Fluorescent and Reflection Stains

*James N. Turner, John W. Swann, Donald H. Szarowski, Karen L. Smith,
David O. Carpenter, and Michael Fejtl*

# CONTRIBUTORS

*Numbers in parentheses indicate the pages on which the authors' contributions begin.*

**Jonathan J. Art** (47), Pharmacological and Physiological Sciences, The University of Chicago, Chicago, Illinois 60637

**Gary E. Baker** (325), W. M. Keck Center for Integrative Neuroscience, Department of Physiology, University of California, San Francisco, San Francisco, California 94143

**T. Clark Brelje** (97), Department of Cell Biology and Neuroanatomy, University of Minnesota Medical School, Minneapolis, Minnesota 55455

**R. Andrew Cameron** (265), Division of Biology, California Institute of Technology, Pasadena, California 91125

**David O. Carpenter** (345), Wadsworth Center for Laboratories and Research, New York State Department of Health, Albany, New York 12201

**Victoria E. Centonze** (1), Integrated Microscopy Resource for Biomedical Research, University of Wisconsin, Madison, Wisconsin 53706

**A. H. Cornell-Bell** (221), Department of Cell Biology, Yale University School of Medicine, New Haven, Connecticut 06520

**Peter DeVries** (1), Integrated Microscopy Resource for Biomedical Research, University of Wisconsin, Madison, Wisconsin 53706

**Cheryl Emmons** (183), Division of Nephrology, Department of Medicine, UCLA School of Medicine, Los Angeles, California 90024

**Michael Fejtl** (345), Wadsworth Center for Laboratories and Research, New York State Department of Health, Albany, New York 12201

**Per-Ola Forsgren** (79), Molecular Dynamics, Sunnyvale, California 94086

**David L. Gard** (241), Department of Biology, University of Utah, Salt Lake City, Utah 84112

**Miriam B. Goodman** (47), Pharmacological and Physiological Sciences, The University of Chicago, Chicago, Illinois 60637

**F. Gumkowski** (221), Department of Cell Biology, Yale University School of Medicine, New Haven, Connecticut 06520

**Irene L. Hale** (289), Department of Biological Sciences, and Neuroscience Research Institute, University of California, Santa Barbara, Santa Barbara, California 93106

**Laurinda A. Jaffe** (211), Department of Physiology, University of Connecticut Health Center, Farmington, Connecticut 06030

**J. D. Jamieson** (221), Department of Cell Biology, Yale University School of Medicine, New Haven, Connecticut 06520

**Ira Kurtz** (183), Division of Nephrology, Department of Medicine, UCLA School of Medicine, Los Angeles, California 90024

**S. Lawrence** (221), Department of Cell Biology, Yale University School of Medicine, New Haven, Connecticut 06520

**Leslie M. Loew** (195), Department of Physiology, University of Connecticut Health Center, Farmington, Connecticut 06030

**Lars Majlof** (79), Molecular Dynamics, Sunnyvale, California 94086

**Brian Matsumoto** (289), Department of Biological Sciences, and Neuroscience Research Institute, University of California, Santa Barbara, Santa Barbara, California 93106

**K. Olsen** (221), Department of Cell Biology, Yale University School of Medicine, New Haven, Connecticut 06520

**L. R. Otake** (221), Department of Cell Biology, Yale University School of Medicine, New Haven, Connecticut 06520

**Stephen W. Paddock** (1), Howard Hughes Medical Institute, Laboratory of Molecular Biology, University of Wisconsin, Madison, Wisconsin 53706

**J. R. Peterson** (221), Department of Cell Biology, Yale University School of Medicine, New Haven, Connecticut 06520

**Benjamin E. Reese** (325), Neuroscience Research Institute and Department of Psychology, University of California, Santa Barbara, Santa Barbara, California 93106

**K. Sadler** (221), Department of Cell Biology, Yale University School of Medicine, New Haven, Connecticut 06520

**Gerald Schatten** (1), Department of Zoology, University of Wisconsin, Madison, Wisconsin 53706

**Karen L. Smith** (345), Wadsworth Center for Laboratories and Research, New York State Department of Health, Albany, New York 12201

**Robert L. Sorenson** (97), Department of Cell Biology and Neuroanatomy, University of Minnesota Medical School, Minneapolis, Minnesota 55455

**Stephen A. Stricker** (1, 265), Department of Biology, University of New Mexico, Albuquerque, New Mexico 87131

**Robert G. Summers** (265), Department of Anatomy and Cell Biology, State University of New York at Buffalo, Buffalo, New York 14214

**John W. Swann** (345), Wadsworth Center for Laboratories and Research, New York State Department of Health, Albany, New York 12201

**Donald H. Szarowski** (345), Wadsworth Center for Laboratories and Research, New York State Department of Health, Albany, New York 12201

**Mark Terasaki** (211), Laboratory of Neurobiology, National Institute for Neurological Disorders and Stroke, National Institutes of Health, Bethesda, Maryland 20892

**P. G. Thomas** (221), Department of Cell Biology, Yale University School of Medicine, New Haven, Connecticut 06520

**James N. Turner** (345), Wadsworth Center for Laboratories and Research, New York State Department of Health, Albany, New York 12201

**Martin W. Wessendorf** (97), Department of Cell Biology and Neuroanatomy, University of Minnesota Medical School, Minneapolis, Minnesota 55455

**Shirley J. Wright** (1), Department of Zoology, University of Wisconsin, Madison, Wisconsin 53706

# PREFACE

The light microscope has always been a major tool of the cell biologist. In preserved cells, it can be used to localize specific proteins with fluorescent antibodies and in live cells, it can be used to follow dynamic processes with vital dyes. With every advance in optical design, the microscopist has had an opportunity to see more and to obtain a greater understanding of cellular structure. Recently, another new advance in optical design has become available to the researcher, the confocal microscope. Its advantages include increased resolution, higher contrast, and greater depth of field. Together these features promise to increase our understanding of the cell's three dimensional structure as well as its physiology and motility.

These advantages can be realized only if the samples are properly prepared for observation. It has been my experience that a major limitation in the effective application of confocal technology does not have to do with the microscope, but with the manner in which the sample has been prepared for imaging. An investigator must first decide whether the sample, if living, can withstand the intense illumination from the incident beam. Or, in fixed preparations, the investigator must ensure that the specimen is properly preserved to yield accurate images of its architecture. Failure to properly prepare the sample may cause the confocal microscopist to obtain images and data that are inferior to that obtained by more conventional techniques. The intent of this volume is to show the proper techniques to yield superior samples.

Additionally, this volume was prepared for the relatively inexperienced microscopist who has limited time to develop his expertise. It is unfortunate that the expense of these microscopes, coupled with the poor funding environment, has restricted the instruments to shared instrumentation facilities. Thus, the majority of new users have less time than they would like to develop their expertise with the microscope and to get feedback about their sample preparation techniques. For such investigators, this volume should prove especially advantageous. To simplify specimen preparation, specific chapters have detailed protocols so that they can be used at the laboratory bench as "cook book" recipes.

It is hoped that the more experienced investigator may also benefit from this volume. By combining the information from different contributors, it is hoped that the knowledgeable researcher can develop "hybrid" protocols for/preparing/samples not specifically described within this volume. Each chapter of this book is an independent unit; however, its utility can be enhanced by reading and collating the information from other parts of the volume. For example, the chapter on multicolor imaging has useful information that is applicable to single-label studies and thus, to nearly all the protocols within this volume.

In closing, I would like to thank the contributors for devoting their time and energy to the completion of this volume. In addition, I wish to acknowledge the staff of Academic Press, especially Dr. Phyllis B. Moses, for showing extraordinary patience and encouragement in this work. Finally, I would like to thank Dr. Leslie Wilson, the series editor, and Dr. Steven K. Fisher for their support in this project.

**Brian Matsumoto**

# CHAPTER 1

# Introduction to Confocal Microscopy and Three-Dimensional Reconstruction

**Shirley J. Wright,**★,1 **Victoria E. Centonze,**†
**Stephen A. Stricker,**‡ **Peter J. DeVries,**†
**Stephen W. Paddock,**§ **and Gerald Schatten**★

★ Department of Zoology
University of Wisconsin
Madison, Wisconsin 53706

† Integrated Microscopy Resource for Biomedical Research
University of Wisconsin
Madison, Wisconsin 53706

‡ Department of Biology
University of New Mexico
Albuquerque, New Mexico 87131

§ Howard Hughes Medical Institute
Laboratory of Molecular Biology
University of Wisconsin
Madison, Wisconsin 53706

[1] Current address: Department of Biology, University of Dayton, Dayton, Ohio 45469.

1

## I. Introduction

Light and electron microscopy have played vital roles in biological research as important tools for analyzing cellular structure, physiology, and function. Although electron microscopy offers superb resolution of ultrastructural details, it is damaging to specimens and suffers from fixation and sectioning artifacts. In addition, transmission electron microscopy provides static two-dimensional images that are difficult to reconstruct three-dimensionally from serial sections. Conventional light microscopy allows examination of living as well as fixed cells and tissues and therefore dynamic processes can be observed and analyzed quantitatively as they actually occur. Ultrastructural details, however, cannot be obtained because of the relatively low resolution (0.2 $\mu$m). Another difficulty with conventional light microscopy is that out-of-focus information often obscures structures of interest, especially in thick specimens with overlapping structures. Video image processing (video-enhanced microscopy and video-intensified fluorescence microscopy) increases contrast and improves detection (Inoue, 1986, 1989; Shotton, 1988), but does not completely eliminate the problem. An alternative method to remove out-of-focus fluorescence involves computer deconvolution techniques (Agard and Sedat, 1983; Agard *et al.*, 1989). Stunning images are produced by mathematical deconvolution algorithms that make use of the point spread function of the imaging system. The out-of-focus fluorescence is calculated and subtracted from the in-focus image. This successful technique, however, is computer intensive, time consuming, and, until recently, was not commercially available (EM Corp., Newton, MA; Vaytek, Inc., Fairfield, IA). Another solution to the problem of out-of-focus fluorescence is confocal microscopy.

This chapter introduces the principle of confocal microscopy, the types of confocal microscopes currently available, and the various applications of confocal microscopy. Methods of specimen preparation for confocal microscopy are provided as guidelines and should be generally applicable to most cell types. Also included is a discussion of three-dimensional reconstruction and four-dimensional imaging (three-dimensional imaging over time). Methodology for producing color prints and slides of confocal data is also presented. This chapter is principally aimed at prospective or novice confocal microscopists. Additional technical information can be found in several excellent reviews (Inoué, 1989; Pawley, 1989; Shotton, 1989; Wilson, 1990).

## A. Why Confocal Microscopy?

Confocal microscopy offers several advantages over conventional light and electron microscopy. First, the shallow depth of field (0.5–1.5 $\mu$m) of confocal microscopes allows information to be collected from a well-defined optical section rather than from most of the specimen as in the conventional light microscope. Consequently out-of-focus fluorescence is virtually eliminated, which results in an increase in contrast, clarity, and detection sensitivity (Wilson and Sheppard, 1984; see also Inoué, 1989; Shotton, 1989). Second, the confocal microscope optically sections specimens so that physical sectioning artifacts observed with light and electron microscopy are eliminated. Because optical sectioning is noninvasive, living as well as fixed cells can be observed with greater clarity. Another advantage of confocal microscopy is that specimens can be optically sectioned not only in the $xy$ plane (perpendicular to the optical axis of the microscope), but also vertically (parallel to the optical axis of the microscope) in the $xz$ or $yz$ plane (Shotton, 1989; Wilson, 1989). With vertical ($xz$ or $yz$) sectioning, cells are scanned in depth ($z$ axis) as well as laterally ($x$ or $y$ axis), generating images in parallel to the optical axis of the microscope. This gives the effect of looking at a focal plane from the side of the specimen and can show variations in specimen height (Wilson, 1989). Stacks of optical sections taken at successive focal planes (known as a $z$ series) can be reconstructed to produce a three-dimensional view of the specimen. Thus confocal microscopy not only bridges the gap between light and electron microscopy, but provides a means to observe structural components and ionic fluctuations of living cells and tissues in three dimensions without fixation or physical sectioning artifacts.

## B. Confocal Principle

In conventional microscopy, much of the depth or volume of the specimen is uniformly and simultaneously illuminated in addition to the plane in which the objective lens is focused (Fig. 1A). This leads to out-of-focus blur from areas above and below the focal plane of interest. Out-of-focus light reduces contrast and decreases resolution, making it difficult to discern various cellular structures. In contrast, the illumination in a confocal microscope is not simultaneous, but sequential (Inoué, 1989; Shotton, 1989; White et al., 1990). The illumination is focused as a spot on one volume element of the specimen at a time (Fig. 1B). Depending on the specific microscope design, wavelength of light, objective lens, and confocal microscope settings, the spot size may be as small as 0.25 $\mu$m in diameter and 0.5 $\mu$m deep. As the illumination beam diverges above and

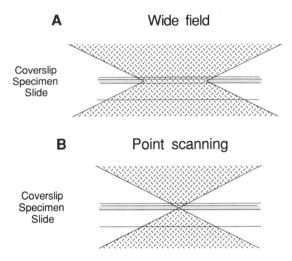

**Fig. 1** Comparison of specimen illumination in conventional and confocal microscopes. (A) and (B) were taken at one instant in time with the same high-numerical aperture oil-immersion objective. In conventional microscopy (A), the whole depth of the specimen is continuously illuminated. Out-of-focus signals are detected as well as the focal plane of interest. In contrast, with a confocal microscope (B), the specimen is scanned with one or more finely focused spots of light that illuminate only a portion of the specimen at one time. Eventually a complete image of the specimen focal plane is produced. Thus conventional fluorescence images of large cells often suffer from out-of-focus information, whereas this problem is reduced in confocal fluorescence images. [From Shotton, D. M. (1989). *J. Cell Sci.* **94,** 175–206, with permission from the Company of Biologists, Ltd., and Shotton, D. M. (1993). *In* "Electronic Light Microscopy: Techniques in Modern Biomedical Microscopy" (D. M. Shotton, ed.). Copyright © 1993, Wiley-Liss, New York. Reprinted by permission of Wiley-Liss, a Division of John Wiley and Sons, Inc.]

below the plane of focus, volume elements away from the focal plane receive less illumination, thus reducing some of the out-of-focus information (Fig. 1B).

Confocal imaging systems are based on the principle of Minsky (1957, 1988), that both the illumination and detection (imaging) systems are focused on the same single volume element of the specimen (Fig. 2). The illuminated volume elements are sampled in such a way that mainly signals from the volume elements in the focal plane are detected, and signals from outside the plane of focus are removed by a spatial filter, which further reduces out of-focus information (Figs. 2 and 3). Thus the illumination, specimen, and detector all have the same focus, that is, they are confocal.

To achieve confocal imaging, excitation light from a laser in laser scanning confocal microscopes is directed toward the specimen (Fig. 4). The beam of light passes through a scanning system and reaches the objective, which focuses the scanning beam as a spot on the specimen. Fluorescence emissions generated by the specimen scatter in all directions. Fluorescence from the focal plane of the

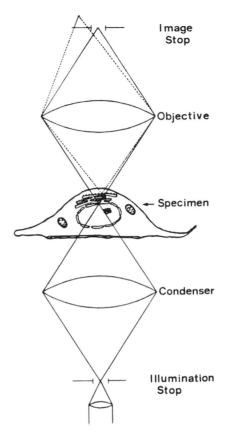

**Fig. 2**  Optics diagram showing the function of apertures in reducing out-of-focus light. Membranes of the cell are labeled with a membrane-permeant fluorescent dye. Although the illuminating beam is focused on the focal plane of the nuclear envelope, structures from above and below also intercept the incident light and fluoresce. Fluorescence emitted from the various focal planes is collected by the objective lens. In-focus light from the nuclear envelope passes through the spatial filter and is detected. Out-of-focus light from other focal planes such as the endoplasmic reticulum is essentially blocked by the spatial filter (image stop), so that mainly in-focus fluorescence is detected. Both the illumination and detection (imaging) systems are focused on the same single volume element of the cell, that is, they are confocal. [Reprinted with permission from Shuman, H., *et al.* (1989). *BioTechniques* **7,** 154–163. Copyright © 1989, Eaton Publishing Co.]

specimen returns via the objective and scanning system, and is reflected off the dichroic mirror and focused on a detector. In front of the detector is a spatial filter containing an aperture (pinhole diaphragm or slit), which defines the image of the spot in the focal plane of the microscope. Most fluorescence originating from above or below the plane of focus of the specimen does not pass through the aperture of the spatial filter and, as a result, little out-of-focus light reaches the detector. Thus the spatial filter not only provides continuous access to the

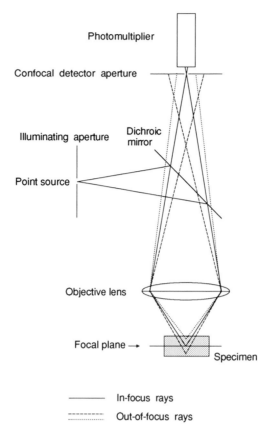

Photomultiplier

Confocal detector aperture

Illuminating aperture          Dichroic
                               mirror

Point source

Objective lens

Focal plane →

Specimen

——————— In-focus rays

---------- Out-of-focus rays

**Fig. 3** Schematic diagram demonstrating the confocal principle in epifluorescence microscopy. Excitation light enters through an illumination aperture, reflects off a dichroic mirror, and is focused on the specimen by the objective lens. The longer wavelength fluorescence emissions generated by the sample return via the objective and pass through the dichroic mirror. Light primarily from the focal plane of the objective passes through the imaging aperture and is detected by a photomultiplier tube. In contrast, light from above and below the plane of focus is not focused on the aperture and is attenuated by it. As a result, out-of-focus light is virtually eliminated from the final confocal image. [From Shotton, D. M. (1989). *J. Cell Sci.* **94**, 175–206, with permission from the Company of Biologists, Ltd., copyright © 1989, and Shotton, D. M. (1993). An introduction to the electronic acquisition of light microscope images. *In* "Electronic Light Microscopy: Techniques in Modern Biomedical Microscopy" (D. M. Shotton, ed.). Copyright © 1993, Wiley-Liss, New York. Reprinted by permission of Wiley-Liss, a Division of John Wiley and Sons, Inc.]

detector for in-focus light, but also effectively suppresses light from nonfocal planes. To form a two-dimensional image, the laser beam scans the specimen in a raster pattern, that is, horizontally and vertically, and the induced fluorescent light is detected and converted to a video signal for display on a computer screen.

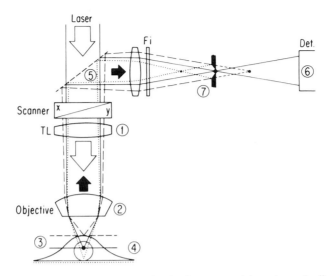

**Fig. 4** Basic design of a laser scanning confocal microscope. A laser beam is directed onto the specimen by a scanning system and is focused on the cell by a high-numerical aperture objective lens. A specimen point in the focal plane of the objective lens, here depicted as a spot in the cell nucleus, is illuminated by the scanning laser beam. Induced fluorescent or reflected light is scattered in all directions. Some of this light is collected by the objective lens and directed through the scanning system toward the beam splitter. In-focus light from the nucleus retraces the incident light path, and is directed by the highly reflective beam splitter, through the imaging aperture to the detector. In contrast, out-of-focus light from the cytoplasm (dotted and dashed lines) has a different primary image plane of focus and is attenuated by the imaging aperture. Thus out-of-focus information is essentially not detected in the final confocal image. 1, Tube lens; 2, objectives; 3, out-of-focus region; 4, focal plane; 5, dichroic reflector; 6, detector; 7, pinhole. (Courtesy of Carl Zeiss, Inc., Thornwood, NY.)

Because of its speed and sensitivity, the detector is usually a low-noise photomultiplier tube that efficiently converts light energy into electrical energy. Light striking a phosphor causes electrons to be released, which are then collected and multiplied into a signal that is amplified and subsequently converted into a video signal for display on a video monitor. The result of confocal imaging provides optical sections with exceptional contrast and often with striking details previously blurred by out-of-focus information.

## II. Anatomy of Confocal Microscopes

Different methods of scanning are employed to achieve confocal imaging and three major confocal instrument designs have emerged to date. Confocal microscopes employ either a laterally moving stage and stationary beam of light (stage scanning), a scanning beam of light and stationary stage (beam scanning), or both a stationary stage and light source (spinning disk). Each has characteristics desirable for various confocal applications.

## A. Stage Scanning Confocal Microscope

The stage scanning type of confocal microscope scans a field of view much larger than the actual field of view of the objective with high resolution (Sheppard and Choudhury, 1977; Brakenhoff, 1979; Wilson and Sheppard, 1984; Wijnaendts van Resandt *et al.*, 1985; see also Shotton, 1989). Because the optical arrangement is stationary and the specimen is scanned with a single beam, the stage scanning confocal microscope has the advantage of constant axial illumination. This minimizes optical aberrations from the objective and condenser, and provides an even optical response across the entire scanned field, which is an important feature for image processing. A limitation is the slow scanning speed, although this can be reduced by scanning a smaller pixel field. Another disadvantage is that specimens on the stage are moved during the scan to produce an image and therefore cells must be firmly fixed to the slide or they may shift during image acquisition, resulting in a distorted image. This is especially apparent with living cells suspended in aqueous media. A stage scanning confocal microscope is commercially available from Meridian Instruments, Inc. (Okemos, MI).

## B. Beam Scanning Confocal Microscope

The beam scanning class of confocal microscopes usually employs rapidly scanning mirrors to scan a laser beam across the specimen. This allows detection either of the induced fluorescence or reflected primary beam (Carlsson *et al.*, 1985; Wilke, 1985; White *et al.*, 1987; see also Shotton, 1989). This type of confocal microscope, known as the confocal laser scanning microscope (CLSM), is the most commonly employed in biological studies to date and is especially useful for confocal fluorescence imaging. The CLSM has superb resolution and a relatively faster scan rate than the stage scanning instruments. It also has the advantage of using conventional epifluorescence microscopy to locate the specimen before confocal fluorescence imaging. This is helpful for localizing the region of interest in the specimen because, when the objective is focused above or below the cell or tissue in a CLSM, the images generated are completely black (because little out-of-focus fluorescence contributes to the focal plane of interest); whereas with conventional imaging, an out-of-focus image is present.

Commonly used lasers for CLSMs include an argon ion laser, which emits at 488 and 514 nm, and a krypton–argon ion laser, which emits at 488, 568, and 647 nm (see also Gratton and van de Ven, 1989, for other laser types). The emission lines of these lasers efficiently excite many fluorochromes that are used in biological applications (Tsien and Waggoner, 1989; Haugland, 1990). With the appropriate excitation filters, observation of cellular structures tagged with fluorescein, rhodamine, and longer wavelength dyes (e.g., cyanine dyes) is possible. However, dyes excited by shorter wavelengths (340–360 nm) such as the ultraviolet (UV)-excitable dyes, Hoechst and 4,6-diamidino-2-phenylindole

(DAPI), cannot be imaged with CLSMs equipped with the longer wavelength argon ion or krypton–argon ion lasers. Optics in the microscope also need to be altered to accommodate the shorter wavelength UV beam. Confocal microscopes equipped with UV lasers and suitable optics to image UV-excitable dyes (Robert-Nicoud *et al.*, 1989; Arndt-Jovin *et al.*, 1990) are becoming commercially available in the United States (Carl Zeiss, Inc., Thornwood, NY; Bio-Rad Microscience, Hercules, CA; Olympus Corporation, Marietta, GA).

There are two types of CLSM: a slow-scan and a video-rate confocal microscope. They differ in the way specimens are scanned and acquired. Each has characteristics that are advantageous for different biological applications.

## 1. Slow–Scan Confocal Laser Scanning Microscope

Slow-scan confocal instruments can be mounted on upright or inverted microscopes and detect both fluorescent and reflected confocal images (Figs. 4 and 5). Thus high-resolution, multiple-labeled specimens are observed with greater clarity than with conventional light microscopes. Most slow-scan CLSMs use software to control the microscope during image acquisition and to further process confocal images. Images are processed either during collection (e.g., by summing or averaging) or after (e.g., contrast enhancement, pseudocoloring, and merging two different images into one double-labeled image). The slow-scan CLSM uses highly reflective, independent galvanometer mirrors to produce the horizontal and vertical patterns of the raster scan (Fig. 5). Mechanical limitations of the galvanometers restrict the speed at which a single frame can be scanned. A full $512 \times 512 \times 8$-bit image may take as long as 2 sec to acquire. As a result, rapid cellular processes, such as ionic changes, cannot be imaged at high resolution without blur, or are entirely missed. Extremely fast events may, however, be resolved at full-screen image size by using a lower pixel resolution, or at a smaller screen size by using full pixel resolution. Slow-scan CLSMs require a digital frame buffer to collect the image line by line and store it in computer memory. This may also reduce acquisition speed of rapid events, but does not pose a problem with fixed specimens. Once assembled, the static image is displayed on the video monitor until a new optical section is collected. Slow-scan CLSMs are available from Bio-Rad Microscience, Carl Zeiss, Inc., Leica, Inc. (Deerfield, IL), Molecular Dynamics (Sunnyvale, CA), and Olympus Corporation.

## 2. Video–Rate Confocal Laser Scanning Microscope

The video-rate CLSM differs from the slow-scan CLSM in its mode of scanning the specimen and image formation (Figs. 6 and 7). Because images are generated at video rates (30 Hz) or faster (up to 120 Hz), rapid, cellular processes can be analyzed as they occur in real time at full-screen image size and resolution. Two CLSM designs are commercially available to achieve video-rate imaging. Each uses a variable slit aperture in conjunction with either an

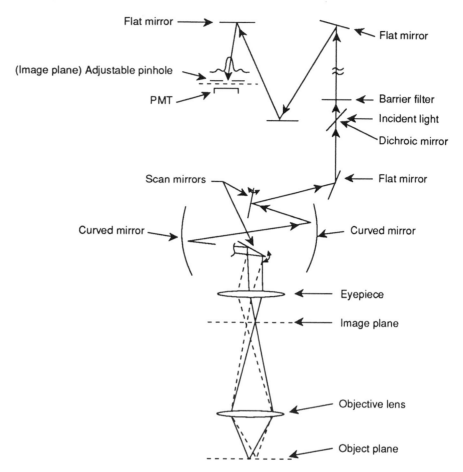

**Fig. 5** Optical light path through a slow-scan confocal laser-scanning microscope (Bio-Rad MRC-500). Light from a multiline argon ion laser passes through an excitation filter that allows selection of either 488-nm light (e.g., blue for fluorescein fluorescence) or 514-nm light (e.g., green for rhodamine fluorescence). The incident laser light is reflected off a dichroic mirror and directed into the scanning unit by highly reflective mirrors. Two oscillating galvanometer mirrors in the scanning unit generate the *x*- and *y*-scanning movements of the laser beam. Two curved mirrors direct the scanning beam between the *x*- and *y*-scanning galvanometer mirrors. The *y* axis-scanning galvanometer mirror directs the beam to the high-numerical aperture objective lens, which focuses the light as a scanning spot moving across the focal plane of the specimen. Induced fluorescence generated by the specimen retraces its path back through the scanning system. The fluorescence then passes through the dichroic mirror and barrier filter, which cuts off wavelengths close to the excitation light source. The longer wavelength fluorescence that passes through the barrier filter is directed by a series of highly reflective mirrors to another dichroic mirror (not shown) that distinguishes between various wavelengths (e.g., fluorescein and rhodamine fluorescence). Fluorescent light of appropriate wavelength then passes through a barrier filter (not shown) and an adjustable pinhole aperture. On the other side of the pinhole aperture is a photomultiplier tube that detects and converts the fluorescence into a video signal that is displayed on the television monitor as a confocal image. [From Webb, W. W., *et al.* (1990). *In* "Optical Microscopy for Biology" (B. Herman and K. Jacobson, eds.). Copyright © 1990, Alan R. Liss, New York. Reprinted by permission of Wiley-Liss, a Division of John Wiley and Sons, Inc.]

acousto-optical deflector (AOD) or a highly reflective, two-sided, scanning mirror element (bilateral scanning). Neither video-rate CLSM requires storage in computer memory to display an image, as do the slow-scan CLSMs.

The optical light path through the video-rate CLSM containing an AOD and a single-sided, scanning galvanometer mirror is shown schematically in Fig. 6. The AOD is an electrically controllable diffraction grating that generates the high-frequency (15.6 kHz) horizontal scan of the laser beam (Draijer and Houpt, 1988, 1993). As piezoelectric transducers attached to the glass AOD cause acoustic waves to propagate throughout the glass, the waves, acting as gratings, diffract the incident laser light. The diffracted beam then strikes a galvanometer mirror that oscillates at the slower 60 Hz to produce the vertical scan. In the reflectance mode, reflected light returns to the detector through the AOD. However, for confocal fluorescence imaging, the induced fluorescent light has an emission wavelength longer than the excitation wavelength (Stokes shift) of the laser beam. As a result, the entire spectral width of the fluorescence emission cannot be descanned back through the wavelength-specific AOD without a significant loss of signal intensity. To compensate for this, the partially de-scanned fluorescence originating from the sample is directed by a dichroic mirror between the galvanometer mirror and the AOD. The fluorescence passes through a barrier filter, and is imaged through a variable-slit aperture before detection with a photomultiplier tube and conversion into a video signal. Thus video output from the microscope can be directly connected to a television monitor to produce live images and does not require computer storage, as do slow-scan CLSMs. A commercial version of this video-rate CLSM is available from Noran Instruments (Middleton, WI).

Another method to achieve video-rate scanning with CLSMs uses bilateral scanning and a variable slit aperture (Fig. 7). In bilateral scanning, the same side of a highly reflective, double-sided, galvanometer-driven mirror is used to scan and descan the specimen, and the other side is used to scan the detector at video rates to generate a confocal image (Brakenhoff and Visscher, 1992). A variable slit aperture placed in an optically conjugate plane with the illumination slit suppresses out-of-focus information. The in-focus light that passes through the slit is scanned by the back surface of the double-sided mirror and directed to either the oculars for viewing by eye, or to a camera [e.g., 35-mm, video, cooled charge-coupled device (CCD) camera]. This allows confocal viewing by eye of fluorescent specimens in their apparent full colors. Direct confocal viewing by eye is possible in the fluorescence mode because the dichroic mirror does not reflect the laser beam to the eyepiece (Fig. 7). In the reflectance mode, direct confocal viewing by eye is not possible. A version of this video-rate CLSM is commercially available from Meridian Instruments.

## C. Spinning Disk Confocal Microscope

The third type of confocal microscope employs a spinning Nipkow disk and stationary light source and stage (Figs. 8 and 9). With the spinning disk confocal

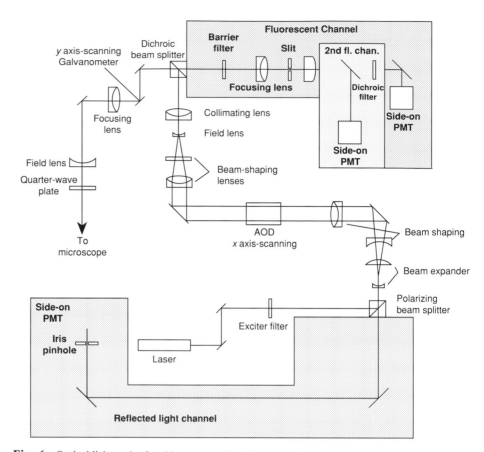

**Fig. 6** Optical light path of a video-rate confocal laser-scanning microscope containing an acousto-optical deflector system (AOD). Light from an argon ion laser is directed by highly reflective mirrors through an excitation filter. The incident laser light is reflected off a polarizing beam splitter and directed toward the scanning system. The scanning system of the video-rate CLSM has an AOD that generates the horizontal $x$ axis-scanning movements of the laser beam. A scanning galvanometer mirror is used to produce vertical, $y$ axis-scanning movements. After passing through the scanning system, the laser light is directed to the objective lens, which focuses the scanning beam on the specimen. Reflected light from the specimen retraces the incident light path (traveling in the reverse direction) back through the scanning system and through the polarizing beam splitter, where it is directed by highly reflective mirrors through an adjustable pinhole aperture. Light that traverses the aperture is detected by a photomultiplier tube that converts the reflected light into an electrical signal. This signal is then converted into a video signal that is displayed on the image monitor. Induced fluorescence from the sample is detected after passing through a different route. Fluorescence from the specimen retraces the illuminating light path until it reaches the dichroic beam splitter. Unlike reflected light, the longer wavelength-induced fluorescence from the sample passes through the dichroic mirror, where some of it is excluded by the barrier filter before entering the slit aperture. A dichroic mirror on the other side of the slit aperture distinguishes between various fluorescence emission wavelengths (e.g., fluorescein and rhodamine) and directs the light beam accordingly. The fluorescence is then directed to a photomultiplier tube where it is converted to a video signal and displayed on the image monitor. (Courtesy of M. Szulczewski and D. Kinser, Noran Instruments, Middleton, WI.)

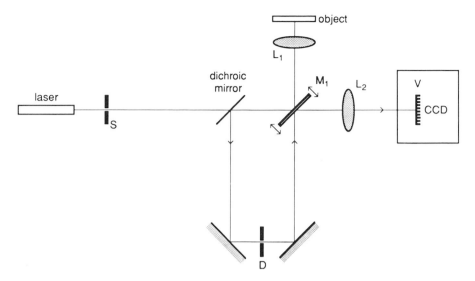

**Fig. 7** Schematic diagram of a video-rate confocal laser-scanning microscope with a bilateral scanning system. This confocal microscope uses a double-sided, rapidly scanning galvanometer mirror (bilateral scanning) to scan the specimen. Light from a laser passes through a slit aperture (S) and dichroic mirror and is scanned onto the specimen by the front surface of mirror $M_1$. The longer wavelength fluorescence emitted by the specimen (object) is descanned by the same mirror surface and reflected by the dichroic mirror. The fluorescence is directed through a variable detection slit aperture (D) and placed in an optically conjugate plane with the illumination aperture to create the confocal effect. The in-focus light that passes through the slit is scanned by the back surface of the double-sided mirror and is directed either to the oculars for direct confocal viewing by eye or to a camera [e.g., 35-mm, video (V), or cooled charge-coupled device (CCD)]. [From Brakenhoff, G. J., and Visscher, K. (1992). *J. Microsc.* (*Oxford*) **165**, 139–146. Reprinted by permission of Blackwell Scientific Publications.]

microscope, cells can be seen directly by eye in color as a confocal image in both reflected and fluorescence modes (Paddock, 1989; Wright *et al.*, 1989; Boyde *et al.*, 1990). This allows direct confocal focusing through the specimen. Unlike CLSMs, which use a single spot of light to scan the specimen, spinning disk confocal microscopes scan the specimen with many spots of light simultaneously. Light from each spot traces a single scan over successive parts of the specimen. Spinning disk confocal microscopes also differ from CLSMs in that instead of using laser light to scan the specimen, a broad-spectrum, noncoherent light (white light) is the illumination source as in conventional light and fluorescence microscopy. This permits full selection of filter combinations typically employed for conventional epifluorescence. Dyes excited by UV, such as DNA fluorochromes, can be imaged confocally in addition to fluorescein, rhodamine, and infrared dyes. Hence, cells labeled with three or more fluorochromes can be imaged confocally (Wright *et al.*, 1989, 1990). However, the Nipkow disk typically transmits only 1% of the illumination, resulting in dim fluorescence images.

Unless fluorescent samples are bright, an intensifying video camera or cooled CCD camera must be used to generate sufficient signals and improve the signal-to-noise ratio. The relatively large aperture size (60 $\mu$m) of the holes in the Nipkow disk as compared to CLSMs compromises optical sectioning so that optical section thickness may be 1 $\mu$m for spinning disk microscopes as compared to 0.5–0.6 $\mu$m for CLSMs with the same objective. The design of the spinning disk confocal microscopes also differs from the CLSMs in that only $xy$ sectioning, not orthogonal $xz$ sectioning, is possible. There are two types of spinning disk microscopes: the tandem scanning and "mono" scanning microscope.

## 1. Tandem Scanning Confocal Microscope

The Nipkow disk of the tandem scanning confocal microscope (TSM) contains thousands of apertures (20–60 $\mu$m in diameter) that are in tandem or diametrically opposed pairs arranged in spirals (Fig. 8) (Egger and Petran, 1967; Petran *et al.,* 1968, 1985). Each aperture on one side of the Nipkow disk serves as an illumination aperture, and acts as a small diffraction-limited spot in the focal plane of the objective, which focuses the multiple illuminating spots on the specimen (Fig. 8). In-focus light from the specimen is detected after passing through the conjugate aperture on the opposite side of the disk. High-speed rotation (up to 2400 rpm) of the Nipkow disk causes the spots of light to scan the specimen many times a second and produce an apparent real-time image. This yields a stable, continuous confocal image in fluorescence and reflectance modes that can be directly viewed by eye in real time. A video camera connected to the microscope also allows direct confocal recording and digital image processing of the specimen. Therefore the TSM offers the advantage of real-time imaging and direct confocal viewing of true image colors by eye in both reflected and fluorescence modes. A TSM is commercially available from Noran Instruments.

## 2. Monoscanning Confocal Microscope

The monoscanning spinning disk confocal microscope also employs a Nipkow disk with spirally arranged apertures (Xiao and Kino, 1987; Xiao *et al.,* 1988; Kino, 1989; Lichtman *et al.,* 1989). It produces images in real time and uses noncoherent white light for illumination. Unlike the TSM, the monoscanning confocal microscope detects light through the same aperture from which a given area of the specimen was illuminated (Fig. 9). Thus illumination and imaging are performed simultaneously through the same aperture. This design permits easier alignment of the Nipkow disk. To eliminate unwanted light reflected by the Nipkow disk, one version of this confocal microscope tilts the Nipkow disk and uses polarized light (Kino, 1989). Commercial versions of the monoscanning spinning disk confocal microscope are available from Newport Bio-Instruments (Fountain Valley, CA) and Technical Instrument Co. (San Jose, CA).

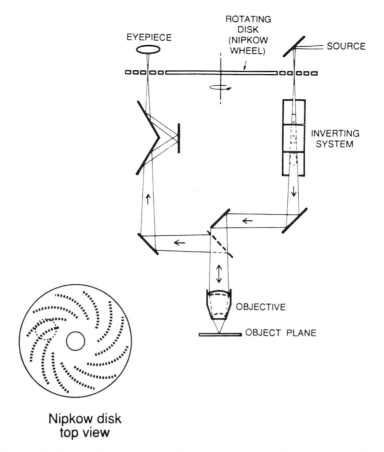

Nipkow disk
top view

**Fig. 8** Schematic diagram showing the optical path through the tandem scanning confocal micro-scope. White light from a conventional light source (typically a mercury or xenon arc lamp) passes through an excitation filter (not shown) before being directed onto a spinning Nipkow disk that contains thousands of 20- to 60-$\mu$m apertures arranged in a precise spiral pattern. As the light falls on one side of the disk, it passes through the apertures. After passing through an inverting system, the spots of light are directed to the objective, where they are focused on the specimen. High-speed rotation (up to 2400 rpm) of the Nipkow disk causes the spots of light to scan the specimen. The induced fluorescent or reflected light produced by the specimen is collected by the objective lens and reflected off a beam splitter and highly reflective mirrors to the conjugate apertures on the other side of the spinning disk. The in-focus fluorescence from the specimen passes through the conjugate apertures and a barrier filter (not shown) before being detected. In contrast, out-of-focus light from the specimen does not have a conjugate aperture to pass through, and is stopped by the disk, contributing little to the confocal image. The time taken to traverse the field of view is so short that an apparent real-time image is produced at the eyepiece. Thus the specimen can be observed confocally by eye if the sample is of sufficient brightness, or with cameras (e.g., 35-mm, video, or cooled charge-coupled device). Because the apertures in the disk are arranged in spirals, an inverting system is placed under the illumination side of the Nipkow disk in order for the conjugate apertures to line up, and a series of mirrors directs the spots of light to the beam splitter. On the detection side of the Nipkow disk, a system of mirrors maintains an equal distance for the optical path on both sides of the disk to create the confocal effect. [From Kino, G. S. (1989). *In* "The Handbook of Biological Confocal Microscopy" (J. Pawley, ed.), IMR Press, Madison, WI, with permission.]

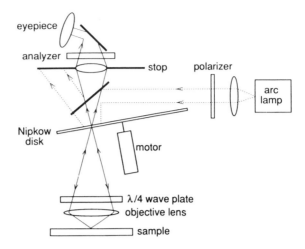

**Fig. 9** Schematic diagram of the optical path in a monoscanning confocal microscope. White light from a conventional light source (e.g., mercury or xenon arc lamp) is passed through a polarizer and directed onto the Nipkow disk. A typical microscope uses a disk with 200,000 pinholes, 20–25 $\mu$m in diameter, rotated at ~2000 rpm to produce a 700-frame/sec 5000-line image. Thus thousands of spots of light are focused by the objective and scan the specimen at any one time. Reflected light or fluorescence emitted from the sample passes through a quarter-wave plate and retraces its path through the same illumination aperture. Light from the focal plane of the specimen passes through an analyzer before being detected at the eyepiece. Out-of-focus light does not enter the apertures and is not imaged. The specimen can be viewed confocally by eye if the sample is sufficiently bright. A camera (35-mm, video, or cooled charge-coupled device) may also be used to observe specimens confocally. To reduce unwanted reflected light from the disk, the disk is made of a low-reflective material, the disk is tilted, and a stop is placed where light reflected from the disk is focused. To eliminate the remaining reflected light, the input light is polarized by the polarizer, rotated 90° by the quarter-wave plate, and observed through an analyzer with its plane of polarization at right angles to that of the input light. [From Kino, G. S. (1990). *In* ''The Handbook of Biological Confocal Microscopy'' (J. Pawley, ed.), Rev. Ed., Plenum, New York, with permission.]

## III. Procedures and Protocols

Eggs and embryos are ideal biological specimens for the analysis of confocal fluorescence imaging because of their relatively large size (~100 $\mu$m in diameter) and overlapping features, which contribute to out-of-focus fluorescence when viewed with conventional epifluorescence microscopy. In addition, eggs undergo ionic fluctuations at fertilization and at various times during the cell cycle (Epel, 1978). Confocal fluorescence microscopy facilitates the full use of ion-indicating dyes at high resolution because information is obtained only from the region of interest. The following methods are specifically designed for preparing fixed and living eggs and embryos for confocal fluorescence imaging and three-dimensional reconstruction. The specimen preparation methods and specific confocal microscope settings provided below worked best for our samples and are meant as guidelines for preparing and imaging other types of specimens. Our methods should be generally applicable to other cell types.

## A. Confocal Microscopic Anatomy of Fixed Cells

Methods are presented to visualize one or more cellular components with fluorescently labeled probes. Protocols are also included for the prevention of artificial flattening of specimens during mounting and confocal viewing.

## 1. Specimen Preparation and Immunocytochemistry

Sea urchin (*Lytechinus pictus*, *Strongylocentrotus purpuratus*) and surf clam (*Spisula solidissima*) eggs and embryos were obtained and fertilized (Costello *et al.*,1957; Lutz and Inoue, 1986). Embryos were either fixed in methanol at −20°C for 10 min and stained for 5 min with 2.5 $\mu m$ thiazole orange (Molecular Probes, Eugene, OR) or processed for immunocytochemistry.

Sea urchin eggs contain an extracellular coat that rises and hardens after fertilization. This coat needs to be removed because it is impermeable to antibodies during immunofluorescence procedures. Several means are available for coat removal (Hinegardner, 1975; Harris, 1986). We treated fertilized eggs with 5 m$M$ aminotriazole, which prevents hardening of the fertilization coat by inhibiting ovoperoxidase activity released during the cortical granule reaction (Showman and Foerder, 1979). Treated eggs were stripped of fertilization coats and either directly fixed in methanol as above or prior to fixation, extracted in microtubule preservation buffer containing 10 m$M$ ethylene glycol-bis($\beta$-aminoethyl ether)-$N,N,N',N'$-tetraacetic acid (EGTA), 0.5 $M$ MgCl$_2$, 25 m$M$ phenylmethylsulfonylfluoride, 25% glycerol, 2% Triton X-100, and 23 m$M$ $N$-2-hydroxyethylpiperazine-$N'$-2-ethanesulfonic acid (HEPES) (pH 6.9) (Balczon and Schatten, 1983). For egg extraction, a 10- to 15-ml aliquot of the egg suspension was gently centrifuged and the pelleted eggs were resuspended in 40–50 ml of extraction buffer at room temperature for 2–4 hr or overnight. The eggs were allowed to settle on polylysine (1 mg/ml)-coated coverslips (Mazia *et al.*, 1975) and processed for immunofluorescence microscopy with specific antibodies (Table I), using anti-tubulin antibody and fluorescein isothiocyanate (FITC)-labeled secondary antibody, followed by anti-centrosome antibody and rhodamine-labeled secondary antibody (Balczon and Schatten, 1983; Schatten *et al.*, 1988) and Hoechst 33258 for DNA (Luttmer and Longo, 1986).

Surf clam eggs were processed for immunocytochemistry with anti-tubulin antibody, FITC-labeled secondary antibody (Kuriyama *et al.*, 1983), and Hoechst 33342 for DNA (Luttmer and Longo, 1986). *Drosophila* embryos were prepared for immunofluorescence according to Kraut and Levine (1991), using anti-*Krüppel* and tetramethylrhodamine isothiocyanate (TRITC)-conjugated second antibody, and anti-*hunchback* and FITC-conjugated secondary antibody.

**Table I**
**Immunolabeling Fixed Sea Urchin Eggs for Confocal Fluorescence Microscopy**

1. Settle fertilized eggs on a polylysine (1 mg/ml)-coated coverslip in a six-well plate for 5–10 min for living eggs and 20–30 min for eggs extracted in microtubule stabilization buffer.
2. To fix the eggs, place the coverslip in a well containing cold (−20°C) 100% methanol and fix for 10 min at −20°C.
3. Rehydrate in phosphate-buffered saline (PBS), pH 7.4, and wash twice (10 min each wash). May be left in second wash for several hours.
4. Touch the edge of the coverslip to a Kimwipe to remove excess fluid prior to placing the coverslip on top of the dividers of a four-compartment, $100 \times 15$ mm petri dish (XPlate, Falcon 1009) containing a moistened Kimwipe in one of the compartments.
5. Add 50–100 $\mu$l of primary antibody to the coverslip and incubate for 1 hr at 37°C.
6. Resuspend in PBS as in step 3.
7. Add the next primary antibody as in steps 4 and 5 and repeat step 6.
8. Incubate the coverslip with 50–100 $\mu$l of a suitable secondary antibody for 1 hr at 37°C, as in step 5.
9. Wash in PBS, as in step 3.
10. The coverslips are now ready to be mounted (see Table II).

## 2. Mounting

Specimens are placed in mounting media to prevent dehydration and fading during storage and confocal viewing. Several types of mounting media are available (Harris, 1986). For our studies, we used buffered glycerol, which is composed of 90% glycerol in 10% phosphate-buffered saline (PBS), pH 7.4. It is important that the mounting medium of choice should contain a suitable antioxidant such as 1,4-diazabicyclo[2.2.2]octane (DABCO; Johnson *et al.*, 1982; Langanger *et al.*, 1983), *p*-phenylenediamine (Johnson and Nogueira Araujo, 1981; Johnson *et al.*, 1982), or *n*-propyl gallate (Giloh and Sedat, 1982) to reduce photobleaching during confocal viewing and loss of fluorescence during storage of samples on slides. The antioxidant we used was either DABCO (100 mg/ml; Aldrich Chemical Co., Milwaukee, WI) or *p*-phenylenediamine (100 mg/ml; Sigma Chemical Co., St. Louis, MO) in 90% glycerol in 10% PBS. Specimens mounted in these media and stored at 4°C were initially well preserved; however, fluorescence in *p*-phenylenediamine tended to fade within 1–3 days, whereas fluorescence in DABCO mounting medium lasted more than 1 month. A stock of DABCO stored at room temperature in an air-tight glass container should last 6 months before yellowing, when it should be discarded. Mounting medium containing *p*-phenylenediamine can be stored at −20°C for 2–3 weeks before it blackens and should be discarded.

To minimize artificial flattening of specimens, spacers were placed between the coverslip and slide prior to mounting (Table II). Spacers were made from broken coverslips (type 0 or 1) or gel (silicone grease, petroleum jelly). Clear nail

**Table II**
**Mounting Coverslips for Confocal Microscopy**
**and Three-Dimensional Reconstruction**

1. To prevent eggs and embryos from being flattened by the coverslip, make spacers by breaking coverslips into long strips to use as supports.
2. Position four spacers on a clean, labeled glass slide to accommodate all sides of the coverslip.
3. With a wooden applicator, place a small drop of mounting medium containing an antioxidant on a slide between the spacers. Mounting medium consists of 1,4-diazabicyclo[2.2.2]octane (100 mg/ml; Aldrich Chemical Co., Milwaukee, WI) in 90% glycerol in 10% PBS.
4. After rinsing the coverslip in distilled water, dry the back and sides with a Kimwipe.
5. Immediately place the coverslip (cell side down) on top of the spacers on the glass slide. The mounting medium should contact the coverslip and spread over its surface.
6. Gently wipe off excess mounting medium with a Kimwipe.
7. Seal the coverslip with clear nail polish.
8. Store the slides in a dark place at 4°C. They should be stable for several months.

polish worked well to seal the coverslips to the slide. Care should be taken to allow the nail polish to dry completely before viewing the samples to prevent it from adhering to the objectives. Excess mounting medium that oozed from underneath the coverslip was removed prior to sealing, as the mounting medium prevented the nail polish from forming a seal around the coverslip.

## 3. Confocal Viewing of Fixed Specimens

Specimens prepared for confocal microscopy were examined with three different types of confocal microscope: a slow-scan CLSM (Bio-Rad), a video-rate CLSM (Odyssey; Noran Instruments), and a spinning disk confocal microscope (TSM; Noran Instruments). For slow-scan confocal microscopy, Bio-Rad MRC-500 and MRC-600 CLSMs were used. Specific settings of the confocal microscopes are given for some of the samples, but may be varied with the application.

Eggs and embryos were examined at a zoom of 2 with a Bio-Rad MRC-600 equipped with either an argon ion or a krypton–argon ion laser set to half-power. In addition, a number 3 neutral density filter was used to attenuate the beam. A Nikon ×60 Plan-Apo numerical aperture (NA) 1.4 oil immersion objective was also used to image the cells. Some samples were examined with a Bio-Rad MRC-500 equipped with an argon ion laser and either a Nikon ×10 Plan-Apo NA 0.45 objective, or a Nikon ×60 Plan-Apo NA 1.4 oil immersion objective. For video-rate confocal microscopy, a video-rate CLSM (Noran Instruments) was equipped with an argon ion laser set to 25% intensity by the AOD system to attenuate the beam, and a ×60 Plan-Apo NA 1.4 oil immersion objective. A TSM (Noran Instruments) equipped with a Photometrics 200 cooled CCD camera (Photometrics, Tucson, AZ), a 200-W Nikon mercury light source, and a

Nikon ×40 fluor NA 1.3 oil immersion objective was used for tandem scanning confocal microscopy as described by Wright *et al.* (1989).

## B. Confocal Physiology of Living Cells

Confocal microscopy coupled with voltage-sensitive and ion-indicating dyes can also be used to study dynamic changes in the physiology of living cells. Two different techniques, confocal ion imaging and four-dimensional imaging (three-dimensional imaging over time), were used to image living embryos (Stricker *et al.*, 1990, 1992). For confocal ion imaging, the same focal plane near the equator of the egg was imaged during the acquisition period. For four-dimensional imaging, a through focal series ($z$ series) was taken at each time point and reconstructed three dimensionally. The following sections describe how the eggs were prepared and how the images were generated with CLSMs.

## 1. Specimen Preparation for Confocal Ion Imaging

Gametes were obtained as described above for fixed cells. Unfertilized sea urchin eggs were gently attached to a coverslip that had been coated with protamine sulfate (10 mg/ml; Sigma Chemical Co.) instead of poly-L-lysine and subsequently glued over a hole drilled in the bottom of a 60-mm petri dish. Eggs were bathed in 20 ml of seawater and the specimen dish maintained at 18°C by a thermoelectric cooling stage (KT controller; United Technology, Whitehouse Station, NJ). Care was taken to calibrate the dish temperature prior to the experiment. The eggs were then microinjected with 5 m$M$ stock of the cell-impermeant form of calcium green, potassium salt (Molecular Probes, Inc.) dissolved in 100 m$M$ potassium aspartate, 10 m$M$ HEPES (pH 7.2). Micro-injections were carried out with a Zeiss Axiovert 10 inverted microscope equipped with an Eppendorf 5170/5242 pressure injection system (Stricker *et al.*, 1992). Calcium green was used as the calcium-indicating probe for four reasons: it is excited by the 488-nm emission line of the argon ion laser, it appears less toxic than fluo-3, it bleaches at a slower rate than fluo-3, and, in contrast to fluo-3, it is fluorescent at low calcium levels.

The microinjected eggs were imaged according to Stricker *et al.* (1990, 1992) with a video-rate CLSM (Noran Instruments) interfaced with a Nikon Diaphot inverted microscope equipped with a Zeiss ×16 (NA 0.32) objective lens. To optimize cell viability, the laser was set at 25% intensity by the acousto-optical deflector system. A fluorescein filter set placed in the optical light path was used to excite calcium green. Eggs were viewed at an optical plane near their equators and the focus, which was fixed by the stepper motor of the confocal microscope, was not changed during acquisition of the sequence. Images were acquired just prior to the addition of sperm by summing 16 frames and recording onto the computer hard disk. Because acquisition and recording took a total of

2–3 sec, optical sections were acquired every 2–3 sec for the first 10 min to document the increase and subsequent decrease in fluorescence observed during fertilization. Cell viability was tested by continued recording every 15–20 min up to the 16-cell stage.

## 2. Specimen Preparation for Four-Dimensional Imaging

Gametes were obtained as described above for fixed cells. At 2 min post-insemination, the fertilized eggs were stained for 2 min with a 5–10 ng/ml seawater stock solution of $DiOC_6(3)$ (Molecular Probes, Inc.) and washed twice in seawater (Stricker *et al.*, 1990). Stained eggs were attached to protamine sulfate-coated coverslips as described above and bathed in 20 ml of seawater at 18°C prior to confocal viewing.

Stained, fertilized eggs were imaged with a Bio-Rad MRC-600 CLSM equipped with an argon ion laser set to one-half power and the beam further attenuated by a 1% transmittance neutral density filter. A fluorescein filter set placed in the optical light path was used to excite $DiOC_6(3)$. Observations were made with a ×25 Leitz NA 0.6 water immersion objective placed directly into the petri dish. Every 8 min, a $z$ series of optical sections was acquired by averaging three full frames for each section and recording to the hard disk of the computer until the embryos had developed to the early blastula stage, prior to hatching.

## 3. Volume Rendering

To produce a three-dimensional reconstruction, stacks of optical sections for each data set were rendered on a Silicon Graphics IRIS 4D-70GT graphics workstation (Silicon Graphics, Mountain View, CA) after transfer via an Ethernet connection from the computer coupled to the microscope. Volume rendering of the stacks of optical sections was performed with Voxel View software (Vital Images, Inc., Fairfield, IA). Images were recorded by photographing the monitor, using a Sony UP-5000 color video printer, a Matrix digital film recorder, or output to videotape. The technique of volume rendering is described in detail in Section V and the various methods to obtain color prints and slides of confocal data sets are described in Section VII.

## IV. Applications of Confocal Microscopy

Confocal microscopy offers a powerful means to address biological problems, giving new understanding of cellular structure and processes (Shotton, 1989). Some of these applications include (1) determining the cellular localization of organelles, cytoskeletal elements, and macromolecules such as proteins, RNA, and DNA, (2) tracing specific cells through a tissue, (3) producing optical

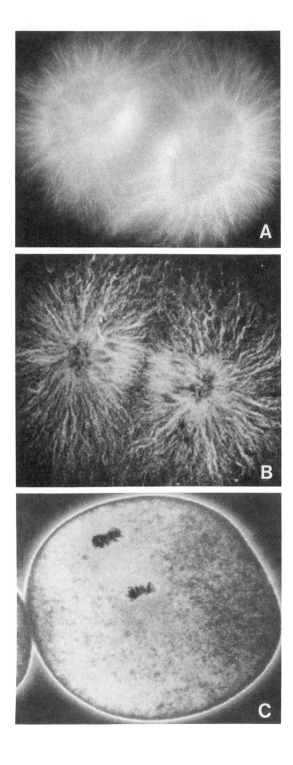

sections for stereo image production and three-dimensional reconstruction, and (4) imaging in four dimensions. Fluorescence recovery after photobleaching and ion imaging are also possible with confocal microscopy. When performed with conventional microscopy, these techniques yield limited information. When used with confocal microscopy, however, they provide a means to determine whether a structure has been photobleached completely and whether ionic changes occur throughout the whole cell or tissue, or only in a specific region. Confocal microscopes can also be used in the reflectance mode. This allows reduction of out-of-focus blur from nonfluorescent labels such as diamino-benzidine reaction products formed during enzyme cytochemical reactions, and from silver grains present in autoradiograms produced during *in situ* hybridization (Robinson and Batten, 1989; Paddock *et al.*, 1991). The images discussed in this section were generated with either a slow-scan CLSM (Bio-Rad Micro-science), a video-rate CLSM (Noran Instruments), or a spinning disk confocal microscope (TSM; Noran Instruments).

## A. Single-Label Imaging

Optical sections of single-labeled specimens taken with a representative conventional microscope, and slow-scan, video-rate, and spinning disk confocal microscopes, are shown in Figs. 10–12. Much information can be gained from a single optical section, because out-of-focus fluorescence is eliminated due to the increase in contrast and apparent resolution. This can be applied to single cells as well as thicker, multicellular specimens. After an optical section is acquired with a CLSM, it can be pseudocolored to highlight various structures and details or colored to mimic the original fluorochrome (e.g, green for fluorescein). In contrast, real-image colors can be observed confocally with the TSM because images are generated and viewed with white light. For example, when the TSM is used in the reflected light mode, real colors of a single optical slice of cultured 3T3 cells stained with Coomassie blue display focal contacts at the cell substratum interface (Color Plate 1).

## B. Multiple-Label Imaging

With multiple labeling, two or more structures can be observed and traced simultaneously in the same cell or tissue. One method to achieve double labeling

---

**Fig. 10** Fluorescence micrographs of sea urchin (*Lytechinus pictus*) embryos in first mitosis, stained for microtubules. (A) Conventional microscope image demonstrating out-of-focus blur. (B) Confocal optical section of a different sea urchin embryo imaged with a Bio-Rad MRC-600 confocal microscope, showing more clearly the arrangement of the mitotic spindle. (C) Confocal image of a surf clam (*Spisula*) embryo in first mitosis, taken with a Bio-Rad MRC-500, revealing that the position of the chromosomes would result in unequal cleavage. [Fig. 10B reprinted from Wright, S. J., *et al.* (1989). *J. Cell Sci.* **94,** 617–624, with permission of The Company of Biologists, Ltd.]

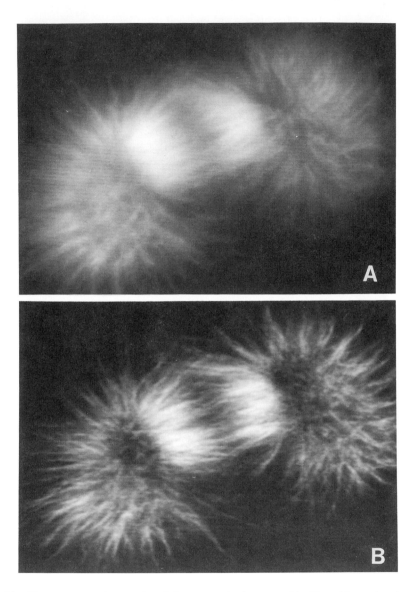

**Fig. 11** Fluorescence micrographs of the same mitotic sea urchin (*Lytechinus pictus*) embryo stained for microtubules and taken with the video-rate CLSM. A conventional image was obtained in (A) by removing the slit aperture, whereas in (B) the slit aperture was present, showing a confocal fluorescence image of a single optical section with improved contrast and resolution.

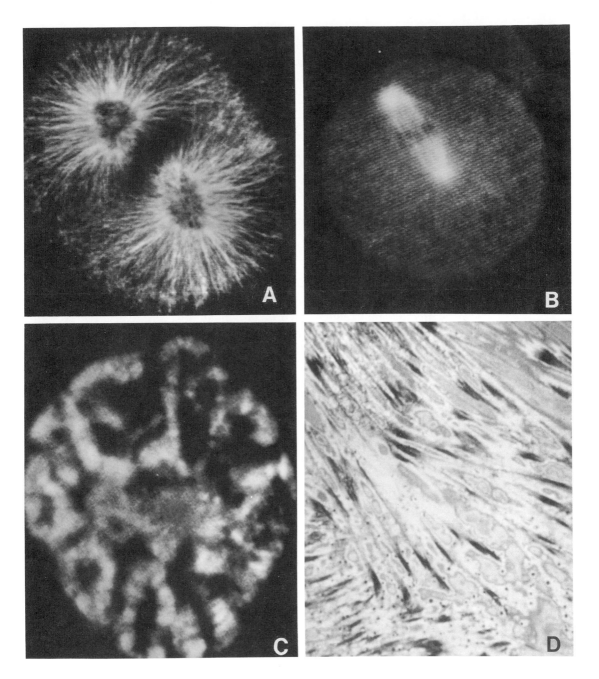

**Fig. 12** Confocal fluorescence micrographs of single optical sections taken with the tandem scanning confocal microscope. (A) Sea urchin (*Strongylocentrotus purpuratus*) embryo in first mitosis, stained for microtubules. (B) Surf clam (*Spisula*) oocyte stained for microtubules, showing an outline of the chromosomes in the meiotic spindle. (C) *Drosophila* salivary gland nucleus stained with ethidium bromide, showing the arrangement of the polytene chromosomes. (D) Cultured Swiss 3T3 cells stained with Naphthol Blue Black, showing dark streaks (focal contacts) at the ends of stress fibers. [Fig. 12A reprinted from Wright, S. J., *et al.* (1989). *J. Cell Sci.* **94**, 617–624, with permission of The Company of Biologists, Ltd.]

with CLSMs uses the 514-nm emission line of the argon ion laser to excite both fluorescein and rhodamine channels. The induced fluorescence is filtered and directed to separate photomultiplier tubes. Alternatively, a krypton–argon ion laser, which has better separation of the fluorescein and rhodamine signals, or two different lasers, can be used to produce the same effect. Color Plate 2 demonstrates this principle by showing the localization of two different gene products within the same *Drosophila* embryo. The relationship between centrosomes and microtubules of a sea urchin embryo in first mitosis is shown in Color Plate 3. Triple labeling with UV-excitable dyes in addition to those excited by fluorescein and rhodamine can be performed with the TSM (Color Plate 4). In CLSMs equipped with krypton–argon ion lasers, longer wavelength dyes excited by 647-nm light, such as cyanine 5.18 and 7.18 (CY5 and CY7) can also be imaged (Haugland, 1990). This permits three or more different fluorochromes to be imaged simultaneously with a single laser so that multiple structures can be examined. A word of caution must be mentioned: multiple-labeled specimens can bleed through from one fluorescent channel to another (Paddock, 1991). Several methods may reduce this problem, including more restrictive excitation and barrier filter sets, dyes with narrower absorbance and emission spectra better suited to the laser, such as BODIPY (Haugland, 1990), and digital image subtraction to remove the bleed-through data.

## C. *z* Series

To obtain three-dimensional information from the specimen, it is common practice to acquire a series of optical sections, referred to as a *z* series, taken at successively higher or lower focal planes along the *z* axis. Each two-dimensional scan of the specimen is called an optical slice or section, and all the slices together comprise a volume data set. The principle of *z* series acquisition is demonstrated schematically in Fig. 13. To obtain three-dimensional information from the *z* series, individual slices from the stack of optical sections may be viewed as a montage. As shown in Fig. 14, the *z* series montage demonstrates the different microtubule arrangements in the mitotic sea urchin embryo.

## D. Stereo Imaging

Although a *z* series montage provides three-dimensional information, stereo pairs produce a more three-dimensional perspective to the specimen. Both CLSM and TSM images can be used to produce stereo images (Boyde, 1985; Shotton, 1989; Wright *et al.*, 1989, 1990; Boyde *et al.*, 1990; Summers *et al.*, 1991). Confocal laser scanning microscopes obtain stereoscopic images by digital manipulation (pixel shifting) of a *z* series. Stereo pairs are also produced by reconstructing a *z* series three-dimensionally and observing two individual views of the rendered volume that are approximately 9° apart. Figure 15 shows the details of the first mitotic spindle in a sea urchin embryo that was volume rendered to produce the three-dimensional stereo view. In addition to pixel

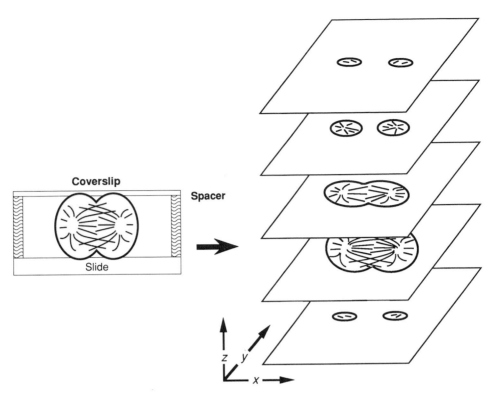

**Fig. 13** Schematic demonstrating the principle of optical sectioning. After the sample is carefully mounted for three-dimensional reconstruction to preserve three-dimensional morphology (as is this mitotic sea urchin egg, which is mounted with spacers to prevent the coverslip from flattening the cell), a through-focal series of optical slices, known as a *z* series, can be taken to generate a volume data set. The volume data set can then be rendered into a three-dimensional reconstruction. Both confocal laser scanning microscopes and spinning disk confocal microscopes can be used to generate the *z* series of optical sections.

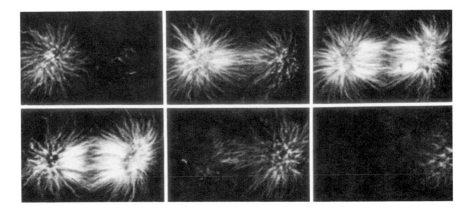

**Fig. 14** Serial, confocal optical sections of a *z* series through a mitotic sea urchin (*Lytechinus pictus*) embryo imaged with a video-rate CLSM. The slices reveal the organization of the spindle in the embryo. Optical sections were taken at 15-$\mu$m intervals.

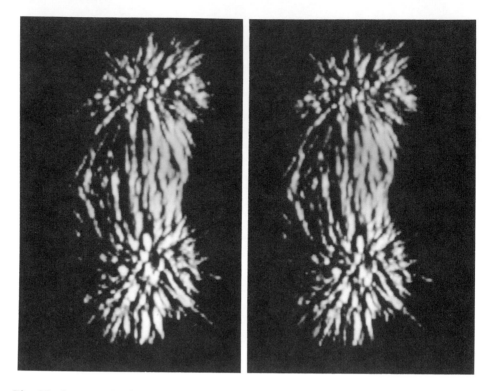

**Fig. 15**  Stereo confocal micrograph of a mitotic sea urchin (*Lytechinus pictus*) embryo stained for microtubules, revealing the three-dimensional organization of the spindle. A *z* series was acquired with a Bio-Rad MRC-600 CLSM and the volume was three-dimensionally reconstructed. The rendered volume was rotated 9° to produce the stereo pair.

shifting, the TSM can produce stereo images by controlling objective movement in both the *x* and *z* axes to generate a left and right image at each focal plane (Boyde, 1985; Boyde *et al.*, 1990). This provides a separate stack of right and left images, which, when compiled, produces a stereo image through two different volumes. Thus each half of the stereo pair can be acquired directly from the specimen without digital manipulation (Boyde, 1985; Wright *et al.*, 1989; Boyde *et al.*, 1990).

## V. Confocal Three-Dimensional Anatomy

Although volumetric information can be obtained from stereo images, it provides only a static view of the specimen from a single direction. Three-dimensional reconstruction offers an improved means of analyzing complex spatial relationships because the data volume can be viewed interactively from any angle (e.g., top, bottom, sides, obliquely). Technology for three-dimensional reconstruction has emerged as a result of technological advances in computer graphics as applied to the biological sciences, and improvements in digital image storage. These developments offer the investigator the ability to dissect the data interactively to develop powerful insights into the complex three-dimensional structure of biological specimens. However, the difficulty in presenting three-dimensionally reconstructed images lies in the lack of appropriate visualization tools because most displays provide a two-dimensional view. To overcome this problem, different perspectives of the specimen are displayed sequentially on the television monitor as a rotating volume, which gives a three-dimensional perspective of the data, provides depth, and brings into view structures otherwise unnoticed.

## A. Definitions

To aid in understanding three-dimensional reconstruction, several terms must be defined. *Rendering* refers to processes, such as rotation, projection, coloring, and shading, that are required to display a specimen on the computer image monitor (Van Zandt and Argiro, 1989). Volume rendering works by taking a *z* series or three-dimensional stack of optical sections, known as a *volume,* and assumes that the three-dimensional objects are composed of volumetric building blocks or cubes called voxels. A *voxel* is defined as a volume element just as a *pixel* is defined as a picture element. A voxel can also be considered a three-dimensional pixel. Each voxel of the volume is assigned a number representing a characteristic of the three-dimensional object such as density or luminosity. At this point, the specimen is summarized by a set of point samples. To generate an image, the three-dimensional array of voxels or points is transferred into computer memory, the volume data is processed, and then displayed on the screen of the image monitor.

## B. Considerations

Several parameters must be considered prior to acquiring a *z* series suitable for three-dimensional reconstruction. Careful attention must be paid to each parameter so that three-dimensional reconstructions are produced with minimal distortions and artifacts.

## 1. Specimen Preparation

Improper specimen preparation can produce distorted three-dimensional images (Bacallao *et al.,* 1989; Paddock *et al.,* 1990; Wright *et al.,* 1990; Holy *et al.,* 1991; Wright and Schatten, 1991). Current fixation and extraction protocols optimized for conventional fluorescence microscopy often result in flattening of specimens. For example, the weight of the coverslip can flatten the specimen if no precautions are taken (Bacallao *et al.*, 1989; Wright *et al.*, 1990; Holy *et al.*, 1991; Wright and Schatten, 1991). In addition, fixation and dehydration protocols can produce distortional artifacts. Hence, it is necessary to employ the greatest care when preparing a sample for three-dimensional reconstruction.

Heterogeneity inherent in specimens can also create problems in acquiring a *z* series (Cheng and Summers, 1989). The intensity of the excitation light and emitted fluorescence can be attenuated by structures situated between the focal plane of interest and the objective lens. This causes self-shadowing of structures and can significantly reduce the image contrast in some areas of the specimen. Often the further one focuses in the *z* axis of a sample, the more prominent loss of contrast and shadowing become so that upper focal planes appear bright whereas lower ones are dim. Increasing the illumination intensity can overcome some of the problem; however, photobleaching may become severe. Hence, antioxidants should be used to reduce photobleaching during acquisition of large data sets. Some procedures to avoid improper specimen preparation are described in Section III.

## 2. Image Registration

A second requirement for effective three-dimensional reconstruction is image registration (Shuman *et al.*, 1989; Pawley, 1989; Paddock *et al.*, 1990; Wright and Schatten, 1991). Each optical section of the *z* series must be in register with its neighbors during image acquisition, otherwise distortion is introduced into the three-dimensional reconstruction. Hence, care must be taken to prevent the specimen from moving during acquisition of the *z* series. Proper image registration can be maintained by fixing cells to a coverslip or slide prior to mounting (as described in Section III), and reducing vibrations of the microscope stage.

## 3. Pixel Resolution

A third important consideration before obtaining a *z* series is the calculation of the "pixel resolution" for the conditions used (objective, magnification, electronic zoom, image size, optical section thickness) so that the proportional dimensions of the specimen are maintained during three-dimensional reconstruction. If relatively too few or too many optical sections are collected, the rendered volume will appear distorted either by being squashed or stretched out, respectively (Wright *et al.*, 1990; Wright and Schatten, 1991). Because the computer (e.g., graphics workstation) bases its calculations on cube-shaped voxels during three-dimensional reconstruction, the *z* depth of each voxel must be of the same dimension as the pixels in the *x* and *y* dimensions of the optical section (Paddock *et al.*, 1990). For example, for the three-dimensional reconstructions discussed in Color Plate 5, a $\times 10$ objective lens was used on the slow-scan CLSM with a zoom of two, and an image size of $256 \times 256$ pixels.

The pixel resolution was calculated to be 1.2 $\mu$m, which is the width of the box calibrated in $\mu$m, divided by the number of pixels across the box (256 pixels). To generate the three-dimensional reconstructions of Color Plate 5, 130–140 optical sections were taken at 1.2-$\mu$m intervals through the depth of the specimen and reconstructed three-dimensionally. If insufficient optical sections are acquired, the computer software can synthesize an image by averaging the section above and below the plane of interest, and insert the interpolated image between the acquired sections. If too many sections are obtained, the program allows sections to be removed from the $z$ series.

## 4. Image Storage

A fourth consideration for collecting images for three-dimensional reconstruction involves image storage (Carrington *et al.*, 1989; Chen *et al.*, 1989; Shuman *et al.*, 1989; Shotton, 1989; Van Zandt and Argiro, 1989; Wright *et al.*, 1990; Holy *et al.*, 1991; Wright and Schatten, 1991). Each optical section may be an 8-bit image, which is 60–384 kbytes, depending on the image size (i.e., $256 \times 256$ pixels vs $768 \times 512$ pixels). When a $z$ series is obtained, 100–200 optical sections are routinely taken, which produces up to ~50 Mbytes of voxel data. Like pixel values in video microscopy, each voxel is associated with a number, ranging from 0 to 255, that is directly proportional to the light intensity for that particular voxel. Storage of these images can be a problem, especially when image processing is needed at a later time. Data can initially be stored on a large, 80- to 90-Mbyte hard disk; however, only one to three $z$ series can be stored at a time. Archival storage on a WORM (write once read many) drive solves the problem of image storage because drives are available that can accept 200–900 Mbytes of data per disk and resolution of the images is not lost because data are stored digitally. Rewritable optical disks or erasable WORM disks are also available if a permanent record of the data is not required. Compression of images by computer is also helpful in reducing image size without losing important information from the image. The advantage of using a high-performance graphics workstation is readily apparent when one considers the impact of both archiving and handling the large data sets during three-dimensional reconstruction to produce a three-dimensional animated sequence of the $z$ series rotating in real time.

## C. Applications

Two major methods are available for the three-dimensional reconstruction and display of a $z$ series of confocal data (Chen *et al.*, 1989; Van Zandt and Argiro, 1989). These systems use either geometric surface rendering (Harris and Stevens, 1989) or volume rendering (Van Zandt and Argiro, 1989). In geometric surface rendering, triangles and two-dimensional polygons are fused together to approximate the surfaces of three-dimensional objects. The method discussed in this section uses volume rendering to generate three-dimensional reconstructions.

Once the *z* series is transferred from the CLSM to the graphics workstation, several manipulations can be performed to reveal particular features of biological interest in the volume. These include changing the view of the volume (i.e., from the top, bottom, obliquely), viewing the entire volume or single optical sections, adjusting the opacity or relative transparency of the volume to reveal structures on the surface or deep within the specimen, obtaining maximal contrast, choosing a background color, pseudocoloring the image within the volume by voxel or gradient values, turning on and positioning a light source to enhance surface features of the specimen, activating antialiasing to prevent formation of linear artifacts (Pawley, 1989; Webb and Dorey, 1989), and compressing the data to eliminate nonrelevant voxels and decrease rendering time. Once these parameters have been set, an animation of the three-dimensional reconstruction is generated by choosing the number of angles (e.g., every 9° of a total of 360°), total rotation, and the axis of rotation. The animation is produced by showing in rapid succession the views taken at different angles of the already rendered *z* series. The animated three-dimensional rotation can then be viewed interactively. It is even possible to cut the volume to reveal hidden information, as demonstrated in Color Plate 6.

### 1. Three-Dimensional Single-Label Imaging

Figure 16 shows four individual optical sections 24 $\mu$m apart taken from a *z* series of $\sim$1430 optical sections taken at 1.2-$\mu$m intervals of a sea urchin pluteus stained for DNA with thiazole orange. This *z* series was used to render the three-dimensional reconstruction in Color Plate 5, which shows several views of the rendered volume. Relationships between internal and external structures are revealed as the specimen rotates (Color Plate 5). The software that generates the rendered volume can accept modifications in parameters such as lighting and opacity that can drastically affect the final image. The volume in Color Plate 5 was also rendered with different pseudocoloring, lighting, opacity, and background color (Wright and Schatten, 1991). When different rendering parameters have been chosen, various features of the three-dimensional reconstruction can be highlighted. This permits analysis of surface detail as well as internal structural components.

### 2. Three-Dimensional Multiple-Label Imaging

*z* series that are collected from two different channels (e.g., fluorescein and rhodamine) can be merged and rendered to highlight desired parameters, as for a single volume data set. The result is a double-labeled three-dimensional data set in which the relationship of two cellular components can be displayed in three dimensions. By rotating the rendered volume, particular nuances of the struc-

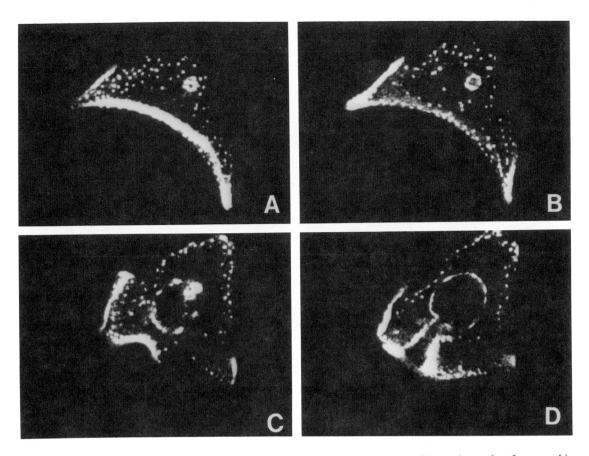

**Fig. 16** Four individual optical sections (A–D), selected at equal 24-$\mu$m intervals, of a sea urchin (*Strongylocentrotus purpuratus*) pluteus stained with thiazole orange to reveal nuclear positions. The optical sections were generated with an MRC-500 confocal microscope equipped with an argon ion laser. These optical sections, from a series of ~130 taken at 1.2-$\mu$m intervals, were used to render the three-dimensional reconstructions in Color Plate 5. Each optical section shows crisp details with no out-of-focus fluorescence from structures above or below the plane of focus.

tures can be revealed. This is illustrated by two different three-dimensional reconstructions of a double-labeled sea urchin embryo in first mitosis: one taken with the fluorescein filter set to show microtubules, and the other with the rhodamine filter set to localize the centrosomes (Fig. 17). Each volume can be displayed in a different color and the two data sets merged to produce a single three-dimensional volume rendering with interlaced optical slices. The merged three-dimensional reconstruction reveals the three-dimensional relationship of the two labeled structures. For example, when the two z series of Fig. 17 are

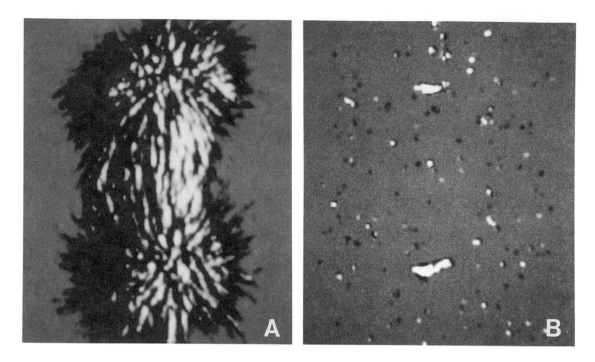

**Fig. 17** Two three-dimensional reconstructions of a mitotic sea urchin (*Lytechinus pictus*) embryo double labeled for microtubules (A) and centrosomes (B). The images were generated on a Bio-Rad MRC-600 confocal microscope equipped with a krypton–argon ion laser, using a separate channel to image each fluorochrome. Optical section increments were every 2 $\mu$m. These two volume data sets can be merged into one volume and rendered to show the three-dimensional relationship of the centrosomes and microtubules.

merged, the microtubules appear to originate from the entire surface of the centrosomes located at each spindle pole.

## 3. Three-Dimensional Confocal Ion Imaging

In addition to imaging cellular structures and organelles it is also possible to observe ionic fluctuations using confocal microscopy. To this end, a large selection of dyes that are sensitive to their local environment and fluoresce at certain ionic (pH, $Ca^{2+}$) concentrations are available that are well suited to illumination from lasers commonly employed in confocal microscopes (Tsien, 1989; Haugland, 1990). At fertilization, sea urchin eggs release a wave of calcium ions inside the cell that triggers various cellular processes, including cortical granule discharge. Because information is gathered from the entire cell with conventional microscopy (Fig. 1A), it is not fully understood whether the rapid burst of free calcium ions occurs as a wave only in the egg cortex or throughout the egg cytoplasm. Hence, this is an ideal system for analysis by confocal microscopy and volumetric reconstruction.

By maintaining the scanning laser beam of the video-rate CLSM at the same focal plane and acquiring images at various time points at this same plane, it is possible to observe the pattern of calcium wave propagation (Stricker *et al.*, 1992). In all eggs examined that had been microinjected with calcium green, a wave of increased fluorescence spread completely across the egg cytoplasm following fertilization (Fig. 18). Surprisingly, even the female pronucleus exhibited an increase in fluorescence (Stricker *et al.*, 1992).

To analyze the calcium waves further, optical sections from a single equatorial plane taken at 2-sec intervals were treated as a volume and rendered to reveal the temporal pattern of fluorescence alterations (Stricker *et al.*, 1992). In this case, time is the third dimension in the three-dimensional reconstruction because the same *z*-axis level was used for all the images. The volume was then cut longitudinally to show the inner cytoplasmic fluctuations in calcium green fluorescence triggered by fertilization (Color Plate 6). After imaging every 2 sec for the first 10 min after fertilization, the eggs were imaged every 15 min to determine egg viability. Under these imaging conditions, the eggs shown in Fig. 18 and Color Plate 6 developed to the 16-cell stage (Fig. 19). Thus, confocal microscopes can be used as a tool to study physiological alterations during development (Stricker *et al.*, 1992).

It is important to note that such confocal studies utilized a single-wavelength type of calcium indicator whose fluorescence emission depends not only upon the free calcium concentration that is supposedly being monitored but also upon various calcium-independent parameters (e.g., dye loading compartmentalization, pathlength, viscosity, etc.). Such factors can artifactually affect the signal that is being detected. These artifacts can in turn make simple comparisons of the absolute fluorescence intensities observed between specimens or across different regions of the same cell unreliable. Hence, in addition to the confocal images of raw fluorescence intensities, such time-lapse studies should also include ratio images that show each time-point divided by a prestimulation image. Alternatively, one should provide normalized data that calculate the change in fluorescence relative to the prestimulation resting level of fluorescence (Cornell-Bell *et al.*, 1990). In either case, it is important that the offset introduced by the imaging system is properly corrected (Finkbeiner, 1992).

## VI. Confocal Four-Dimensional Anatomy

The technique of generating three-dimensional reconstructions becomes even more powerful when *z* series of the same living sample are taken at periodic intervals over time and reconstructed three dimensionally. This method is referred to as *four-dimensional imaging* and produces a consecutive series of three-dimensional reconstructions over time (Stricker *et al.*, 1990). Four-dimensional imaging is especially striking for the analysis of embryonic development because positions and lineages of various cells can be traced back to their origins. In Fig. 20, a fertilized sea urchin egg labeled with $DiOC_6(3)$ was imaged and volume rendered up to the early blastula stage. This technique provides a noninvasive method of monitoring mitotic events, cleavage patterns, and migration patterns of individual cells.

## VII. Presentation of Confocal Data

Several methods are available to reproduce confocal images from the image monitor for publication, poster sessions, and slide presentations. Black-and-white and color images can be recorded with a photographic camera (e.g., 35 mm, Polaroid), video printer, or film recorder. Methods available for image reproduction have been published in detail (Inoué, 1986). This section briefly discusses procedures that work well for confocal images.

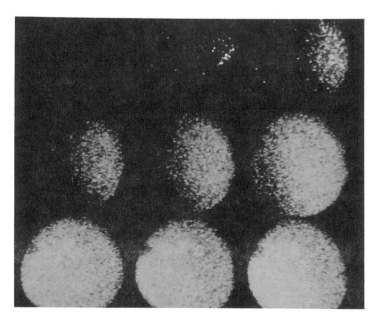

**Fig. 18**  Individual optical sections through the same focal plane of a sea urchin (*Lytechinus pictus*) egg microinjected with the calcium-indicating dye, calcium green. The same equatorial plane of the egg was imaged at 2-sec intervals with a video-rate CLSM over a period of 10 min, during which time the egg was fertilized. The wave of increased fluorescence spread across the egg. The female pronucleus also exhibited an increase in intensity. Optical sections were taken every 15 min and the embryo continued to develop to the 16-cell stage, as shown in Fig. 19.

## A. Photographic Recording from the Monitor

Before recording an image photographically from the television monitor, several parameters must be considered (Table III). These include the type of monitor, camera, lens, and film to be used.

## 1. Image Monitor

A relatively high-resolution, black-and-white or color monitor with a flat screen is preferred because a curved screen will distort the images. Video scan lines that limit the vertical resolution of the image from the monitor also cause image distortion. Because images are formed line by line by a rapidly moving electron beam, video scan lines appear. To prevent them from being prominent, the vertical hold (V-HOLD) control knob on the monitor should be adjusted so that the scan lines are as close together as possible (i.e., a 2 : 1 interlace). This is achieved just before the image becomes unstable. Other means of reducing

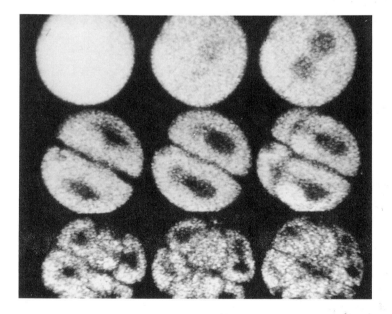

**Fig. 19** Individual optical sections at the same focal plane of the same sea urchin (*Lytechinus pictus*) egg as in Fig. 18, microinjected with calcium green. The same equatorial plane of the egg shown in Fig. 18 was imaged at 15-min intervals after the initial 10 min of imaging at 2-sec intervals. Under these imaging conditions, the embryo developed to the 16-cell stage, demonstrating that confocal microscopy can be used as a tool to image ion fluctuations. [Reprinted with permission of Academic Press from Stricker, S. A., *et al.* (1992). *Dev. Biol.* **149,** 370–380].

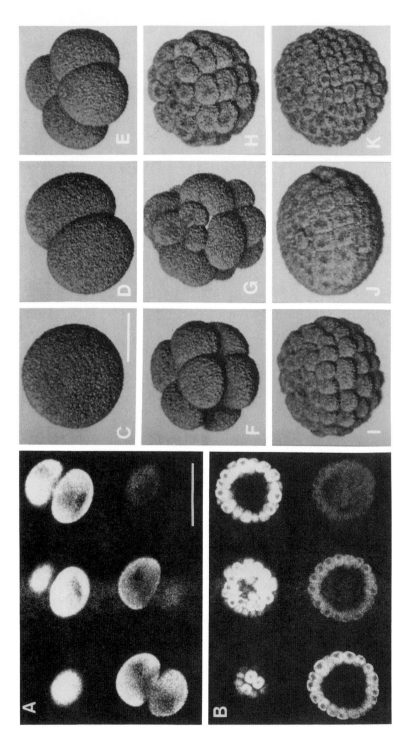

**Fig. 20** Optical sections and three-dimensional reconstructions over time (four-dimensional imaging) of the same developing sea urchin (*Lytechinus pictus*) embryo stained with DiOC$_6$(3). The embryo was imaged with a Bio-Rad MRC-600 equipped with an argon ion laser. A *z* series of optical sections was taken every 8 min through the embryo as it developed. Each *z* series, which consisted of ~30 optical sections taken at 5-$\mu$m steps through the embryo, was rendered with interpolated sections to obtain the appropriate pixel resolution. Optical sections taken approximately 15 $\mu$m apart from a *z* series through the embryo at the two-cell stage (A) and the late morula/early blastula stage (B). (C–K) Three-dimensional reconstructions of the same embryo as in (A) and (B), corresponding to the following developmental stages: (C) zygote; (D) 2-cell stage; (E) 4-cell stage; (F) 8-cell stage; (G) ~16-cell stage, with elongated blastomeres in the process of division; (H) early morula; (I) morula; (J) late morula/early blastula stage, prior to hatching. Scale bars: (A and B) 100 $\mu$m; (C–K) 50 $\mu$m.

**Table III**
**Photographing the Image Monitor**

1. Center the image on the television monitor.
2. Remove the protective monitor cover if present and clean the screen with soft, nonabrasive cloth moistened with 95–100% ethanol to remove fingerprints, etc.
3. Adjust V-HOLD of monitor; use a magnifying glass if necessary. Set to underscan, if the whole image is to be photographed.
4. Set up a tripod and 35-mm camera equipped with a 55-mm microlens so that the monitor face is orthogonal to the camera axis, that is, the face of the camera lens is parallel to the monitor face. If images are displayed on a curved monitor, use a macrolens and set the tripod farther away from the monitor to prevent image distortion.
5. Load film in the camera, set ASA and $f$ stop, and set to automatic exposures. Disable or cover the flash on the camera.
6. If film is to be commercially processed and mounted, take the first shot of a bright area so that the position of the negatives on the film is known before cutting in the automatic slide maker. When all the images are dark, it is difficult to determine where to cut them.
7. With the room dark, adjust the brightness and contrast of the image monitor to below the setting for normal viewing for black-and-white images and for color images, so that the image is visually pleasing.
8. Frame the area of interest in the camera viewfinder and adjust the focus; focusing on linear structures helps.
9. Determine whether exposure is at least greater than or equal to 1 sec and adjust the $f$ stop on the camera if necessary.
10. Take an exposure. To insure a suitable exposure is obtained, take a series of exposures to either side of the original exposure. To overexpose and underexpose one full stop from the chosen stop, take a series of exposures at one-third- to one-half-stop increments.

video scan lines (e.g., Ronchi grating) have also been described (Inoué, 1986). During photographic printing, one must keep in mind that a negative of a television or video image differs from a negative of a regular photograph. Scan lines and loss of resolution can become prominent in positive prints of television or video images if the negative is overly enlarged in the dark room. To photograph the entire image, the monitor should be set in the underscan mode. To photograph a portion of the image, normal mode is usually best (Table III).

## 2. Camera and Lens

To photograph the monitor, the camera (standard- or instant-type format) should be mounted on a stable tripod or platform to reduce vibration, because the exposures may be long (Table III). The camera should be equipped with a lens so that it can focus the image on the monitor to nearly or completely fill the camera format. We commonly use a Nikon N2000 35-mm camera with a Nikon 55-mm Micro-Nikkor lens for flat-faced monitors and a 70- to 210-mm Sigma Macro-Zoom lens for curved screen monitors because a lens of longer focal length minimizes effects of screen curvature. Care must be taken to orient the camera properly because image distortions will occur if the face of the camera lens is not parallel to the face of the monitor.

## 3. Contrast and Brightness

It is important to photograph the monitor in a darkened room (Table III). This prevents reflections of bright objects and room lights from being duplicated in the photograph. In addition, the room lights decrease contrast of the displayed images. A flash is not used to illuminate the screen because it also overpowers the screen image and may be reflected in the monitor image. Once the room is dark and the camera positioned, the contrast and brightness of the image should be optimized (Table III). Then reducing the contrast of the image to slightly below the optimal setting usually works well.

## 4. Exposure Time

The contrast and brightness should be reevaluated to verify enough light is available to expose the camera for ~1 sec at the optimal $f$ stop setting (Table III). A television image is composed of 525 horizontal scan lines scanned at 60 fields/sec (U.S. standard) or 625 scan lines scanned at 50 fields/sec for other countries (Inoué, 1986). A complete U.S. scan takes 1/30 of a second (1/60 of a second for odd-numbered lines and 1/60 of a second for even-numbered lines). Thus exposures shorter than 1/30 of a second will not capture the entire image. Too short an exposure will result in an upper or lower portion of the photograph being darker than the rest because it was exposed to fewer video scans. To obtain a properly exposed picture the exposures should be greater than 1 sec and a series of photographs should be taken to bracket each exposure by slightly overexposing or underexposing the image (Table III).

## 5. Films

A fine-grain black-and-white film (e.g., Kodak Technical Pan, T-MAX 100 film) will produce excellent halftone reproductions. Kodak Technical Pan film is often used because the resulting contrast of the images can be altered by using Kodak developer HC-110 at various dilutions. A test strip of the various exposures can be processed in different developer dilutions to optimize the image in the negatives. For color prints, a fine-grain color slide film such as Kodak Ektachrome 200 or 400 daylight is suitable. Once the color slide is made, a color internegative is used to produce a print from the slide, with a slight loss of resolution. This method is preferred over the use of color print film, in which some colors lose their brightness and hue during processing and printing. Editors of journals will often accept color slides for the final reproduction of the confocal image. This avoids the resolution lost by using a color internegative and minimizes color distortions.

Confocal fluorescence images often have a large area of black background. Frequently the position of the exposures on the slide film is difficult to determine and sometimes structures of interest can be mistakenly cut by automatic slide mounters during commercial film processing. To avoid this problem, take the roll of film's first exposure of a bright object (e.g., bright wall or book) with the room lights on (Table III). The position of each exposure can then be determined before the strip is placed in the automatic slide mounter.

## B. Electronic Photography

Alternatives to standard photographic recording media have become available with the recent renaissance in technology. These include video printers and film recorders that rapidly produce prints and slides in color and black-and-white with little or no loss in resolution as compared to photography.

## 1. Video Printers

Video printers accept input signals from NTSC video (National Television System Committee; 525-line 60-fields/sec color video standard), RGB (red, green, and blue) video, and digital sources (e.g., from a frame grabber). Thus the video printer connects to the image monitor or image frame grabber, and records the image in analog onto special paper. Both black-and-white and color video printers are commercially available from numerous sources and are easy to use. Black-and-white video printers use thermal paper, in which an element of the printing head is heated according to the image signal. Color video printers often use thermal sublimation dye transfer methods, in which dye from an ink ribbon is sublimated (vaporized) onto special color print paper in proportion to the thermal energy of the print head. After pressing the print button, an image is captured and a print is obtained within ~1–2 min. For RGB video with black-and-white printers, the printer is usually hooked up to the green line of the image monitor. To obtain suitable continuous-tone colors for RGB video with color printers, each red, green, and blue line of the image monitor is separately connected to the corresponding red, green, and blue lines of the printer. This allows more faithful reproduction of color tones. Many video printers provide prints with ~500-line resolution and 16.7 million color choices per pixel (dot) on the print. Video printers also allow adjustment of the brightness, color balance, and contrast to a limited extent in their memory. Often video printers have the added advantage of serving as an RGB-to-NTSC converter, which allows color recording of color images to video tape because RGB video signals cannot be recorded directly onto a regular VCR.

## 2. Film Recorders

An alternative to photographic recording and video printers is film recorders that process computer images and record them on photographic film such as 35-mm black-and-white and color slide film (Poor, 1991). Both analog and digital film recorders are commercially available. Analog film recorders record images by displaying a video signal from the computer on a small cathode ray tube (CRT) contained in a case. A camera on the case then takes a picture of the full-color screen image. Thus analog film recorders have the same resolution as the image source (e.g., monitor or video adapter of the computer).

Digital film recorders also have a CRT and camera, but they work differently than analog film recorders. Instead of displaying and photographing a full-color screen image, a digital recorder exposes the red, green, and blue components of the image separately through colored filters. Here, the resolution of the image depends on the rasterizer of the recorder rather than the video card of the computer. The rasterizer, which converts the image into a pattern of pixels that is then split into red, green, and blue components, may divide the image into $4096 \times 2732$ pixels, or 4000-line resolution. Because of the size of 35-mm film, the horizontal measure is larger. Many digital film recorders support 24-bit color (8 bits assigned per pixel for each red, green, and blue component, resulting in 16.7 million possible colors). The result is a much greater resolution than with an analog film recorder. Thus a digital film recorder can produce a color slide that often exceeds the resolution of the image display monitor. For example, a significant difference is observed when a print made with a video printer from an image displayed on a 525-line image monitor is compared with a photograph printed from a 35-mm slide that was recorded with a 4000-line resolution digital film recorder using the same computer image file.

Most popular personal and workstation computers can be interfaced to film recorders, although image files often need to be converted to the native control language (e.g., SCODL language) of the digital film recorder. Once the image file has been converted, rasterized, and sent to the film recorder, the red, green, and blue components of the image are displayed line by line on a monochrome CRT and passed through a filter of the appropriate color before striking the film. Unlike a video printer, in which a full color print is produced in ~2 min, a digital film recorder may take 10–20 min or more to expose the film. Once the image has been captured on film by the digital film recorder, the film is developed and processed as for conventional color slide film. Most film recorders have camera backs for creating instant color transparencies, prints, and slides in addition to conventional color slides. However, the quality of instant images is often poorer than conventional film.

## VIII. Future Prospects

Confocal microscopy is a powerful new instrument for biologists to examine cellular structure and function, and complements light and electron microscopy. The CLSMs and spinning disk confocal microscopes offer a convenient means of examining both living and fixed specimens labeled with multiple probes to determine the three-dimensional organization of various cellular components. The capabilities of these confocal microscopes are proving invaluable in studying fluorescently labeled structures of thick specimens in three dimensions. New advances in computer technology have produced powerful computers that can display and analyze three-dimensional data. The potential for this combination of technologies is enormous, especially when considering three-dimensional volume renderings of living cells and tissues over time. Future advances in the field include more powerful computers and imaging software that will aid in manipulating the voluminous data so that it will be possible to construct volumes rendered three dimensionally in real time from living specimens. Advances in archival media will allow more data to be saved faster and in a more compact form. Other future advances include improvements in confocal microscope design and sensitive dyes and probes for use in biology. Application of these new technologies will permit cell biologists to observe previously unseen phenomena, and explore the subtle relationships between cellular structure and function quantitatively in a dynamic volume.

## Acknowledgments

We thank Drs. S. Carroll, J. Langeland, and S. Attai (Howard Hughes Medical Institute) for preparing the *Drosophila* embryo. We gratefully acknowledge Dr. J. McCarthy, J. Walker, D. Kinser, J. Aeschbach, and M. Szulczewski for making a video-rate CLSM and TSM available and for their helpful discussions. We also thank Dr. D. J. Wright for critical reading of the manuscript. Research described herein was funded by grants from the NIH, and S.J.W. is supported as an NIH-NRSA Postdoctoral Fellow. The Integrated Microscopy Resource is supported by the NIH as a Biomedical Research Technology Resource.

## References

Agard, D. A., and Sedat, J. W. (1983). *Nature (London)* **302**, 676–681.
Agard, D. A., Hiraoka, Y., Shaw, P., and Sedat, J. W. (1989). *Methods Cell Biol.* **30**, 353–377.
Arndt-Jovin, D. J., Robert-Nicoud, M., and Jovin, T. M. (1990). *J. Microsc. (Oxford)* **157**, 61–72.
Bacallao, R., Bomsel, M., Stelzer, E. H. K., and De Mey, J. (1989). *In* "The Handbook of Biological Confocal Microscopy" (J. Pawley, ed.), pp. 181–187. IMR Press, Madison, Wisconsin.
Balczon, R., and Schatten, G. (1983). *Cell Motil.* **3**, 213–226.
Boyde, A. (1985). *Science* **230**, 1270–1272.
Boyde, A., Jones, S. J., Taylor, M. L., Wolfe, A., and Watson, T. F. (1990). *J. Microsc. (Oxford)* **157**, 39–49.
Brakenhoff, G. J. (1979). *J. Microsc.* (Oxford) **117**, 233–242.
Brakenhoff, G. J., and Visscher, K. (1992). *J. Microsc. (Oxford)* **165**, 139–146.
Carlsson, K., Danielsson, P. E., Lenz, R., Liljeborg, A., Majlog, L., and Aslund, N. (1985). *Opt. Lett.* **10**, 53–55.
Carrington, W. A., Fogarty, K. E., Lifschitz, L., and Fay, F. S. (1989). *In* "The Handbook of Biological Confocal Microscopy" (J. Pawley, ed.), pp. 137–146. IMR Press, Madison, Wisconsin.
Chen, H., Sedat, J. W., and Agard, D. A. (1989). *In* "The Handbook of Biological Confocal Microscopy" (J. Pawley, ed.), pp. 127–135. IMR Press, Madison, Wisconsin.
Cheng, P. C., and Summers, R. G. (1989). *In* "The Handbook of Biological Confocal Microscopy" (J. Pawley, ed.), pp. 163–179. IMR Press, Madison, Wisconsin.
Cornell-Bell, A. H., Finkbeiner, S. M., Cooper, M. S., and Smith, S. J. (1990). *Science* **247**, 470–473.

Costello, D. P., Davidson, M. E., Eggress, A., Fox, M. H., and Henley, C. (1957). "Methods for Obtaining and Handling Marine Eggs and Embryos." Lancaster Press, Lancaster, Pennsylvania.

Draijer, A., and Houpt, P. M. (1988). *Scanning* **10**, 139–145.

Draijer, A., and Houpt, P. M. (1993). *In* "Electronic Light Microscopy: Techniques in Modern Biomedical Microscopy" (D. M. Shotton, ed.), pp. 273–288. Wiley-Liss, New York.

Egger, M. D., and Petran, M. (1967). *Science* **157**, 305–307.

Epel, D. (1978). *Curr. Top. Dev. Biol.* **12**, 185–246.

Finkbeiner, S. (1992). *Neuron* **8**, 1101–1108.

Giloh, H., and Sedat, J. W. (1982). *Science* **217**, 1252–1255.

Gratton, E., and van de Ven, M. J. (1989). *In* "The Handbook of Biological Confocal Microscopy" (J. Pawley, ed.), pp. 47–59. IMR Press, Madison, Wisconsin.

Harris, K. M., and Stevens, J. K. (1989). *J. Neurosci.* **9**, 2982–2997.

Harris, P. J. (1986). *Methods Cell Biol.* **27**, 243–262.

Haugland, R. P. (1990). *In* "Optical Microscopy for Biology" (B. Herman and K. Jacobson, eds.), pp. 143–157. Alan R. Liss, New York.

Hinegardner, R. (1975). *In* "The Sea Urchin Embryo" (G. Czihak, ed.), pp. 10–25. Springer-Verlag, Berlin.

Holy, J., Simerly, C., Paddock, S., and Schatten, G. (1991). *J. Electron Microsc. Tech.* **17**, 384–400.

Inoué, S. (1986). "Video Microscopy." Plenum, New York.

Inoué, S. (1989). *In* "The Handbook of Biological Confocal Microscopy" (J. Pawley, ed.), pp. 1–13. IMR Press, Madison, Wisconsin.

Johnson, G. D., and de C. Nogueira Araujo, G. M. (1981). *J. Immunol. Methods* **43**, 349–350.

Johnson, G. D., Davidson, R. S., McNamee, K. C., Russel, G., Goodwin, D., and Holbrow, E. J. (1982). *J. Immunol. Methods* **55**, 231–242.

Kino, G. S. (1989). *In* "The Handbook of Biological Confocal Microscopy" (J. Pawley, ed.), pp. 92–97. IMR Press, Madison, Wisconsin.

Kraut, R., and Levine, M. (1991). *Development* **111**, 601–609.

Kuriyama, R., Borisy, G. G., and Masui, Y. (1983). *Dev. Biol.* **114**, 151–160.

Langanger, G., De Mey, J., and Adam, H. (1983). *Mikroskopie* **40**, 237–241.

Lichtman, J. W., Sunderland, W. J., and Wilkinson, R. S. (1989). *New Biol.* **1**, 75–82.

Luttmer, S. J., and Longo, F. J. (1986). *Gamete Res.* **15**, 267–283.

Lutz, D. A., and Inoue, S. (1986). *Methods Cell Biol.* **27**, 89–110.

Mazia, D., Schatten, G., and Sale, W. (1975). *J. Cell Biol.* **66**, 198–200.

Minsky, M. (1957). U.S. Pat. 3,013,467.

Minsky, M. (1988). *Scanning* **10**, 128–138.

Paddock, S. W. (1989). *J. Cell Sci.* **93**, 143–146.

Paddock, S. W. (1991). *Proc. Soc. Exp. Biol. Med.* **198**, 772–780.

Paddock, S., DeVries, P., Holy, J., and Schatten, G. (1990). *Proc. Soc. Photo-Opt. Instrum. Eng.* **1205**, 20–28.

Paddock, S., Mahoney, S., Minshall, M., Smith, L., Duvic, M., and Lewis, D. (1991). *BioTechniques* **11**, 486–493.

Pawley, J. (1989). *In* "The Handbook of Biological Confocal Microscopy" (J. Pawley, ed.), pp. 15–22. IMR Press, Madison, Wisconsin.

Petran, M., Hadravsky, M., Egger, D., and Galambos, R. (1968). *J. Opt. Soc. Am.* **58**, 661–664.

Petran, M., Hadravsky, M., Benes, J., Kucera, R., and Boyde, A. (1985). *Proc. R. Microsc. Soc.* **20**, 125–129.

Poor, A. (1991). *PC Mag.* **10**, 305–322.

Robert-Nicoud, M., Arndt-Jovin, D. J., Schormann, T., and Jovin, T. M. (1989). *Eur. J. Cell Biol.* **48**, Suppl. 25, 49–52.

Robinson, J. M., and Batten, B. E. (1989). *J. Histochem. Cytochem.* **37**, 1761–1765.

Schatten, G., Simerly, C., Asai, D. J., Szoke, E., Cooke, P., and Schatten, H. (1988). *Dev. Biol.* **130**, 74–86.

Sheppard, C. J. R., and Choudhury, A. (1977). *Opt. Acta* **24,** 1051–1073.

Shotton, D. M. (1988). *J. Cell Sci.* **89,** 129–150.

Shotton, D. M. (1989). *J. Cell Sci.* **94,** 175–206.

Shotton, D. M. (1993). *In* "Electronic Light Microscopy: Techniques in Modern Biomedical Microscopy" (D. M. Shotton, ed.), pp. 1–38. Wiley-Liss, New York.

Showman, R. M., and Foerder, C. A. (1979). *Exp. Cell Res.* **120,** 253–255.

Shuman, H., Murray, J. M., and DiLullo, C. (1989). *BioTechniques* **7,** 154–163.

Stricker, S. A., Paddock, S., and Schatten, G. (1990). *J. Cell Biol.* **111,** 113a.

Stricker, S. A., Centonze, V. E., Paddock, S. W., and Schatten, G. (1992). *Dev. Biol.* **149,** 370–380.

Summers, R. G., Musial, C. E., Cheng, P.-C., Leith, A., and Marko, M. (1991). *J. Electron Microsc. Tech.* **18,** 24–30.

Tsien, R. Y. (1989). *Methods Cell Biol.* **30,** 127–156.

Tsien, R. Y., and Waggoner, A. (1989). *In* "The Handbook of Biological Confocal Microscopy" (J. Pawley, ed.), pp. 153–161. IMR Press, Madison, Wisconsin.

Van Zandt, W., and Argiro, V. (1989). *Unix Rev.* **7,** 52–57.

Webb, R. H., and Dorey, C. K. (1989). *In* "The Handbook of Biological Confocal Microscopy" (J. Pawley, ed.), pp. 37–45. IMR Press, Madison, Wisconsin.

Webb, W. W., Wells, K. S., Sandison, D. R., and Strickler, J. (1990). *In* "Optical Microscopy for Biology" (B. Herman and K. Jacobson, eds.), pp. 73–108. Alan R. Liss, New York.

White, J. G., Amos, W. B., and Fordham, M. (1987). *J. Cell Biol.* **105,** 41–48.

White, J. G., Amos, W. B., Durbin, R., and Fordham, M. (1990). *In* "Optical Microscopy for Biology" (B. Herman and K. Jacobson, eds.), pp. 1–18. Alan R. Liss, New York.

Wijnaendts van Resandt, R. W., Marsman, H. J. B., Kaplan, R., Davoust, J., Stelzer, E. H. K., and Stricker, R. (1985). *J. Microsc. (Oxford)* **138,** 29–34.

Wilke, V. (1985). *Scanning* **7,** 88–96.

Wilson, T. (1989). *Trends Neurosci.* **12,** 486–493.

Wilson, T. (1990). "Confocal Microscopy." Academic Press, New York.

Wilson, T., and Sheppard, C. J. R. (1984). "Theory and Practice of Scanning Optical Microscopy." Academic Press, New York.

Wright, S. J., and Schatten, G. (1991). *J. Electron Microsc. Tech.* **18,** 2–10.

Wright, S. J., Walker, J. S., Schatten, H., Simerly, C., McCarthy, J. J., and Schatten, G. (1989). *J. Cell Sci.* **94,** 617–624.

Wright, S. J., Schatten, H., Simerly, C., and Schatten, G. (1990). *In* "Optical Microscopy for Biology" (B. Herman and K. Jacobson, eds.), pp. 29–43. Alan R. Liss, New York.

Xiao, G. Q., and Kino, G. S. (1987). *Proc. Soc. Photo-Opt. Instrum. Eng.* **809,** 107–113.

Xiao, G. Q., Corle, T. R., and Kino, G. S. (1988). *Appl. Phys. Lett.* **53,** 716–718.

**CHAPTER 2**

# Rapid Scanning Confocal Microscopy

## Jonathan J. Art and Miriam B. Goodman

Department of Pharmacological and Physiological Sciences
University of Chicago
Chicago, Illinois 60637

## I. Introduction

The renaissance in biological light microscopy is due in part to advances in dye chemistry, digital signal processing, and, especially, in microscope design that markedly improve image quality. As physiologists, one of our goals is to examine variations in structure, ion concentration, or potential within living cells or among cells in tissues. In general, it is difficult to combine high-speed acquisition and high spatial resolution while preserving maximum sensitivity at low light levels. One corollary is that the light signal may be increased with intense illumination, but only at the risk of radiation damage that may modify the cellular behavior under study. The development of fluorescent dyes that rapidly indicate small variations in voltage (Fluhler *et al.*, 1985) and ion concentration (Grynkiewicz *et al.*, 1985) has made it possible to follow cellular events on a millisecond time scale. These dyes, in conjunction with video-imaging techniques appropriate for low light levels (Spring and Lowy, 1989), allow simultaneous measurement of the activity of multiple cells as well as the observation of heterogeneity within a single cell. However, the complex three-dimensional nature of biological structures presents additional challenges. One goal is to observe the variation in response between individual cells in a tissue. The problem in fluorescence microscopy is that contributions arising from individual cells arrayed in depth are projected into the same image plane. This is a consequence of the design of conventional epifluorescence microscopes (see Section III,A). More generally, it means that optical signals from out-of-focus object planes are included in the resulting image. It is, therefore, impossible to determine what cell or subcellular region in depth gives rise to the optical signal for a given portion of the image. Many of the difficulties in resolving complex tissues can be overcome by either numerical (Agard and Sedat, 1983) or optical techniques (Amos *et al.*, 1987).

In this article we seek to evaluate to what extent scanning confocal microscopy at video rates achieves the goal of joining sensitivity with high spatial and temporal resolution. In the process, we describe the physical and theoretical limits imposed by optics, photochemistry, and light detection on reaching this goal. In addition, this article discusses currently available technology for video-rate confocal microscopy, with particular attention to the specific requirements of the analysis of physiological behavior. Included in the discussion is an analysis of the performance of one commercially available device (Odyssey; Noran Instruments, Middleton, WI). Other, more specialized instruments, such as rotating prism confocal microscopes (Koester, 1980) used in ophthalmology, operate at video rates but will not be considered in detail here. Finally, we suggest criteria for assessing the new technologies.

## II. Video–Rate Confocal Microscopes

The history and theory of confocal microscopy has been extensively reviewed elsewhere (Pawley, 1990, and this volume) and will be addressed in more detail in Section III. In short, the object is illuminated and observed so that the light from out-of-focus planes is eliminated from the image. This is accomplished by illuminating a single diffraction-limited volume in the object and observing the light transmitted, reflected, or emitted by that point. A full image is generated as either the specimen or the light beam is moved sequentially to examine each point in the object. Multiple points can be simultaneously scanned if they are spaced widely enough that interference between adjacent points is eliminated. These three general strategies, shown schematically in Fig. 1, are termed object

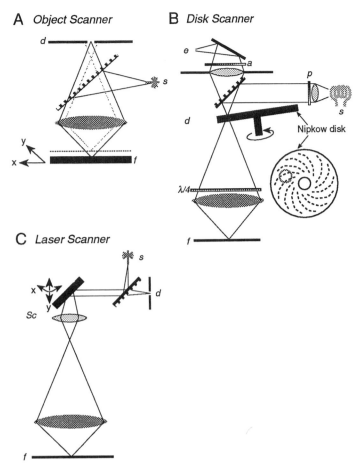

**Fig. 1** Schematic drawings of three types of scanning confocal microscopes. (A) Object scanner: image is formed by moving object through a stationary spot of light focused in the object plane; (B) disk scanner: image is formed by simultaneous illumination by multiple spots focused in the object plane. Each spot is the image of a pinhole aperture in the Nipkow disk; (C) laser scanner: image is formed by moving a diffraction-limited spot of light across the object plane in a rectangular raster pattern. *f,* Focal plane in object; *s,* point source; *d,* detector aperture; *e,* eyepiece; *a,* analyzer; *p,* polarizer; *Sc,* laser scanner. The detector aperture is placed in a conjugate image plane in all cases.

scanning (Fig. 1A), disk scanning (Fig. 1B), and laser scanning (Fig. 1C) confocal microscopy. Evaluation of the performance of a given microscope for a particular application includes an estimate of the image quality and overall signal-to-noise ratio (SNR). In addition, the choice between the three depends, in part, on considerations peripherally related to image quality. These include (1) the speed of the scanning device, (2) the intensity and wavelength of the light source, and (3) the nature of the detector. The secondary issue of whether the instrument is to be used solely for imaging factors in the decision.

The simplest confocal microscope suitable for fluorescence and reflectance imaging is the object-scanning configuration depicted in Fig. 1A. The object may be scanned by moving the entire microscope stage or the specimen alone with stepping motors or piezoelectric movers. Although the latter technique is faster, it is unlikely that the object would be light enough to be scanned at video rates. Also, because physiological studies often employ additional apparatus attached to the specimen, such as microelectrodes, scanning by this technique would require movement of the accessory equipment as well. Confocal microscopes that employ moving light sources are more readily incorporated into physiological studies and will, therefore, be discussed in considerable detail.

## A. Disk Scanning Microscopes

The earliest video-rate confocal technique, reduced to practice shortly after the Minsky (1961) patent, was the rotating disk technology of Petran *et al.* (1985; Petran and Hadravsky, 1968) with later developments and improvements by Xiao *et al.* (1988). Devices employing this technology are commercially available [e.g., the TSM (Tracor Northern, now Noran Instruments), VX100 (Newport Instruments), and K2S-Bio (Technical Instrument Company)]. Two features of this device make it the best choice for universal high-speed imaging. First, these devices are fast; acquisition rates can exceed 640 frames/sec with 7000-line resolution (Xiao *et al.*, 1988). Second, they permit broadband illumination; white light sources like high-pressure mercury or xenon arc lamps can be used. These lamps, coupled with band-pass filtering, are capable of exciting most conventional fluorescent dyes.

Other features tend to reduce the overall SNR in the image and make disk scanners less attractive for fluorescence microscopy. First, the intensity of the illumination is limited by the reduced light transmission through the apertures of the spinning disk. To maximize spatial resolution (both lateral and axial), the separation between the pinholes on the disk is large. Generally, not more than 1 or 2% of the disk is open to the passage of light. If we assume that 1 mW focused to a diffraction-limited spot will saturate a fluorescent dye (White and Stryer, 1987), and 4000 points are being simultaneously scanned (Xiao *et al.*, 1988), then a total of 4 W of power is required. Because only 2% of the field is open, a light source that can provide 50 times this or 200 W at the relevant wavelength is needed. This is a large number, considering that a 150-W Xenon arc lamp produces ~1 W at 500 nm (Oriel, 1990). To image weakly fluorescent specimens, it is possible to trade spatial resolution for intensity. This is achieved by increasing the pinhole size, decreasing the separation between them, or both. Details concerning the effect of either manipulation on spatial resolution are found in the theoretical treatment of Wilson and Hewlett (1991). The net effect is to increase the fraction of the total power that reaches the specimen as well as the fraction of emitted light that is collected.

The images produced by disk scanning systems may be observed directly, either by eye or with a camera. Although the images are produced at rates that far exceed video rates, a camera is required to record the images. It is the camera, not the microscope, that determines the acquisition rate, light sensitivity, and the overall SNR. The sensitivity, linearity, speed, and spatial resolution of currently available cameras are discussed in detail in Vol. 29 of this series. The reader is referred to the chapters by Spring and Lowy (1989) and Aikens *et al.* (1989) for in-depth discussions. To increase sensitivity at low light levels, one common solution is to amplify the signal with a microchannel plate (MCP) and record the image with a video-rate charge-coupled device (CCD) camera. The overall SNR in the recorded image is limited by the low (0.1) quantum efficiency (QE) of the MCP and the high noise levels of the CCD. Better SNRs and QEs, up to 0.8, can be realized with slow-scan CCDs, but the cost is a further decrease in temporal resolution.

The overall SNR of disk scanning confocal microscopes is limited not only by the camera used, but also by the method of illumination. The rotating disk, placed in the image plane, is a partially reflective surface. Incident light reflected by the disk produces a high background and subsequent loss of contrast. The problem is pronounced in fluorescence applications, in which intense illumination is often needed to excite the fluorophore. Even if the disk reflected one-millionth of the incident photons, the resultant flux might be comparable to that produced by the fluorophore. One solution is to use a quarter-wave ($\lambda/4$) plate placed immediately behind the objective. The $\lambda/4$ plate is oriented so that it converts plane-polarized light into circularly polarized light and vice versa. When the circularly polarized light is reflected, it reverses polarization. As it returns from the specimen and passes through the $\lambda/4$ plate, it is converted back into plane-polarized light oriented 90° to the polarization of the incident illumination (Hecht, 1987). An analyzer (polarizer) whose plane of polarization is parallel to that of the light reflected from the object is placed just under the eyepiece (Fig. 1B). Oriented and placed in this way, it will reject light reflected from the disk and other optical components in the microscope, and enhance the SNR in the image. Unfortunately, because fluorescent light emitted from the specimen is randomly polarized, a fraction of the desired signal will also be eliminated from the image.

Disk scanning confocal microscopes are ideal when fast, full-field images of highly reflective objects are desired. With a light source that is sufficiently powerful, they are a good choice for use with most fluorescent dyes. As faster cameras with better SNRs and higher QEs are developed, disk scanning systems will become more attractive for fluorescence applications. There are subsidiary issues, however, that demand attention. For example, it may be desirable to illuminate a small region of the entire field so that photodamage is restricted to a portion of the specimen. Collecting images from a smaller region is also useful because the amount of data to be stored and processed is likewise reduced. Because disk scanners are designed for generating full-field images, scanning subregions is not easily arranged. A second concern is the range over which intensity of both the incident and emitted light may be controlled. As noted earlier, the intensity may be increased by using disks with larger and/or more closely spaced apertures. The VX100 (Newport Instruments) achieves this with a single disk with five different aperture tracks: one that is open, two with slits, and two with pinholes. Although this approach is more flexible than using a disk with a single aperture array, the range over which intensity may be controlled is necessarily limited by the small number of options.

## B. Laser Scanning Microscopes

An intense, coherent light source is obtained if a laser is substituted for the arc lamp. Unfortunately, the laser limits the number of wavelengths that can be used (Gratton and vandeVen, 1990). For example, the low power, air-cooled argon ion laser common in confocal microscopy has only two principal lines (488 and 514 nm). A laser may be used as the light source for a disk scanning unit (Xiao *et al.*, 1988) or serve as the basis for a laser-scanning confocal microscope (LSCM). At 30 frames/sec, video rate (Inoué, 1986) is a modest 1/20 of that achieved by disk scanning units. Yet it is sufficiently fast to produce an image that appears continuous to the human eye and allow measurement of ion concentration with single-frame resolution of 33 msec. To build an image at this rate, the beam must sweep across the field extremely rapidly (left to right in 52 $\mu$sec). Here, we describe the various techniques currently employed to steer the laser, the limitations of each, and what strategies could be used to achieve video-rate acquisition.

## 1. Mechanical Scanning

Most beam steering confocal microscopes use a pair of mirrors, each mounted on the shaft of a separate galvanometer, to create a raster-like scan of a stationary object. The pattern is produced by moving the horizontal scan mirror rapidly from left to right; at the end of each scan it returns abruptly to the original position. The vertical scan mirror is simultaneously moved slowly from the top to the bottom of the field to create the full-frame image. The angular position of the shaft and attached mirror is determined by the current through the galvanometer. More precisely, the position of the mirror as a function of driving current is described as a simple second-order mechanical system. Typical scanners used for *xy* positioning can be driven by sawtooth, triangle, or sine waves at frequencies up to 5% of the resonant frequency (General Scanning, 1984). The galvanometer pair used in the MRC-600 (Bio-Rad, Richmond, CA) generates a 768 × 512 pixel raster at a maximum rate of 1 frame/sec.

Higher scan rates can be attained with existing galvanometer scanners in two ways. First, reduce the field of view. It is possible to collect images at the respectable rate of 16 frames/sec with an MRC-600 if the field is reduced to 192 × 128 pixels and every fourth line is scanned. Second, move the mirrors faster. If operated in resonance mode they can be driven sinusoidally up to 85% of the natural frequency of the galvanometer (11 to 10 kHz). Speed is increased further if the object is scanned in both horizontal directions: left to right followed immediately by right to left. This complicates image formation somewhat, as the pixel order on alternate lines must be reversed to produce a coherent image. This is the strategy adopted by Tsien (1990) to achieve video-rate acquisition. There is no theoretical limit to the speed of galvanometer mirror scanners save those imposed by engineering constraints. If less massive mirrors and drive shafts could be built, the acquisition rate of mechanical scanners might be significantly enhanced.

Regardless of whether they are used as resonance or *xy* scanners, the long-term stability of galvanometers is a serious concern for confocal microscopy. Most scanners are not optimized for long-term reproducibility because they are used in applications in which the image is acquired in a single pass, such as copiers and desktop scanners. Confocal microscopy often requires averaging over several frames in order to improve the SNR and image quality. Whether or not the image improves with averaging is critically dependent on the assumption that each pixel is collected from the same position in each frame. In this way, random noise due to both photon statistics and the detector is averaged out of the image. Positional error produced by the beam-steering system may be random, systematic, or both. Random error tends to blur the object so that the lateral resolution is reduced compared to that expected from diffraction-limited optics. This can be observed by comparing the image of a highly reflective or fluorescent object acquired in a single frame with that generated by an average of many frames. The extent to which features in the averaged image remain crisp and distinct is a measure of the random error in galvanometer position. Systematic error arises due to drift in the positional accuracy of the mirror and is manifested by blurring of the image in the direction of the drift. This error is most acute with galvanometer mirrors that show significant drift with temperature, because they will heat during use.

## 2. Acousto–optic Scanning

Acousto-optical deflectors (AODs) are used in at least three laser scanning confocal microscopes (Draaijer and Houpt, 1988; Goldstein *et al.,* 1990; Suzuki and Horikawa, 1986). Acousto-optical deflectors are attractive for beam steering because they are solid-state devices that permit rapid scanning and have no moving parts. Briefly, incident light is deflected by a diffraction grating acoustically generated in the AOD. The physics of producing and modulating this diffraction grating constrains the application of AODs as beam scanners. Because their behavior is quite complex compared to the mechanical systems discussed previously, the theory of their operation is discussed in detail.

As shown schematically in Fig. 2A, ultrasonic acoustic waves within a medium result in alternating regions of rarefaction and condensation (Yariv and

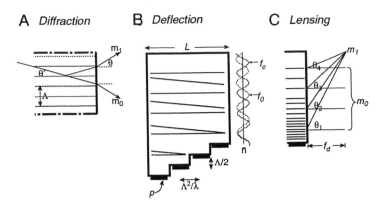

**Fig. 2** Theory of acousto-optical deflectors (AODs). (A) Diffraction in the AOD. Horizontal lines represent maxima and minima in the index of refraction, $n$, produced by the acoustic wave. Incident light is diffracted by regions where the index of refraction is maximal. A single incident light ray and the undeviated ($m_0$) and first-order ($m_1$) diffracted beams are shown. $\theta$ is the angle formed by $m_1$ with respect to a normal to the crystal surface. (B) Deflection by the AOD. Shown is an array of piezoelectric drivers where $\Lambda^2/\lambda$ is the width and $\Lambda/2$ is the rise of each step. The drivers in the array run at a single acoustic frequency, but alternate elements are driven $\pi$ radians out of phase. Horizontal lines represent maxima of $n$ produced at the center acoustic frequency, $f_c$, and angled lines are those produced at a lower frequency, $f_0$. The grid spacing is shown to scale. (C) Lensing produced by AOD. Horizontal lines represent maxima of $n$ at a single point in time when the AOD is driven by a rapid, linear acoustic frequency sweep. $\theta_1$–$\theta_4$ are the Bragg angles for selected grid spacings. Note that the first-order diffracted beams come to a single focal point at a distance of $f_d$. $m_0$, Zeroth-order diffraction beam; $m_1$, first-order diffraction beam; $\theta$, Bragg angle; $\Lambda$, acoustic wavelength; $L$, crystal thickness; $p$, piezoelectric driver; $\lambda$, center optical wavelength; $\bar{n}$, mean index of refraction; $f_c$, center acoustic frequency; $f_0$, acoustic driving frequency less than $f_c$; $f_d$, focal length of AOD lens.

Yeh, 1984). This corresponds to regions of lower and higher indices of refraction about a mean value, $n$, for the material used to construct the AOD. Because the speed of sound in the material is about five orders of magnitude slower than the speed of light in the same material, the medium behaves as a stationary diffraction grating for light. The grid spacing is equal to the acoustic wavelength, $\Lambda$, which is the acoustic frequency, $f$, divided by the velocity of sound, $V$, in the medium ($\Lambda = f/V$). If light of wavelength $\lambda$ passes through a grating of thickness $L$, where $L > \Lambda^2/\lambda$, the interaction between the light and sound is in the Bragg domain (Debye and Sears, 1932), and light is diffracted only into the first order, $m_1$. Light incident on the grating at the Bragg angle, $\theta$, will be diffracted as shown in Fig. 2A, by an angle governed by the relation

$$\theta \approx \sin \theta = \lambda/2\Lambda = \lambda f/2V \qquad (1)$$

The angle between the undeviated beam $m_0$ and the diffracted beam $m_1$ will be $2\theta$. Because the angles are less than a degree, the approximation $\theta \approx \sin \theta$ is applied. From Eq. (1) it is clear that the angle of diffraction is determined by the acoustic wavelength and, hence, the driving frequency. Therefore the beam can be deflected through different angles by changing the acoustic frequency. Unfortunately, the power in the diffracted beam $m_1$ drops sharply as the angle of the incident light departs from the Bragg angle, severely limiting the angular range over which a stationary AOD can steer the light beam. Korpel *et al.* (1966) devised a scheme that uses a phased array of transducers to compensate for the change in Bragg angle, $\Delta\theta$, associated with varying the acoustic wavelength (see Fig. 2B). At the acoustic center frequency, $f_c$, the grating produced is perpendicular to the axis of sound propagation. As the acoustic frequency is changed, the angle of the grating is rotated to compensate for $\Delta\theta$ precisely, and the intensity of the diffracted beam is held constant. If the acoustic drive frequency is changed by $\Delta f = f_1 - f_0$, the beam is deflected through an angle $\Delta\theta$ given by

$$\Delta\theta = \lambda \Delta f / 2V \qquad (2)$$

To deflect the beam along a line, the phased array of transducers is driven by linearly sweeping the acoustic frequency from $f_0$ to $f_1$ for a total deflection angle, $\Delta\theta$, given by Eq. (2) above.

### a. Wavelength Dependence

By using a phased transducer array, the AOD becomes a suitable device for beam steering. As is clear from Eq. (2), the angle of deflection is proportional to wavelength $\lambda$. Generally, the design of an AOD is optimized for particular optical and acoustic wavelengths. The AOD used in the Noran Odyssey is optimized for $\lambda_c = 488$ nm. Table I lists the angle of beam deflection for a number of incident wavelengths.

Two features of the AOD that depend on wavelength are immediately apparent. First, the position of the beam at $f_c$ shifts with wavelength. This results in a wavelength-dependent pan of the image. Second, the range of angles through

**Table I**
**AOD Deflection as a Function of Wavelength**

| Wavelength (nm) | $2\theta$ at $f_0$ ($10^{-3}$ radians)[a] | $2\theta$ at $f_c$ ($10^{-3}$ radians)[b] | $2\theta$ at $f_1$ ($10^{-3}$ radians)[c] | Magnification (*re* field at 488 nm) | Overlap (% field at 488 nm) |
|---|---|---|---|---|---|
| 363 | 8.83 | 13.25 | 17.67 | 1.34 | 49 |
| 400 | 9.73 | 14.60 | 19.47 | 1.22 | 66 |
| 457 | 11.12 | 16.68 | 22.42 | 1.07 | 87 |
| 488 | 11.88 | 17.81 | 23.75 | 1.00 | 100 |
| 529 | 12.87 | 19.30 | 25.75 | 0.92 | 92 |
| 726 | 17.66 | 26.49 | 35.24 | 0.67 | 51 |

[a] The lowest acoustic driving frequency, $f_0$, is 100 MHz
[b] The center acoustic driving frequency, $f_c$, is 150 MHz
[c] The highest acoustic driving frequency, $f_1$, is 200 MHz

which the illuminating beam rotates during the frequency sweep is expanded for wavelengths longer than $\lambda_c$ and is reduced for shorter wavelengths. If the number of pixels in an image is constant, then this is equivalent to a wavelength-dependent zoom of the object. The magnification relative to that at $\lambda_c = 488$ nm is given in the fifth column of Table I. Correction for these effects is incorporated in the design of the microscope. If images of a single object collected at well-separated, multiple illumination wavelengths are to be combined, then the position of the field (pan) is determined by the shortest wavelength and the magnification (zoom) that must be used is determined by the extent of overlap between the longest and shortest wavelength fields.

### b. Video-Rate Scanning with Acousto-optical Deflectors

For maximum compatibility, video-rate image acquisition should match existing video standards (e.g., EIA RS-170). The faster horizontal component determines the minimum acceptable speed of AOD operation. Specifically, the AOD must be able to (1) reposition the beam during the retrace and (2) steer the beam across the entire horizontal scan line during the time devoted to the active scan. For RS-170 video, then, the AOD must be able to reposition the beam from the end of a scan line in the $\sim10$ $\mu$sec devoted to retracing. This is equivalent to requiring that the initial wavefront of a new acoustic frequency must propagate across the incident laser beam in the same time interval. This time ($\tau$) for a beam diameter, $D$, and acoustic velocity, $V$, is

$$\tau = D/V \tag{3}$$

The acoustic velocity in the Odyssey AOD is $4.1 \times 10^3$ m/sec, and for the beam diameter of 40 mm, a change in the diffraction grating across the beam can be accomplished in the required 10 $\mu$sec.

Recall that scanning the beam along a line is accomplished by driving the AOD with a linear sweep of acoustic frequencies. The second requirement for RS-170 video-rate scanning is met if this frequency sweep is complete in 52 $\mu$sec. When the frequency is changed this rapidly, the diffraction grating spacing at any moment varies across the diameter of the beam. As shown in Fig. 2C, the result is that different parts of the beam will be deflected through different angles. Because the spacing and, hence, deflection angle varies linearly across the diameter of the beam, this will bring the beam to a focus. It has been shown (Gerig and Montague, 1964) that for a sweep duration, $\Delta t$, with a frequency change of $\Delta f$, the first-order diffracted light $m_1$ will be focused at a distance, $f_d$, where

$$f_d = V^2 \Delta t / \lambda \Delta f \tag{4}$$

The Odyssey AOD steers the laser beam across a scan line by sweeping the acoustic frequency through the range $\Delta f = 100$ MHz. For light at 488 nm, the AOD produces a lens with a focal length of 19.6 m. Introducing another lens after the AOD compensates for this effect. Poor placement of this lens results in either under- or overcompensation. Failure to compensate correctly for the AOD lens effect will result in an astigmatic image (see Fig. 3). Equation (4) shows that $f_d$ will vary with wavelength and $\Delta f$. Reducing $\Delta f$, the range of the acoustic frequency sweep, reduces the total angle, $\Delta\theta$, through which the beam is deflected and produces zoom in the image [see Eq. (2)]. To ensure proper correction for the AOD lensing effect, the correction lens must be repositioned whenever either the illumination wavelength or zoom is changed (see Fig. 4).

Clearly, AODs are more than adequate for scanning at video rates. There are two additional properties of AODs that are relevant to laser scanning confocal microscopy. First, beam deflection by AODs limits the number of resolvable points along a line. There are approximately 1000 of these points per horizontal scan line in the Odyssey, more than twice the number required for compatibility with video frame grabbers. Second, the diffraction efficiency of the AOD is proportional to the magnitude of the acoustic drive. Attenuating the light intensity provided to the specimen is a simple matter of modulating this signal. Unfortunately, the maximum diffraction efficiency is small ($\sim$60%) compared to galvanometer mirror systems (up to 99% with coated mirrors). If the AOD is used both to illuminate the object (scan) and detect light from points in the object (descan), the total loss through the optical path is doubled. For this and the added reason that AOD deflection is wavelength dependent, these units are suitable only for both scanning and descanning light at a single wavelength. Fluorescence microscopy can use AODs to produce the illumination scan, but must rely on other strategies such as image dissector tubes (Goldstein *et al.*, 1990) or slit apertures (Draaijer and Houpt, 1988), for descanning and detection. This is a slight disadvantage because slit apertures decrease the axial as well as

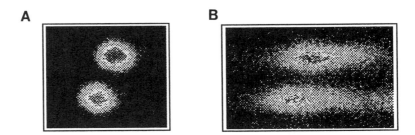

**A**　　　　　　　　　　**B**

**Fig. 3** Improper correction of AOD lensing effect produces astigmatism in the image. Shown are fluorescent images of two 1-$\mu$m latex beads (Cat. No. 18660; Polysciences). (A) Correction lens is placed properly; the beads appear circular at plane of maximum focus. (B) Lens is displaced slightly along the light path; the same two beads at the same focal depth are blurred along one axis. These images were collected with the Odyssey, a Nikon Optiphot microscope, Zeiss ×40 NA 0.75 water immersion objective, 364-nm excitation wavelength, and a 420-nm barrier filter, slit width = 15 $\mu$m. The raw images fill 60 of a total of 255 gray levels. This intensity range was expanded by histogram equalization (Pratt, 1978) to fill all 255 gray levels for display purposes. The blocky appearance is due to the shallow pixel depth of the output device (a 300-dpi Adobe PostScript-based laser printer).

some lateral resolution (see Section III,A). Another disadvantage is that images collected at multiple illumination wavelengths must be corrected for the wavelength-dependent pan, zoom, and focal length characteristics of the AOD before building a single composite image. The problems associated with the wavelength-dependent pan and zoom are minimized when the AOD is calibrated during manufacture and the appropriate corrections are applied in the acoustic drive signal. In any case, polychromatic fluorescent beads should be used as test objects to calibrate and define the registration between images acquired with different wavelengths of illumination (Waggoner *et al.*, 1989).

### c. Fastest and Brightest

We have discussed the disadvantages associated with both mechanical and acousto-optical methods of generating a faster scan of an object at video rates. The best features of each can be exploited with a combination of both technologies. Because video frame rates are modest, a galvanometer can easily generate the slower vertical component of the scan, leaving the faster horizontal component to be scanned with an AOD. This hybrid approach can be used directly for reflected light (Fig. 4). Here, a single light path is used both to illuminate the object and to collect reflected light through a pinhole detector aperture. As noted above, the wavelength dependence of the AOD precludes descanning emitted fluorescent light along the horizontal scan line. The fluorescent light is descanned only along the vertical component and the emitted light returns along a separate path shown as dashed lines in Fig. 4. It is projected as a line at the detector, and a slit aperture must be used in place of the usual pinhole. In this way, video rates are achieved for both fluoresence and reflectance without resort to continually oscillating mirrors. Another approach is to dispense with scanning in the horizontal direction entirely and scan the object vertically at video frame rates with a diffraction-limited bar of light. One instrument (InSight; Meridian Instruments, Okemos, MI) does this by scanning a bar of light across the object with one side of a double-sided galvanometer mirror, the other side is used to collect light from the object. This permits rapid scanning (up to 120 frame/sec), direct viewing, and, like disk scanners, is designed for use with a camera detector (Brakenhoff and Visscher, 1990).

## III. Confocal Slice

The optical sectioning property of confocal microscopy has been exploited to generate three-dimensional images of cellular features (Bertero *et al.*, 1990; Carlsson *et al.*, 1989; Schormann and Jovin, 1990). Because it is not yet possible to capture an entire three-dimensional image set at video rates, we will confine our analysis to a single confocal plane. The role of confocal microscopy in this case is to maximize sensitivity and the SNR in the image by eliminating interference from light scattered from out-of-focus planes and the optics of the micro-

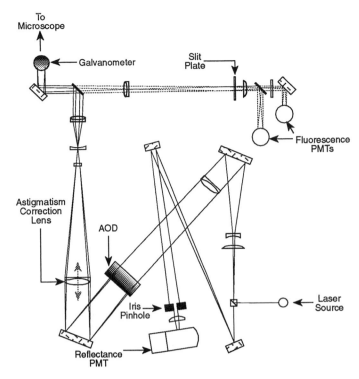

**Fig. 4** Schematic drawing of the light path of the Noran Odyssey. The incoming laser beam is spread into a line by a cylindrical lens, projected onto the AOD for producing the horizontal scan. The line is focused to a spot by another cylindrical lens and steered by a dichroic and plane mirror in series to a galvanometer mirror. The galvanometer is responsible for producing the vertical scan. From here, the light is directed through a quarter-wave plate into a camera port on the microscope (not shown). Reflected light gathered from the object follows the light path shown by the solid lines, and fluorescent light follows that shown by the dashed lines.

scope. To evaluate the utility of video-rate confocal microscopy for time-resolved physiological measurement, we will consider three issues. First, we will determine the thickness of the confocal slice and the relevant volume over which the response is measured. Second, we will estimate the rate at which photons are produced, and how rapidly we will be able to detect responses with the desired SNR. Third, we will address the effect of focused, high-intensity laser light on fluorescent dyes.

## A. Physical Basis of Optical Sectioning

The familiar technique of Köhler illumination is employed in conventional microscopy to achieve uniform illumination in the face of a nonuniform light source (Inoué, 1986). For transmission imaging, the condenser determines the illumination level and, to a some extent, the coherence of the illuminating light. If the condenser iris is stopped down fully, the illumination reduces to a point source in the back focal plane of the objective. A point source in this position produces parallel light in the object (see Fig. 5A). Or, equivalently, the illumination is constant throughout the depth of the specimen. This is identical to the situation in conventional epifluorescence microscopes, save that the objective now serves as the condenser (Taylor and Salmon, 1989). Because biological specimens are generally transparent, constant illumination through depth will excite fluorophores throughout. A fraction of the fluorescence produced in planes above and below the focal plane will be collected by the objective and, hence, combined with the in-focus light to produce the image. This is largely responsible for the hazy appearance of fluorescence images (flare).

The reduced flare achieved by confocal microscopy is the direct result of focusing the illumination on the fluorophores in the focal plane while, simultaneously, restricting the light collection (detection) to the same plane. More generally, this implies that imaging is a combined function of the method of illumination and detection. Illumination in the confocal case is acheived by a point source in an image plane. A point source here produces focused light in the object (see Fig. 5B). The three-dimensional intensity distribution is given by the function $I(r,w)$; where $r$ and $w$ are normalized, optical units defined in Table II. Similarly, a point detector in a second, conjugate image plane creates a detector sensitivity function in the object, which we designate $D(r, w)$ (after Sheppard

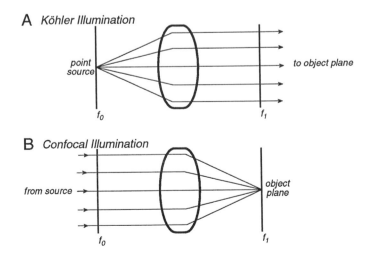

**Fig. 5** Köhler vs confocal illumination. (A) Köhler illumination in epifluorescence microscopes produces an effective point source in the back focal plane of the objective, resulting in parallel light in the object. (B) Confocal illumination uses a point source and lens (not shown) to produce parallel light at $f_0$, resulting in a focused spot of light in the object plane at $f_1$. $f_0$, Back focal plane of the objective; $f_1$, front focal plane of the objective.

**Table II**
**Normalized Optical Coordinates**[a]

| Cartesian | Cylindrical |
| --- | --- |
| $u = (2\pi x/\lambda)n\sin\alpha$ | $r^2 = u^2 + v^2$ |
| $v = (2\pi y/\lambda)n\sin\alpha$ | $\therefore r = (2\pi/\lambda)n\sin\alpha \, (x^2 + y^2)^{1/2}$ |
| $w = (2\pi z/\lambda)n\sin^2\alpha$ | $w = (2\pi w/\lambda)n\sin^2\alpha$ |

[a] See Brakenhoff (1989) and Born and Wolf (1980), p. 436.

and Mao, 1988). When an image is formed, the response recorded at any point in the object is the weighted average over the product of $I(r, w)$ and $D(r, w)$. This product is termed the confocal response function or $C(r, w)$ (Brakenhoff *et al.*, 1989).

The volume defined by $C(r, w)$ is the minimum resolvable element, or resel, in a confocal image (Webb and Dorey, 1990). This definition arises by analogy with the commonplace picture element or pixel. The thickness of the confocal slice is determined by the extent of this volume along the optical axis. The response function for both illumination, $I(r, w)$, and detection, $D(r, w)$, is determined by the detector geometry, wavelength of light, and numerical aperture of the optics employed. The simplest case is the reflected light confocal microscope, using a point source for illumination and an infinitely small pinhole for detection. Here, $I(r, w)$ and $D(r, w)$ are identical because a single wavelength, objective, and aperture geometry are used so that $C(r, w) = I^2(r, w)$. The theoretical intensity distribution in three dimensions for a point source is well known (Born and Wolf, 1980, Chap. 8). First calculated by Zernike and Nijboer (1949), it is shown in Fig. 6 as contour lines of equal intensity. In the Odyssey, in which the detector apertures for fluorescence are narrow slits rather than pinholes, the analysis is somewhat more complex (Wilson, 1989).

Heuristically, an analytical treatment of the optical sectioning and image enhancement achieved by confocal techniques can be derived from a knowledge of $C(r, w)$. Because this is a product of $I(r, w)$ and $D(r, w)$, the analysis can be generalized for arbitrary source and detector geometries given an analytical expression for each aperture (Sheppard and Mao, 1988). Deriving an expression for $I(r, w)$ in the focal plane ($w = 0$) begins with the notion that the intensity distribution for an incoherent light source, $S(r)$, focused by a lens with an amplitude point spread function (PSF), $h_s(r)$ is given by the convolution

$$I(r, 0) = S(r) \otimes |h_s(r)|^2 \tag{5}$$

For point illumination of a planar object, the intensity distribution in the object is simply the three-dimensional PSF of the lens used to image the light as shown in Fig. 6. The analysis is simplified if we divide $I(r, w)$ into two components: (1) an axial component, $I_a(0, w)$, equal to the transect along the optical axis, and (2) a lateral component, $I_l(r, 0)$, equal to the intensity in the focal plane.

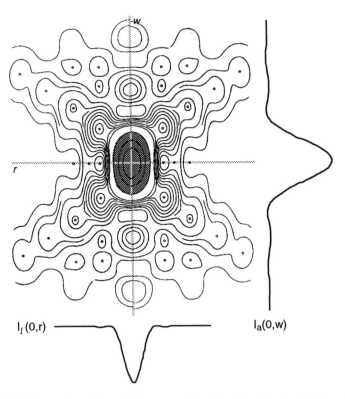

**Fig. 6**  Light intensity produced by a point source and an aberration-free lens in three dimensions. Because a lens of this type is cylindrically symmetric, the Cartesian coordinates (x, y, z) can be collapsed into two cylindrical coordinates (r, w), where r is the radial distance from optical center and w is the distance from the focal plane along the optical axis (see Table II). The volume described by this function can be visualized by rotating the figure about the w axis. Each contour represents a surface of equal intensity or isophote. The shaded area in the center is the volume at which the intensity has fallen to half of its value, $I_0$, at the origin. This volume is termed a "resel." $I_1(0, r)$ is the intensity at the focal plane and $I_a(0, w)$ is the intensity along the optical axis. (Contour plot adapted from Zernike and Nijboer, 1949.)

It can be shown (Born and Wolf, 1980) that $I_a(0, w)$ for a circular, aberration-free objective is given by

$$I_a(0, w) = I_0 \left[ \frac{\sin(w/4)}{(w/4)} \right]^2 \tag{6}$$

as shown on the right side of Fig. 6. Here, $I_0$ is the intensity in the focal plane at $w = 0$. The same treatment reveals that $I_1(r, 0)$ is given by

$$I_1(r, 0) = I_0 \left[ \frac{2 J_1(r)}{r} \right]^2 \tag{7}$$

as shown at the bottom of Fig. 6, where $J_1$ is a first-order Bessel function.

When a point detector is used, a similar detector sensitivity function is created in the object proportional to the PSF of the lens used to focus light on the detector. The detector sensitivity function has the form

$$D(r, 0) = R(r) \otimes |h_d(r)|^2 \tag{8}$$

where the detection sensitivity, $D(r)$, is the convolution of the lens amplitude PSF, $h_d(r)$, with the detector response distribution, $R(r)$. By symmetry, the sensitivity function for a plane source/point detector combination has the same form as that given above for the point source/plane object combination. We need only substitute the detector sensitivity at the origin, $D_0$, for $I_0$. Finally, we divide the confocal response function into analogous axial and lateral components and find, for a point source and a point detector,

$$C_a(0, w) = \text{const.} \left[ \frac{\sin(w/4)}{(w/4)} \right]^4 \tag{9a}$$

and

$$C_l(r, 0) = \text{const.} \left[ \frac{2 J_1(r)}{r} \right]^4 \tag{9b}$$

## B. Dimensions of Confocal Volume

Recall that the confocal response function $C(r, w)$ defines a volume in the object that is the smallest resolvable element, or resel. Because most of the energy in $C(r, w)$ is concentrated about the optical axis and the focal plane, the resel is a volume shaped by the surface at the first minimum of $C(r, w)$. This volume can be approximated as a cylinder whose diameter is the full width at half-maximum (FWHM) of $C_l(r, 0)$, and whose height is the FWHM of $C_a(0, w)$ (see Fig. 6). For a reflected light confocal microscope with a point source and a point detector, the dimensions of this cylinder are given in Eqs. (10a–d). Expressed in terms of illumination wavelength, $\lambda$, objective lens numerical aperture (NA), and the index of refraction, $n$, the dimensions are

$$\Delta r = \text{FWHM of } C(r, 0) = 0.61\lambda/\text{NA} \tag{10a}$$

$$\Delta w = \text{FWHM of } C(0, w) = 2n\lambda/(\text{NA})^2 \tag{10b}$$

$$a_r = \text{area of } C(r, 0) = \pi(\Delta r/2)^2 = 0.292\lambda^2/(\text{NA})^2 \tag{10c}$$

$$V_r = \text{volume} = a_r\Delta w = 0.584\lambda^3/(\text{NA})^4 \tag{10d}$$

These expressions apply only to point illumination and detection at a single wavelength. To analyze the confocal response volume generated in fluorescence mode by the Odyssey, two corrections must be applied: one for the wavelength of the emitted light, and a second for the detector aperture, which is a slit rather than a pinhole. Because the PSF of the objective is wavelength dependent, separate formulas are needed for the excitation and emission wavelengths. For our purposes, it is sufficient to use the wavelength of maximum fluorescence as the emission wavelength. Because this is always longer than the excitation wavelength, the net effect of fluorescence is to make the detection volume larger than the illumination volume. Accordingly, we rewrite Eqs. (9a) and (9b) by defining $r_{em} = r_{ex} (\lambda_{ex}/\lambda_{em})$, $w_{em} = w_{ex} (\lambda_{ex}/\lambda_{em})$, and $\beta = \lambda_{ex}/\lambda_{em}$, for excitation and emission wavelengths. Then, expressed in the coordinate system of the illumination wavelength, the appropriate formulas are

$$C_l(r, 0) = I_l(r, 0)D_l(r, 0) = \text{const.} \left[ \frac{2J_1(r)}{r} \right]^2 \left[ \frac{2J_1(r\beta)}{(r\beta)} \right]^2 \quad (11a)$$

$$C_a(0, w) = I_a(0, w)D_a(0, w) = \text{const.} \left[ \frac{\sin(w/4)}{(w/4)} \right]^2 \left[ \frac{\sin(w\beta/4)}{(w\beta/4)} \right]^2 \quad (11b)$$

The axial component of the fluorescent confocal response function given by Eq. (11b) is shown in Fig. 7B. For fluorescein with $\lambda_{ex} = 488$ nm and $\lambda_{em} = 520$ nm, the FWHM has expanded by 3.4% compared to the reflectance case, in which $\lambda_{ex} = \lambda_{em}$ (Fig. 7A).

The general effect of modifying either $I(r, w)$ or $D(r, w)$ is illustrated in the following way. $D(r, w)$ can be viewed as a weighting function over which the available light will contribute to image formation. This implies that little additional light will be captured if the detector sensitivity function is bigger than the illumination intensity function (see Fig. 8B). If the opposite situation obtains (i.e., that the illumination function is larger than the detector function), then object regions that fall inside the illumination volume, but outside the detector

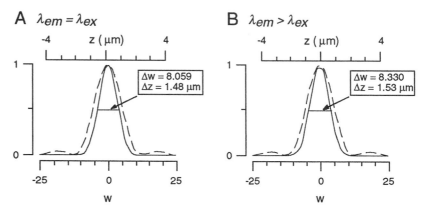

**Fig. 7** Axial component of the theoretical confocal response function. The bottom axis is the distance along the optical axis in normalized optical units, and the top axis is the distance along the optical axis for a water-immersion, NA 0.75 objective used with excitation illumination at $\lambda_{ex} = 488$ nm. Dashed curves in both figures are the illumination function at $\lambda_{ex} = 488$ nm. The full width at half-maximum (FWHM) is given in both normalized optical units and real distances. (A) Confocal response for reflected light imaging, $\lambda_{ex} = \lambda_{em}$ (solid curve). (B) Confocal response for fluorescence imaging, $\lambda_{em} > \lambda_{ex}$ (solid curve); for this example, $\lambda_{ex} = 488$ nm and $\lambda_{em} = 520$ nm. This value for $\lambda_{em}$ was chosen because it is the peak emission wavelength of fluorescein excited at 488 nm.

volume, are subject to damaging exciting light but do not contribute proportionally to image formation (see Fig. 8A). In the limit, this is identical to Köhler illumination and the SNR is similarly decreased. The best image for the least illumination is achieved when the illumination intensity distribution, $I(r, w)$, matches the detector sensitivity function, $D(r, w)$. This is illustrated in Fig. 8C, in which the FWHM of the product of these two, $I_a^2(0, w)$, is reduced. Also shown in Fig. 8C is the fact that the side lobes are reduced to less than 1% of the peak.

The second correction, for the aperture geometry, may be applied using the expression given by Sheppard and Mao (1988) for the PSF of a slit aperture. Here, $I(r, w)$ is the same as before, but the required detector sensitivity function depends on the orientation of a feature in the object with respect to the detector. Along the axis parallel to the slit, the response is equivalent to a full-field (or Köhler illumination) response, whereas perpendicular to this axis the detector function incorporates a Struve function, $H_1$,

$$C_1(r, 0) = I_1(r, 0)D_1(r, 0) = \text{const.}\left[\frac{\sin(w/4)}{(w/4)}\right]^2\left[\frac{3\pi H_1(2u)}{8u^2}\right] \tag{12}$$

which is almost as sharp as the pinhole function (Sheppard and Mao, 1988; Wilson and Hewlett, 1990).

An estimate of the thickness (i.e., $\Delta w$) of the confocal volume is obtained by measuring the reflectance from a plane mirror. The behavior obtained with a slit aperture in place of a pinhole is found by comparing the axial response function recorded by the Odyssey reflectance (or pinhole) channel with that recorded by the fluoresence (or slit) channel (Fig. 9). Direct comparison between the two channels is not possible with fluorescence because of the wavelength dependence of the AOD. However, the axial response function for fluoresence may be measured by using a planar, uniformly fluorescent object. Suitable objects are a thin film of fluorophore dissolved in oil sandwiched between a microscope slide and coverslip, or a fluorophore dissolved in a thin agar gel. We recommend measuring the axial response functions because the thickness of the optical section is determined by the PSF of the lens actually used. Aberrations in the objective (Wilson and Carlini, 1989) as well as the confocal attachments can result in a $C(r, w)$ that departs significantly from theory. For example, if the astigmatism due to the AOD lensing effect is improperly corrected, then the axial response function splits into two peaks (Cogswell et al., 1990). For a well-corrected objective lens, these problems are less acute for the lateral response function.

## IV. Estimating Number of Fluorescent Photons

Knowledge of the size of the confocal volume and the intensity of illumination allows us to estimate the number of photons that are produced during a single frame. Fluorescent emission at low light levels is described by Poisson sta-

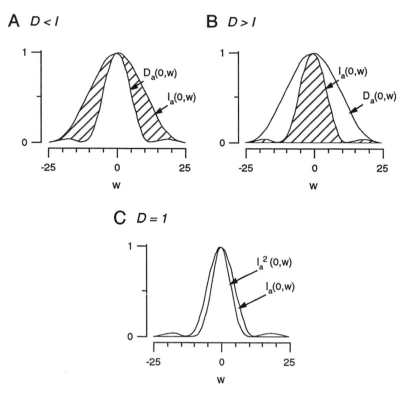

**Fig. 8** Matching the illumination and detection volumes. For clarity we show only the transect along the optical axis, normalized to unity at $w = 0$. The effect in the focal plane is qualitatively the same. (A) Detection volume is smaller than the illumination volume. The shaded area is the illumination intensity transect along the $w$ axis, and the open area is the detection sensitivity function along the same axis. The detector function serves as a weighting function for light collection. This implies that only a fraction of the light reflected or emitted by object regions in the shaded area will contribute to the image while receiving full illumination. (B) Detector volume is larger than the illumination volume. The shaded area shows the illumination intensity and the open area is the detector sensitivity function. This reduces the SNR and widens the confocal response function. (C) Confocal response when the illumination and detection volumes are precisely matched. The confocal response for both cases (A) and (B) lies between the $I_a(0, w)$ and $[I_a(0, w)]^2$ curves shown in (C).

tistics. For such processes, the SNR increases as the square root of the number of photons. For example, 100 photons are needed to distinguish 1 level in 10 and 10,000 photons are required to make a measurement with 1% precision. As a result, the ability to create an image rapidly and detect variations in the object with the desired precision depends on maximizing the number of photons collected per pixel. Designing appropriate scanning strategies and experimental protocols depends on estimating the number of photons that result from illumi-

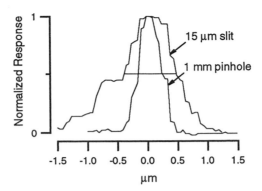

**Fig. 9** Experimental axial confocal response function of a Zeiss ×63 Plan-Apochromat NA 1.4 oil immersion objective. The microscope was aligned, and care was taken to insure that AOD-induced astigmatism was compensated. Data were collected as a flat (to $\lambda/10$), plane mirror was moved through focus and the reflected light along either the reflected (pinhole) or fluorescent (slit) light path of the Odyssey was recorded. Curves are normalized to unity at the maximum intensity and adjusted along the $z$ axis so that the peaks lie at $z = 0$. Note that the pinhole was set at its minimum setting (1 mm) and the slit used (15 $\mu$m) collects 82% of the central peak of the intensity function in the focal plane. FWHM with the pinhole detector is 0.453 $\mu$m (compare to theoretical value of 0.25 $\mu$m), and with the slit detector it is 0.9 $\mu$m.

nating fluorescent molecules within the confocal volume. With knowledge of the thickness of the confocal slice, the dye concentration, and estimates of the dye quantum efficiency and photodestruction rates, it is possible to predict the number of photons produced by a fluorophore during the pixel dwell time. The analysis of the feasibility of any experiment, therefore, begins with a calculation of the expected number of photons produced.

## A. Theory

When a molecule absorbs a photon it will be converted from a lower to a higher energy level, for example, from the ground state, $S_0$, to the first excited state, $S_1$ (see Fig. 10). In decaying back to $S_0$, the energy may be released in a variety of ways. The decay to $S_0$ is termed fluorescent if the molecule emits light within 1 $\mu$sec of absorption. The transition from $S_1$ need not be fluorescent, and may result in conversions to triplet states ($T$), for example. We can estimate the number of photons emitted by a fluorophore from the rate constants of the transitions between electronic states of the molecule. In our analysis we assume that the dye is sufficiently dilute that neither the illuminating nor emitted energy is absorbed by nearby fluorophores. We also assume that the fluorescent transitions of interest as well as photodestruction or bleaching occur from the first excited state, $S_1$. Further, in many cases, the transition rate to the triplet state, $k_I$, is small and can be ignored.

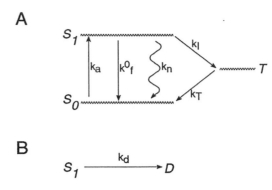

**Fig. 10** Electronic state diagram of a fluorophore. (A) Transitions between $S_0$, $S_1$, and $T$. (B) Photodestruction. For the model considered here, photodestruction is defined as the conversion from $S_1$ to another, nonfluorescent chemical species, $D$. $k_d$ is the rate constant of this transition. $S_0$, Ground singlet state; $S_1$, first excited singlet state; $T$, triplet states; $k_a$, rate constant of the transition for $S_0$ to $S_1$; $k_f^0$, rate constant of fluorescence; $k_n$, rate constant of nonradiative decay, $k_l$, rate constant of transition from $S_1$ to $T$, also known as intersystem crossing; $k_T$, rate constant of transition from $T$ to $S_0$.

Mathies *et al.* (1990) present expressions for the number of photons emitted from a dilute solution of fluorophore flowing past a focused laser beam as a function of the intensity and duration of illumination. Their analysis includes the effect of photodestruction, and is relevant to the confocal case in which the sample is fixed and the illumination is moving. If $k_f^0$ is the rate constant of fluorescent emission, and $\{S_1\}$ is the fraction of time spent in the excited state, then the number of photons, $n$, emitted by a molecule illuminated for time $\Delta t_{dwell}$ is given by

$$n = k_f^0 \{S_1\} \Delta t_{dwell} \tag{13}$$

Because dye molecules may leave $S_1$ by an irreversible chemical reaction and be destroyed, we can define a probability that a given molecule is intact after being illuminated for a time $t$ as $p(t)$. The total number of photons emitted by a single molecule during an interval would be the integral of the product of $n$ and $p(t)$,

$$n_f = \int np(t) \, dt \tag{14}$$

If $k_d$ is the rate constant of photodestruction, then assuming first-order kinetics,

$$dp/dt = -k_d\{S_1\} \tag{15}$$

and integrating yields

$$p(t) = \exp(-k_d\{S_1\}) \tag{16}$$

$k_d$ can be determined by measuring its reciprocal, the time constant of fluorescent decay, $\tau_d$, under constant illumination.

An expression for $\{S_1\}$ is found by assuming the steady state is achieved quickly compared to $\Delta t_{\text{dwell}}$ and that the state transitions diagrammed in Fig. 10 can each be described by first-order kinetics

$$\{S_1\} = k_a \bigg/ \left( k_a + k_f + \frac{k_a k_I}{k_T} + \frac{k_I^2}{k_T} \right) \tag{17}$$

where $k_a$ is the rate constant from $S_0$ to $S_1$, and $k_f$ is the sum of the rate constants for all pathways from $S_1$ and is equal to the reciprocal of the excited state lifetime, $\tau_f$, as given below

$$k_f = k_f^0 + k_n + k_I = 1/\tau_f \tag{18}$$

Measurement of the fluorescent decay in response to pulsed illumination (Lakowicz, 1986) yields $\tau_f$, which is generally on the order of $10^{-9}$ sec. If the transition to the triplet state is small, the last term in Eq. (17) may be neglected, resulting in

$$\{S_1\} = k_a \bigg/ \left( k_a + k_f + \frac{k_a k_I}{k_T} \right) \tag{19}$$

Substituting for $n$, $p(t)$, and $\{S_1\}$ into Eq. (14), and integrating yields

$$n_f = \left( \frac{k_f^0}{k_d} \right) \left[ 1 - \exp\left( \frac{-k_d k_a \Delta t_{\text{dwell}}}{k_a + k_f + k_a k_I/k_T} \right) \right] \tag{20}$$

This equation can be simplified by introducing the variables $k = k_a/k_f$ and $\tau = \Delta t_{\text{dwell}}/\tau_d$ and terms for the quantum yield of fluorescence, $Q_f$, and the quantum yield of photodestruction, $Q_d$. Both $Q_f$, the fraction of energy released as light ($Q_f = k_f^0/k_f$) and $Q_d$, the fraction of molecules photodestroyed ($Q_d = k_d/k_f$), are measurable properties of the fluorophore (Mathies and Stryer, 1986). Substituting $Q_f/Q_d$ for $k_f^0/k_d$ and $k_d$ and $\tau$ into Eq. (20) yields

$$n_f = \left( \frac{Q_f}{Q_d} \right) \left\{ 1 - \exp\left[ \frac{-k\tau}{k(k + k_I/k_T) + 1} \right] \right\} \tag{21}$$

When the triplet state is unimportant ($k_I/k_T \ll 1$), Eq. (21) reduces further to

$$n_f = \left( \frac{Q_f}{Q_d} \right) \{ 1 - \exp[-k\tau/(k + 1)] \} \tag{22}$$

This is the result of Mathies et al. (1990) and reduces to that given by Hirschfeld (1976) if saturation is ignored ($k \ll 1$). The only variable that remains unspecified is the absorption rate constant, $k_a$. Because we have assumed that the fluorophore is dilute, $k_a$ is the product of the absorption cross section, $\sigma_a$ (molecules $\cdot$ cm$^2$), and the illumination intensity, $I_{\text{ex}}$

$$k_a = \sigma_a I_{\text{ex}} \tag{23}$$

where, $\sigma_a$ is related to the molar absorption or extinction coefficient, $\varepsilon$ $(M^{-1}cm^{-1})$ by $\sigma_a = 3.83 \times 10^{-21}\ \varepsilon$. Because $\varepsilon$ is wavelength dependent, it must be measured at the illumination wavelength. From Eq. (22), we see that the mean number of photons, $n_f$, emitted from a fluorophore is an exponential function of both the intensity ($k$) and duration ($\tau$) of illumination, and that $n_f$ asymptotes to a maximum of $Q_f/Q_d$.

## B. Estimate for Video–Rate Confocal Microscopy

Equation (22) gives an estimate of the number of photons, $n_f$, emitted per molecule contained within a resel for a given intensity and duration of illumination. To estimate $n_f$ we need

$$k = k_a/k_f = \sigma_a I_{ex} \tau_f \tag{24a}$$

$$\tau = \Delta t_{dwell}/\tau_d \tag{24b}$$

As is shown in Table III, values for $k$ and $\tau$ can be calculated from measurable properties of the fluorophore and the microscope.

We will perform the calculation for the following example: a specimen uniformly stained with 10 $\mu M$ fluorescein viewed with an NA 0.75 water immersion objective. Fluorescein is a convenient choice because its fluorescent behavior is

**Table III**
**Fluorophore Chemistry**

| Parameter | Symbol (units) | Value for fluorescein[a] | Common method of measurement |
|---|---|---|---|
| Absorption cross section | $\sigma$ (cm²·molecule) | $3.06 \times 10^{-16}$ | absorption in solution[b] |
| Quantum efficiency of fluorescence | $Q_f$(none) | 0.99 | ratio of integrated fluorescence of test dye solution to that of a standard dye solution with the same absorbance[c] |
| Fluorescence lifetime | $\tau_f$(s) | $4.4 \times 10^{-9}$ | fluorescence relaxation in response to flash illumination |
| Time constant of photodestruction | $\tau_d$(s) | $700 \times 10^{-6}$ | fluorescence decay under constant illumination |
| Quantum efficiency of photodestruction | $Q_f$(none) | $2.7 \times 10^{-5}$ | fluorescence as a function of flow rate in a fluid column illuminated by a focused laser beam[d] |

[a] Values from Mathies and Stryer (1986), except $\tau_d$ which is from Mathies *et al.* (1990).
[b] $\sigma$ is the molar absorption coefficient, $\varepsilon$ (cm$^{+1}$·M$^{+1}$), multiplied by $3.82 \times 10^{-21}$ (molecules·cm$^{-3}$). $\varepsilon$ is defined as the absorption of a 1 $M$ solution through a 1-cm pathlength.
[c] Rhodamine B ($Q_f = 0.97$) is a common standard (see Minta *et al.*, 1989).
[d] See Mathies and Stryer (1986) for details of method.

well known (see Table III) and it is easily excited with 488-nm light. Furthermore, we choose the water immersion objective in accord with our emphasis on studies of thick living tissues. The theoretical dimensions of the resel are determined from the expressions given previously in Eqs. (10a–d)

$$\Delta r \approx 0.61\lambda/NA = 4 \times 10^{-5} \text{ cm} \tag{25a}$$

$$\Delta w \approx 2\lambda n/NA^2 = 2.3 \times 10^{-4} \text{ cm} \tag{25b}$$

$$a_r \approx 0.292\lambda^2/(NA)^2 = 1.24 \times 10^{-9} \text{ cm} \tag{25c}$$

$$v_r \approx 0.584\lambda^3/(NA)^4 = 2.9 \times 10^{-16} \text{ liters} \tag{25d}$$

Bear in mind that these values hold for the case in which $\lambda_{em} = \lambda_{ex}$. Because they are within 3% of the values for the fluorescein case ($\lambda_{em} = 520$ nm, $\lambda_{ex} = 488$ nm), the error introduced by this simplification is small.

At half-maximum intensity, the power in the object plane is 72.8 $\mu$W. The intensity of illumination, $I_{ex}$, per resel is $5.87 \times 10^4$ W/cm$_2$, which is equivalent to $1.45 \times 10^{23}$ photons/(sec · cm$^2$) at 488 nm. For a full-field scan, the resel dwell time, $t_{dwell}$, is 100 nsec. From Eq. (24) we estimate that $k = 1.95 \times 10^{-1}$ photons/molecule, $\tau = 1.42 \times 10^{-4}$, and $Q_f/Q_d = 3.67 \times 10^4$. From Eq. (22), then, $n_f = 0.85$ photons/molecule. The mean number of photons emitted from a single resel in a single pass, $N_f$, is the simply the product of $n_f$ and the number of molecules per resel, $m$.

$$N_f = n_f m \tag{26}$$

In this example, $m$ is 1745 molecules/resel and $N_f = 1486$ photons/resel. Only 8.7% of the photons will be captured by an objective with an NA of 0.75, and so we expect to collect only 129 of these photons. This estimate is valid only so far as the triplet state of fluorescein may be neglected. Its accuracy is also limited by the extent to which the parameters listed in Table III are the same *in situ* as they are in the solution in which they are measured. All of these parameters depend to some extent on the solvent or local environment. At one extreme is the fast membrane-bound voltage-sensitive dye, di-4-ANEPPS, whose absorption coefficient, $\varepsilon$, in lipid environments is 1.6 times that in water. In addition, di-4-ANEPPS and related compounds appear nonfluorescent in aqueous solution because the $Q_f$ in water is one-sixth the $Q_f$ in lipid (Fluhler *et al.*, 1985).

## C. On Maximizing the Fluorescent Signal

The number of photons collected may be increased by increasing the fraction of $N_f$ captured by using a higher NA objective. Higher NA (up to 1.4) is achieved with oil immersion objectives. However, the net result may be to decrease $N_f$. This may arise from the lower throughput of multielement objective lenses. In addition, the confocal volume is smaller, so fewer molecules are contained in the resel. Reworking the example above for a Zeiss ×63 NA 1.4 oil immersion objective, we find that $n_f$ is 1.76 photons/molecule, $m$ is 161, and $N_f$ is 283 photons/resel. $N_f$ for this high-NA objective is approximately 20% of that obtained with the lower NA objective. Note that 30% or 85 of these photons will be captured as compared to 8.7% or 129 in the example above. Examination of Eqs. (10a) and (10d) reveals that $\Delta w$ decreases with the square of the NA and the resel volume, $v_r$, decreases with the fourth power of the NA. Thus, using high-NA objectives will increase axial resolution, but is likely to decrease the total number of photons captured. In this example, the axial resolution is increased by a factor of 2.75 and the the number of photons captured is decreased by 30%. An alternative strategy is to double the solid angle of capture by replacing the usual microscope condenser with a second objective and mirror (Art *et al.*, 1991).

How can $N_f$ be maximized? From Eq. (26) we note that $N_f$ will be increased when $m$, $n_f$, or both are increased. Consider, first, ways to increase $m$. Most obviously, the dye concentration may be increased. This route may be undesirable for a variety of reasons. Absorption of exciting light by concentrated dye may lead to differences in effective $I_{ex}$ with depth that are difficult to predict, although one study suggests a method for compensating for these effects (Visser *et al.*, 1991). Additionally, if the fluorophore is an ion-indicator dye, increasing its concentration may interfere with cell function by buffering the ion of interest. $m$ may also be increased by increasing the effective illumination and/or detection volume. This is realized by using larger apertures. As discussed previously (see Section III,A), the best results are obtained when the two functions are matched. In disk scanning microscopes, the illumination and detector apertures are the same so that the illumination distribution and detector sensitivity functions are always matched. In contrast, laser scanning microscopes do not normally permit any adjustment of the illumination distribution and the confocal volume is increased by increasing the size of the detector aperture. Brakenhoff *et al.* (1990) have suggested that the light capture would increase as the fourth power of the loss in axial resolution. For many purposes, the increase in signal more than compensates for the decreased axial resolution.

Next, consider ways to increase the number of photons emitted per molecule, $n_f$. From Eq. (22) we note that $n_f$ is increased when either the intensity ($k$) or duration ($\tau$) of illumination is increased. The cost of increasing $\tau$ is, of course, a concomitant decrease in temporal resolution. The cost of increasing $k$ is a decrease in the SNR due to increased number of background photons. This issue is considered in detail in the next section.

## D. Signal-to-Noise Ratio and Optimal Intensity

The primary sources of noise or background photons, $n_b$, are Rayleigh and Raman scattering. Rayleigh scattering is simple elastic scattering of the illumination from molecules and optical surfaces. These photons are not completely eliminated by the chromatic beam splitter and barrier filter and contribute noise to the image. Raman scattering is produced when a fraction of the energy of the incident photon is absorbed by a molecule and the remainder is released as light of a different wavelength. The energy absorbed usually fits the energy gap between two vibrational or rotational states (Castellan, 1964). Proteins may produce Raman emission bands close to the excitation wavelength (488 nm), which cannot easily be distinguished from fluorescence (Tsien and Waggoner, 1990). $n_b$ from both sources is proportional to $I_{ex}$. As shown by the discussion above, the signal, $n_f$, increases with illumination intensity. For small $k$ and $\tau$, $n_f$ is approximately proportional to the product $k\tau$. When $k\tau$ is large, this relationship no longer holds [see Eq. (22)]. In contrast, $n_b$ is directly proportional to $k\tau$ for all values. Increasing $k$, therefore, may increase the noise to a greater extent than the signal, thereby decreasing the SNR. The SNR is given by the ratio of $n_f$ to its standard deviation, SD. This is proportional to

$$\text{SNR} = n_f/\text{SD} \propto n_f/\sqrt{n_b} \qquad (27)$$

When the triplet state may be ignored, $n_f$ is proportional to $k_a/(k_a + k_f)$ [see Eq. (22)]. Because $n_b$ is proportional to $I_{ex}$ and $k_a = \sigma_a I_{ex}$, then $n_b$ is proportional to $k_a$. So,

$$\text{SNR} \propto /\sqrt{k_a}/(k_a + k_f) \qquad (28)$$

As noted by Tsien and Waggoner (1990), this reaches a maximum when $k_a = k_f$ or $k = 1$. Substituting for $k_a$ ($k_a = 4\sigma_a P/\pi \Delta r^2$), and for $k_f$ ($k_f = 1/\tau_f$), and solving for $P$, we find that the optimal SNR is achieved when the power is

$$P = a_r/\tau_f \sigma_a = \pi \Delta r^2/4\tau_f \sigma_a \qquad (29)$$

For the example considered here ($\tau_f = 4.4$ nsec; $\sigma_a = 3.06 \times 10^{-16}$; $\Delta r = 0.4$ $\mu$m), this implies that the best SNR is achieved when

$$P = 9.33 \times 10^{14} \text{ photons/sec} = 0.34 \times 10^{-3}\text{W}.$$

Using this illumination power would produce 7756 photons/resel in our example, with 8.7% or 675 captured by the objective. The optimal power is reduced to ~12.8% of this value when the triplet state is considered (Tsien and Waggoner, 1990).

An optimistic view of the preceding analysis is that sufficient photons are produced to permit fluorescence imaging with acceptable SNR at video rates. The realist, however, remains skeptical because intensities of this order are difficult to achieve and may damage the specimen. Even if the illumination intensity required for maximal SNR does not irreversibly damage the preparation, it may temporarily alter its physiology (Sheetz and Koppel, 1979). For this reason, it is important to have an independent measure of cell function, and compare cell behavior in the presence and absence of illumination. Also, the investigator should explore ways to reduce the energy focused on the specimen. This can be accomplished by reducing the illumination intensity, using longer wavelengths, or reducing the dwell time. In addition, a large fraction of the photons captured by the objective will not be detected by low-QE PMTs (Art, 1990). Our estimate shows that with optimal illumination intensities only ~60 photons/resel would be detected. Although this signal is large enough to follow movements of a fluorescent particle at video rates, it is not sufficient to monitor small changes in ion concentration. Specifically, an average of at least 2 frames would be needed to capture a total of 100 photons/resel to detect a 10% change in fluorescence.

The photon estimate is only as accurate as the estimate of dye concentration. In addition, it depends on a uniform distribution of fluorophore molecules within the resel. With ion-sensitive dyes the concentration may be known because the impermeant salt is often introduced directly into the cell with a micropipette. In this instance, the concentration is also reasonably uniform throughout the cytosol. Other dyes, such as those used to mark and track receptors, will necessarily have a heterogeneous distribution. For this reason, a conventional definition of concentration within the resel is meaningless. The photon estimate may be further compromised by the fact that some fluorophores have a preferred orientation for photon absorption. Membrane-bound voltage-sensitive dyes are an example of this type (Loew and Simpson, 1981). Throughout our analysis, we have ignored such complicating issues. Given these uncertainties, an expedient technique may be to prepare a specimen and scan it with a wide detector aperture. By increasing the illumination until a signal is detected, the minimum intensity is found. To increase axial resolution, the detector aperture must be reduced with a concomitant decrease in the number of photons. If this can be accomplished with illumination intensities that do not alter the behavior of the specimen, then optical sectioning may be exploited.

## V. Conclusions

In this article, we sought to evaluate to what extent scanning confocal microscopy at video rates achieves the goal of joining sensitivity with high spatial and temporal resolution. Of the currently available methods, LSCMs offer flexibility not available with other types of scanning microscopes. Principal among these is the ability to steer the beam so that the area scanned is restricted to a small region in the object field. This has three benefits alluded to earlier: (1) photodamage is limited to the portion illuminated, (2) the quantity of data is reduced, and (3) the effective acquisition rate is increased. This ability may also be exploited for other purposes. For example, a high-intensity beam can be steered to bleach an area of interest selectively (Axelrod et al., 1976; Peters et al., 1974), or to release caged compounds (Lester et al., 1979; Gurney and Lester, 1987). Finally, photometry rather than imaging could be realized, in principle, by integrating the response while randomly scanning points distributed in a Gaussian manner about a mean position. To achieve video rates with the LSCM, AODs are convenient devices for rapid scanning. The costs of choosing such devices are the wavelength dependence of the angle of deflection and the reduced efficiency of beam deflection. The inability to scan and descan multiple wavelengths simultaneously forced the use of a slit aperture in front of the detector. Even with this geometry, it is possible to define and measure the confocal volume and estimate the number of photons for a given intensity of illumination.

In future, we expect three areas of development, with improvements in beam steering, detector technology, and the ability to modulate the confocal volume. In principle, faster mirror-scanning systems can be built. With their advent, it will be possible to avoid the compromises imposed by AODs. The use of solid-state diode detectors with QEs between 0.6 and 0.8 will increase the sensitivity by an order of magnitude. The SNR will not be compromised, because at high pixel rates the noise in detection is limited by photon statistics rather than instrumentation noise. For maximum sensitivity and axial resolution, the illumination intensity and detector sensitivity functions should match. By varying the illumination and detector apertures in tandem on the LSCM as they do per force on the disk scanning units, image acquisition with the highest SNR at the greatest speed could be achieved.

## Acknowledgments

This work is supported by DC00454–04 (NIH), N00014–88 (ONR), Brain Research Foundation grant, and an A. P. Sloan Fellowship to J.J.A., and a Howard Hughes predoctoral fellowship to M.B.G. The authors thank Jim Aeschbach, Jamie Collier, Dave Kinzer, Mike Szulczewski, and Jim Walker of Noran Instruments.

## References

Agard, D. A., and Sedat, J. W. (1983). *Nature (London)* **302**, 676–681.

Aikens, R. S., Agard, D. A., and Sedat, J. W. (1989). *Methods Cell Biol.* **29**, 291–313.

Amos, W. B., White, J. G., and Fordham, M. (1987). *Appl. Opt.* **26**, 3239–3243.

Art, J. J. (1990). *In* ''Handbook of Biological Confocal Microscopy'' (J. B. Pawley, ed.), Rev. Ed., pp. 127–139. Plenum, New York.

Art, J. J., Goodman, M. B., and Schwartz, E. A. (1991). *Biophys. J.* **59**, 155a.

Axelrod, D., Koppel, D. E., Schlessinger, J., Elson, E., and Webb, W. W. (1976). *Biophys. J.* **16**, 1055–1069.

Bertero, M., Boccacci, P., Brakenhoff, G. J., Malfanti, F., and van der Voort, H. T. M. (1990). *J. Microsc. (Oxford)* **157**, 3–20.

Born, M., and Wolf, E. (1980). ''Principles of Optics.'' Pergamon, Oxford.

Brakenhoff, G. J., and Visscher, K. (1990). *Trans. R. Microsc. Soc.* **1**, 247–250.

Brakenhoff, G. J., van Spronsen, E. A., van der Voort, H. T. M., and Nanninga, N. (1989). *Methods Cell Biol.* **30**, 379–398.

Brakenhoff, G. J., Visscher, K., and van der Voort, H. T. M. (1990). *In* ''Handbook of Biological Confocal Microscopy'' (J. B. Pawley, ed.), Rev. Ed., pp. 87–91. Plenum, New York.

Carlsson, K., Wallen, P., and Brodin, L. (1989). *J. Microsc. (Oxford)* **155**, 15–26.

Castellan, G. W. (1964). ''Physical Chemistry.'' Addison-Wesley, Reading, Massachusetts.

Cogswell, C. J., Sheppard, C. J. R., Moss, M. C., and Howard, C. V. (1990). *J. Microsc. (Oxford)* **158**, 177–185.

Debye, P., and Sears, F. W. (1932). *Proc. Natl. Acad. Sci. U.S.A.* **18,** 409–414.

Draaijer, A., and Houpt, P. M. (1988). *Scanning* **10,** 139–145.

Fluhler, E., Burnham, G., and Loew, L. (1985). *Biochemistry* **24,** 5749–5755.

"Galvanometer Scanners." General Scanning, Inc. (1984). Watertown, Massachusetts.

Gerig, J. S., and Montague, H. (1964). *Proc. IEEE* **52,** 1753 (corr).

Goldstein, S. R., Hubin, T., Rosenthal, S., and Washburn, C. (1990). *J. Microsc. (Oxford)* **157,** 29–38.

Gratton, E., and vandeVen, M. J. (1990). *In* "Handbook of Biological Confocal Microscopy" (J. B. Pawley, ed.), Rev. Ed., pp. 53–67. Plenum, New York.

Grynkiewicz, G., Poenie, M., and Tsien, R. Y. (1985). *J. Biol. Chem.* **260,** 3440–3450.

Gurney, A. M., and Lester, H. A. (1987). *Physiol. Rev.* **67,** 583–617.

Hecht, E. (1987). "Optics." Addison-Wesley, Reading, Massachusetts.

Hirschfeld, T. (1976). *Appl. Opt.* **15,** 3135–3139.

Inoué, S. (1986). "Video Microscopy." Plenum, New York.

Koester, C. J. (1980). *Appl. Opt.* **19,** 1749–1757.

Korpel, A., Adler, R., Desmares, P., and Watson, W. (1966). *Proc. IEEE* **54,** 1429–1437.

Lakowicz, J. R. (1986). *In* "Applications of Fluorescence in the Biomedical Sciences" (D. L. Taylor, A. S. Waggoner, F. Lanni, R. F. Murphy, and R. R. Birge, eds.), pp. 29–67. Alan R. Liss, New York.

Lester, H. A., Krouse, M. E., Nass, M. M., Wassermann, N. H., and Erlanger, B. F. (1979). *Nature (London)* **280,** 509–510.

Loew, L. M., and Simpson, L. L. (1981). *Biophys. J.* **34,** 353–365.

Mathies, R. A., and Stryer, L. (1986). *In* "Applications of Fluorescence in the Biomedical Sciences" (D. L. Taylor, A. S. Waggoner, F. Lanni, R. F. Murphy, and R. R. Birge, eds.), pp. 129–140. Alan R. Liss, New York.

Mathies, R. A., Peck, K., and Stryer, L. (1990). *Anal. Chem.* **62,** 1786–1791.

Minsky, M. (1961). U.S. Pat. 3,013,467.

Minta, A., Kao, J. P. Y., and Tsien, R. Y. (1989). *J. Biol. Chem.* **264,** 8171–8178.

Oriel. (1990). "Light Sources, Monochromators, Detection Systems." Stratford, Connecticut.

Pawley, J. B., ed. (1990). "Handbook of Biological Confocal Microscopy," Rev. Ed. Plenum, New York.

Peters, R., Peters, J., Tews, K. H., and Bahr, W. (1974). *Biochim. Biophys. Acta* **367,** 282–294.

Petran, M., and Hadravsky, M. (1968). *J. Opt. Soc. Am.* **58,** 661–664.

Petran, M., Hadravsky, M., and Boyde, A. (1985). *Scanning* **7,** 97–108.

Pratt, W. K. (1978). "Digital Image Processing." Wiley, New York.

Schormann, T., and Jovin, T. M. (1990). *J. Microsc. (Oxford)* **158,** 153–164.

Sheetz, M. P., and Koppel, D. E. (1979). *Proc. Natl. Acad. Sci. U.S.A.* **76,** 3314–3317.

Sheppard, C. J. R., and Mao, X. Q. (1988). *J. Mod. Opt.* **35,** 1169–1185.

Spring, K. R., and Lowy, R. J. (1989). *Methods Cell Biol.* **29,** 269–289.

Suzuki, T., and Horikawa, Y. (1986). *Appl. Opt.* **25,** 4115–4121.

Taylor, D. L., and Salmon, E. D. (1989). *Methods Cell Biol.* **29,** 207–237.

Tsien, R. Y. (1990). *Proc. R. Microsc. Soc.* **25,** S53.

Tsien, R. Y., and Waggoner, A. (1990). *In* "Handbook of Biological Confocal Microscopy" (J. B. Pawley, ed.), Rev. Ed., pp. 169–178. Plenum, New York.

Visser, T. D., Groen, F. C. A., and Brakenhoff, G. J. (1991). *J. Microsc. (Oxford)* **163,** 189–200.

Waggoner, A., DeBaisio, R., Conrad, P., Bright, G. R., Ernst, L., Ryan, K., Nederlof, M., and Taylor, D. (1989). *Methods Cell Biol.* **30,** 449–478.

Webb, R., and Dorey, C. K. (1990). *In* "Handbook of Biological Confocal Microscopy" (J. B. Pawley, ed.), Rev. Ed., pp. 41–51. Plenum, New York.

White, J. C., and Stryer, L. (1987). *Anal. Biochem.* **161,** 442–452.

Wilson, T. (1989). *J. Microsc. (Oxford)* **154,** 143–156.

Wilson, T., and Carlini, A. R. (1989). *J. Microsc. (Oxford)* **154,** 243–256.

Wilson, T., and Hewlett, S. J. (1990). *J. Microsc. (Oxford)* **160,** 115–139.
Wilson, T., and Hewlett, S. J. (1991). *J. Microsc (Oxford)* **163,** 131–150.
Xiao, G. Q., Corle, T. R., and Kino, G. S. (1988). *Appl. Phys. Lett.* **53,** 716–718.
Yariv, A., and Yeh, P. (1984). "Optical Waves in Crystals." Wiley (Interscience), New York.
Zernike, F., and Nijboer, B. R. A. (1949). *Colloq. Int. C. N. R. S.* No. 1, 227–235.

## CHAPTER 3

# Confocal Microscopy: Important Considerations for Accurate Imaging

## Lars Majlof and Per-Ola Forsgren

Molecular Dynamics
Sunnyvale, California 94086

## I. Introduction

Confocal microscopy is a powerful tool for visualization and quantification of three-dimensional structures that were previously impossible to capture. During the first few years of the existence of confocal microscopes the emphasis was indeed on visualization, and many of the issues we discuss here were of minor importance. Now, as demands for quantitative measurements are commonplace, it is becoming more and more important to understand the limitations of the confocal microscope as a measurement tool.

The commercially available confocal microscopes can essentially be divided into two categories: spinning disk type and laser scanning. We will not specifically address any of these types of instruments, but will rather deal with general issues encountered when using a confocal microscope for fluorescence imaging.

However, because the laser-scanning instrument type is dominating this field, we have also included a section on detector characteristics for photomultiplier-type detectors. (Spinning disk instruments typically use conventional video-type cameras to digitize the images.)

We investigate the influence of refractive index in immersion and mount media on depth measurements and show that one can easily make systematic errors of 30% or more if care is not taken. This article also addresses lens performance and selection criteria and presents depth resolution measurements for a selection of objectives. The conversion of a continuous optical image into a digital image is a process known as spatial sampling. Information may be lost in this process, unless appropriate measures are taken. We present basic rules of thumb for correct spatial sampling.

## II. Factors Affecting Confocal Imaging

### A. Refractive Index Differences and Their Effect on Focus

The refractive index of a medium determines the speed of light in it. At the interface between two media with different indices of refraction, light adheres to Snell's law of refraction, that is, rays that come in at an angle other than perpendicular change their direction in the new medium. A rather nonintuitive consequence, that has been known at least since the 1950s (Galbraith, 1955), is that the movement of the focal plane in a microscopic specimen does not always correspond to the movement of the specimen stage. A full treatment of the phenomenon is complicated but one can use ray optics and Snell's law of refraction to derive an approximate formula for correction of focus movement. Figure 1 illustrates the ray paths in a microscope objective.

The reason that the plane of focus moves a different distance than the specimen stage is that the immersion medium between objective and coverslip has a different index of refraction than the medium in which the specimen is mounted. The distance traveled by the plane of focus is larger than the stage movement if the mount medium has a higher refractive index than the immersion medium. A higher refractive index in the immersion medium than in the mount medium gives the opposite result.

The following formula is derived from geometry and from Snell's law of refraction:

$$d/D = (n/n_0)(\cos a/\cos b) \qquad (1)$$

where $d$ is the movement of the focus plane, $D$ is the movement of the lens, $n$ is the refractive index of the mounting medium, $n_0$ is the refractive index of the immersion medium, and $a$ and $b$ are the angles of incident light. The equation shows that the correction of focus movement $d$ is dependent both on $n/n_0$ and the incident angles of the rays from the objective. (The angles $a$ and $b$ are related by Snell's law and thus also depend on the refractive indices $n_0$ and $n$.) Microscope

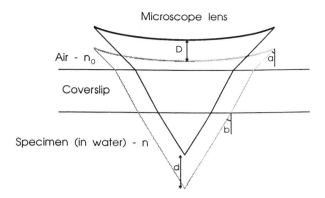

**Fig. 1** The optical rays of a microscope lens in two positions above the specimen. D, The physical movement of the stage; d, the movement of the plane of focus. The rays in the figure are drawn for air as immersion medium and water as mount medium. Water has a higher refractive index than air, therefore the distance traveled by the focal plane is greater than the distance traveled by the objective.

objectives for biological use are optimized for a certain combination of immersion and mount media. They can, however, if the refractive indices are different, give only a single optimally thin plane of focus for one depth in the specimen. Typically, well-corrected objectives are constructed to trade optimal resolution at a single depth for less optimal but good resolution over a range of depths. A rigorous treatment of the depth correction would call for an integration of the above equation over all angles $a$, with a weight function for different light intensities at different angles. It would also require knowledge about the particular optimizations for the objective, data that are generally known only by the manufacturer. Furthermore, the analysis so far has been performed on axis (points in the middle of the field); if off-axis imaging points are considered, the treatment becomes even more complicated.

Restricting the analysis to close-to-axis rays and making a zero-order approximation in which both angles $a$ and $b$ are small, the ratio of the cosines can be assumed to be 1. Under these limitations, the ratio of distances becomes

$$d/D = n/n_0 \qquad (2)$$

In Table I a number of different combinations of immersion and mount media are listed, showing how large the discrepancies may be between stage and focal plane movements.

The two images in Fig. 2 illustrate the depth correction effect. The sample contains fluorescent beads, 6.5 $\mu$m in diameter. They were dried onto a coverslip and then placed on an object glass with glycerol in between. This produced a monolayer of beads at an optimal imaging distance for the lens. The images were scanned in the vertical direction with a $\times$40 NA 0.95 air objective. To the right is

**Table I**
**Examples of Corrections for Some Combinations of Immersion and Mount Media**

| Immersion medium | Mount medium | Correction |
|---|---|---|
| Air | Water | 1.33 |
| Air | Glycerol | 1.47 |
| Oil | Air | 0.66 |
| Oil | Water | 0.88 |
| Oil | Glycerol | 0.97 |

a bead scanned without taking refractive index differences into account and to the left the correction has been performed. Large beads were used to reduce the influence of the point-spread function of the lens.

The conclusion derived from Table I, Fig. 2, and the preceding discussion is that to make any type of accurate measurement that includes the depth dimen-

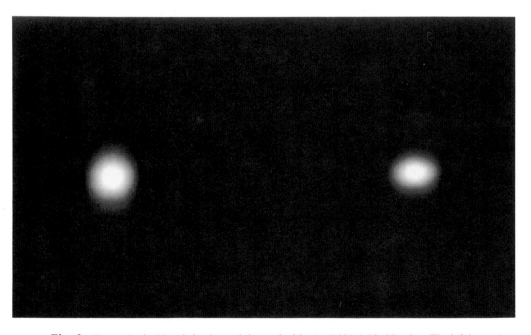

**Fig. 2** Two spherical beads in glycerol, imaged with a ×40 NA 0.95 objective. The left image has been corrected for refractive index differences, giving the correct round shape of the bead, whereas the right image shows the distortion when no correction is used.

sion, it is imperative to compensate for the refractive index variations. Otherwise, errors of up to 50% are possible.

The previous discussion serves as a good starting point to analyze spherical aberrations. As indicated by Eq. (1), paraxial (close to the center axis) and marginal (furthest away from the axis) rays will have focuses at different depths. Let us consider a theoretical objective with one optimal focus plane at the top of the specimen, where all rays intersect at the same point. As indicated in Fig. 3, the paraxial and marginal rays do not coincide as we go further into the specimen. If we assume that paraxial and marginal rays have the same plane of focus at the top of the specimen, the difference in focal depth between the two rays is (Carlsson, 1990)

$$\delta = z\left(\frac{n}{n_0} - \frac{\sqrt{n^2 - NA^2}}{\sqrt{n_0^2 - NA^2}}\right) \tag{3}$$

where $\delta$ is the difference in focal point for paraxial and marginal rays, $z$ is the distance from the optimal focus plane, $n$ is the refractive index of the mount medium, $n_0$ is the refractive index of the immersion medium, and NA is the numerical aperture of the lens.

One can thus see that the width of the point-spread function in the depth direction depends both on the numerical aperture of the lens and the distance into the specimen.

Figure 4 shows vertical cross-sections of 0.5 $\mu$m beads at 5, 30, and 115 $\mu$m from the coverslip. A common way to describe the resolution of an optical system is to measure the FWHM (full width at half-maximum) values of a point source. Figure 5 shows a diagram of measured vertical FWHM for 0.5-$\mu$m fluorescent latex beads as a function of depth below the coverslip for a ×40/NA 0.95 Plan Apo objective. The results reveal the strong widening of the point-spread function caused by the spherical aberration.

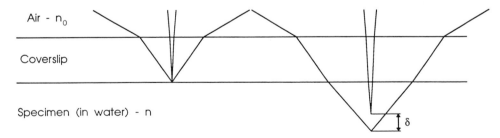

**Fig. 3**  The optical rays in a theoretical microscope objective. Both paraxial and marginal rays are shown for two different locations of the objective with respect to the specimen. The spherical aberration is evident in the difference of focal depth of the two rays for the lower position of the objective.

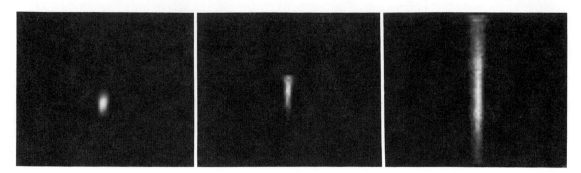

**Fig. 4** Projections from the side of 0.5-$\mu$m beads at different distances from the coverslip. The beads are in water and were scanned with a ×40 NA 0.95 lens. *Left:* 5 $\mu$m from coverslip. *Middle:* 30 $\mu$m from coverslip. *Right:* 115 $\mu$m from coverslip.

Another consequence of the spherical aberration is that the measured intensity in the image is reduced. The reason is that the effective gathering angle for fluorescent light from a particular point becomes smaller with increasing spherical aberration. Marginal rays collect fluorescence only from points excited by marginal rays of incident light whereas in a nonaberrated situation they would also collect fluorescence excited by paraxial incident light. In Fig. 6 we show the maximum intensity in the same beads that were the basis for the FWHM measurement (see Fig. 5) as a function of distance into the specimen. The specimen consisted of a sparse distribution of beads in gelatin.

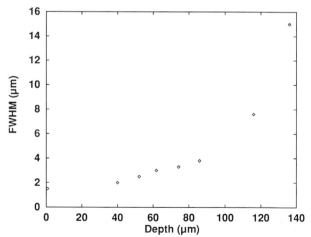

**Fig. 5** Vertical full width at half-maximum (FWHM) measurement of 0.5-$\mu$m beads as a function of distance (in water) below the coverslip. A ×40 NA 0.95 lens was used in the experiment and the correction collar was set for actual coverslip thickness.

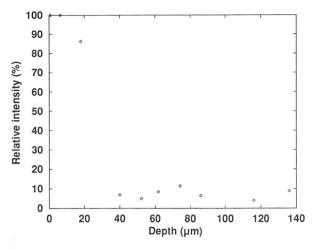

**Fig. 6**  Measured intensity of the brightest section of 0.5-$\mu$m beads as a function of distance (in water) below the coverslip. A ×40 NA 0.95 lens was used in the experiment and the correction collar was set for actual coverslip thickness.

Large variations in index of refraction within a specimen will make it difficult to image it correctly. To illustrate this effect we prepared two specimens with 6.5-$\mu$m latex beads. In one the beads were in water and in the second they were in glycerol. The difference in refractive index between bead and medium is larger in water than in glycerol. Figure 7 shows the difference between the imaged vertical cross section for a single bead in the two samples.

## B. Lens Selection

The selection of the right lens has always been crucial to high quality-microscopic imaging. The partially new requirements imposed by confocal microscopy have made the choice even more critical. Now the proper choice of lens may well make the difference between a successfully collected data set or no data at all. In this section we highlight some of the most important factors to consider when making the choice.

The classic criterion for lens selection (Taylor and Salmon, 1989) (after having determined the needed magnification) is the numerical aperture (NA) of the lens. The NA is a measure of the light-gathering power of the lens and is defined by

$$NA = n \sin \theta \qquad (4)$$

where $n$ is the index of refraction for the immersion medium and $\theta$ is the angle between the optical axis and the greatest marginal ray entering the lens. The NA is also a measure of the resolving power of the lens, as shown below.

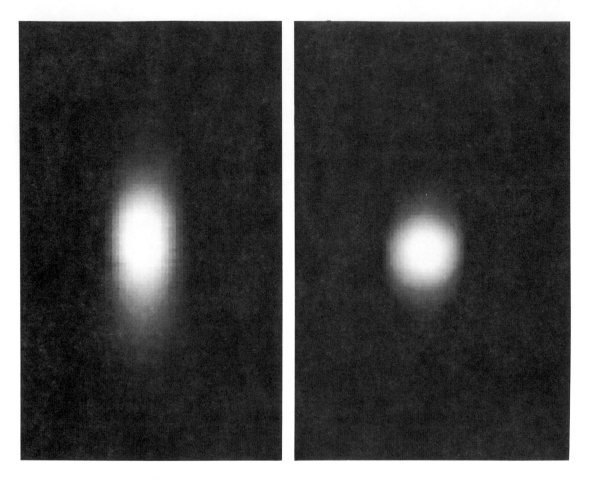

**Fig. 7**  Two 6.5-$\mu$m latex beads, the left in water and the right in glycerol, which has a refractive index more similar to that of the latex bead. The bead measured in water acts as a lens and changes the image of itself.

The image brightness for conventional epifluorescence microscopy is related to the NA and the magnification according to

$$\text{Brightness} \cong \text{NA}^4/\text{magnification}^2 \qquad (5)$$

This, and the fact that the in-plane, two-point resolution (according to the Raleigh criterion) can be expressed as

$$R_f = 0.61\lambda/\text{NA} \qquad (6)$$

clearly show why the practical rule for conventional microscopy is to select the lens with the highest numerical aperture. (Even a small increase in NA has a large impact on light collection and makes it possible to resolve smaller details in the specimen.)

In confocal microscopy similar relationships apply. Here, because of the optical properties of the scanning system, the resolution criteria are more critically dependent on the NA. In the confocal fluorescence case the theoretical two-point resolution is defined by

$$R_f = 0.46\lambda/\text{NA} \tag{7}$$

which is a 30% improvement over the conventional case. Figure 8 shows how the NA affects the intensity and in-plane resolution when imaging close to the coverslip, well within the design parameters for the lenses used.

## C. Depth Discrimination

The discussion above relates to lens performance in two-dimensional imaging. In confocal microscopy the depth dimension is, however, also important. One can theoretically derive an expression for the thickness of the confocal sections, at least for the limiting case of an infinitely small confocal aperture (Carlsson and Aslund, 1987). This expression,

$$R_d = 1.4 n_0 \lambda/\text{NA}^2 \tag{8}$$

shows that a high NA may be favorable; the higher the NA, the thinner the slice that can be cut from the specimen. Note, however, that the index of refraction of the immersion medium is part of the expression. This means that the nominal vertical resolution of an NA 0.95 dry objective is better than that for an NA 1.0 oil immersion objective (although the resolution of the latter is better in the planar image)!

It is also important to remember that this expression applies close to the coverslip (and close to the optical axis). The discussions above about spherical aberrations make it clear that performance can be expected to decrease farther from the coverslip. Nevertheless, it is interesting to calculate the theoretical resolution to obtain an understanding of the limitations of the technique. Table II shows data for some typical lenses (assuming that the wavelength is 500 nm, i.e., green fluorescence).

Although high-NA lenses seem to be the preferred choice, they may not be practical in all experimental situations. A basic limitation is the short working distance they possess (one cannot image past the point where the lens runs into the coverslip). A thinner than normal coverslip may provide a way to add several tens of microns of useful depth range. This may seem harmless, especially when used with a oil immersion objective, but will in fact always lead to reduced depth resolution due to spherical aberration (Keller, 1990).

A potentially valuable option is the use of water and glycerol immersion lenses. Because the entire optical path between the specimen and the front lens of the objective is composed of the same medium (no coverslip is used) no depth correction issues arise and the spherical aberration with depth is minimized.

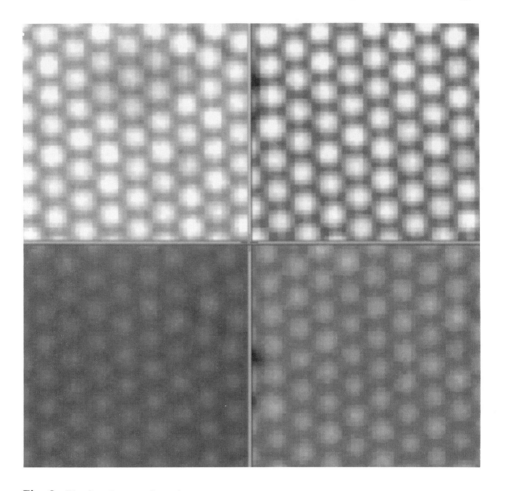

**Fig. 8**   The four images show the same monolayer of fluorescent latex beads (1.6-$\mu$m diameter) imaged through four different $\times$40 lenses. The lenses used were as follows: (*lower left*) $\times$40 NA 0.70, (*lower right*) $\times$40 NA 0.85, (*upper left*) $\times$40 NA 0.95, and (*upper right*) $\times$40 NA 1.0 oil. The images represent the best confocal section for each lens. The laser power and detector sensitivity used were the same for each image to allow direct comparisons of intensities.

## D. Behavior of Real Lenses

To investigate the three-dimensional imaging properties of different types of microscope lenses, we created slides with fluorescent latex beads suspended in a water-based gel. The bead concentration was kept low to minimize the influence of laser absorption on the measurement. (Using a $\times$40 lens there would be only a few beads in focus within the full field of view of the microscope.) In the preparation of the slides we also made sure to have a few beads adhere to the

**Table II**
**Theoretical Lateral and Depth**
**Resolutions (at 500 nm) of Typical High-**
**Quality Microscopy Objectives**[a]

| Objective | $R_f$ ($\mu$m) | $R_d$ ($\mu$m) | $R_d/R_f$ |
|---|---|---|---|
| ×40 NA 0.85 dry | 0.27 | 0.97 | 3.5 |
| ×40 NA 0.95 dry | 0.24 | 0.78 | 3.2 |
| ×40 NA 1.0 oil | 0.23 | 1.06 | 4.6 |
| ×60 NA 1.4 oil | 0.17 | 0.54 | 3.3 |
| ×100 NA 1.4 oil | 0.17 | 0.54 | 3.3 |

[a] $R_f$, Lateral two-point resolution; $R_d$, full-width
half-maximum (FWHM) of the point-spread function in depth. The last column shows the ratio between lateral and axial resolving power.

coverslip (thus serving as markers for the position of the coverslip), making for
reliable depth measurements with respect to the coverslip position.

We have chosen to investigate ×40 lenses, basically because there is a wide
range of choice for this magnification, but also because it is a representative
magnification for many types of biological work. Table III lists the lenses used in
our study.

For each of these lenses, we scanned series of sections that covered the entire
useful depth range (as limited by the thickness of the sample) of the lenses. In the
resulting data sets (200–250 sections, 512 ×512 pixels) we then measured the
vertical diameter of the beads, as well as their intensities as a function of depth
below the coverslip.

**Table III**
**Working Parameters of ×40 Objectives**
**Investigated**[a]

| Type | NA | Working distance (mm) | $n/NA^2$ |
|---|---|---|---|
| Plan Achro | 0.70 | 0.50 | 2.04 |
| Fluor | 0.85 | 0.39 | 1.38 |
| Plan Apo | 0.95 | 0.13 | 1.11 |
| Plan Apo-oil | 1.0 | 0.1 | 1.52 |

[a] Listed are their numerical apertures (NA),
their working distance, and the ratio between intended immersion medium and the square of the
numerical aperture.

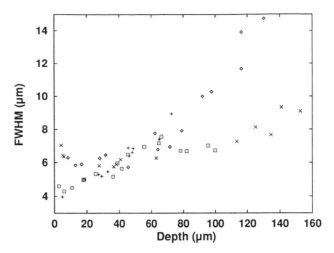

**Fig. 9** Diagram showing the full-width half-maximum vertical diameter of fluorescent latex beads as a function of the depth below the coverslip for four different objectives. ◇, ×40 NA 0.70; +, ×40 NA 0.85; □, ×40 NA 0.95; ×, ×40 NA 1.0.

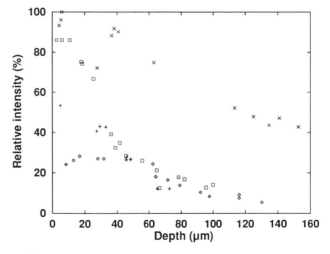

**Fig. 10** Diagram of relative measured fluorescence intensity as a function of the depth below the coverslip for each lens. All intensity values are scaled with respect to the brightest average bead image (right under the coverlip) for the Plan Apo 1.0/oil lens. ◇, ×40 NA 0.70; +, ×40 NA 0.85; □, ×40 Na 0.95; ×, ×40 NA 1.0.

It is interesting to note that the ×40/NA 0.95 Plan Apo that theoretically has the best vertical resolution only does so within a reasonably short distance from the coverslip. The extremely rapid decay in measured fluorescence intensity for this lens is even more astonishing. This does not correlate with the normal fluorescence image; beads are perceived as quite bright throughout the entire working range of the lens. We can only speculate as to the reason for this, but it is possible that this particular lens design sacrifices axial chromatic aberration to achieve other corrections.

## E. Detector Characteristics

The detector system in all current laser-scanning confocal microscopes is based on the photomultiplier tube. This device is a vacuum tube with a photosensitive cathode and a set of secondary electrodes (dynodes). It is capable of high amplification with excellent signal-to-noise characteristics, and can be used to measure a large dynamic range (several orders of magnitude) of photon flux.

Unfortunately not every incident photon is detected. The wavelength of the

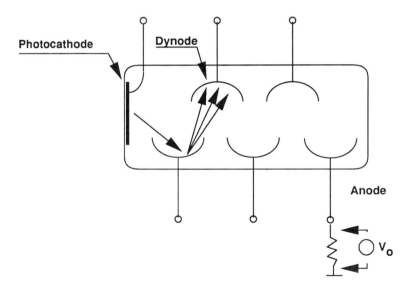

**Fig. 11** Photomultiplier tube. Photons with energy above a certain threshold (which depends on the material in the photocathode) may excite electrons enough to let them escape from the cathode. An electric field between the cathode and the following dynode accelerates the free electrons from the cathode toward the dynode. The electrons accumulate enough energy before striking the dynode to create several free secondary electrons in the dynode. This process is repeated throughout the dynode chain, resulting in high multiplication factors, that is, for every photon that results in a primary electron, the photomultiplier tube can generate a pulse of electrons that may easily be measured and quantified.

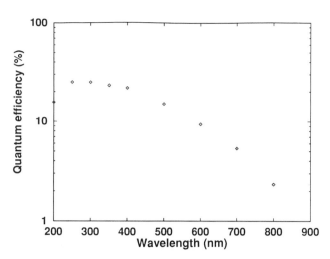

Fig. 12  Quantum efficiency for a "red-enhanced" photocathode as a function of wavelength.

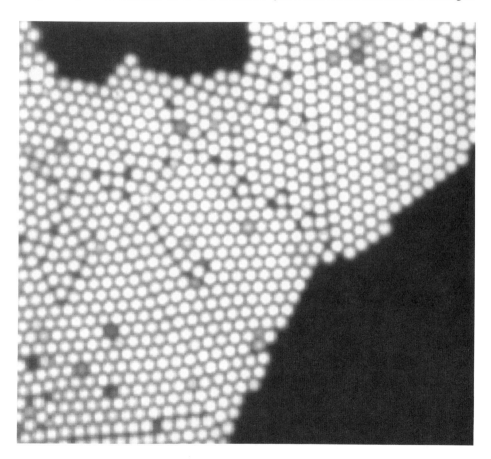

Fig. 13  Example of insufficient discrete sampling. *Left:* Image shows a specimen of 1.6-μm beads sampled every 0.25 μm. *Right:* The same specimen sampled every 1.0 μm, which is not enough to resolve the beads accurately.

light (i.e., its energy) strongly affects the probability of detection. Figure 12 shows the quantum efficiency (i.e., the probability that an incident photon will generate an electron) as a function of the wavelength for a typical photo-multiplier tube.

Two observations can immediately be made: the response is highly nonlinear over the visible area, and the overall sensitivity is poor (typically less than 10% of the photons are detected). More specifically, the sensitivity to green fluorescence is two to three times larger than the sensitivity to red. The most important consequence of this is that direct comparisons of measured fluorescent intensities are difficult. This is especially true when comparing intensities from multiple dyes (the fluorescence of which are from different parts of the spectrum and thus measured with different sensitivities). Caution may also be in order when comparing intensities from samples in which the sample environment (pH, etc.) may affect the fluorescence distribution of the dye during the course of the experiment. If the fluorescence is in the area where the quantum

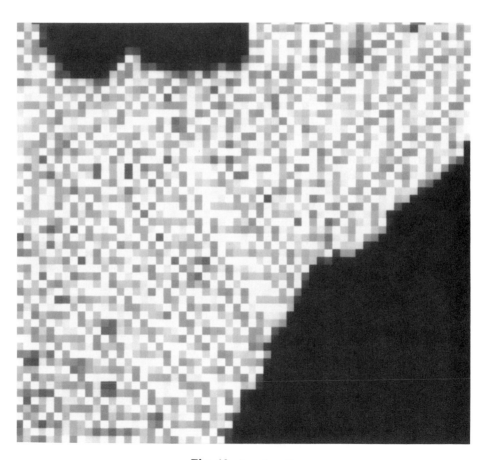

**Fig. 13** (*continued*)

sensitivity changes rapidly, small shifts in the peak fluorescence wavelength may result in comparatively large changes in the measured value.

In light of the poor sensitivity for the red part of the spectrum, optical filters and beam splitters for the detection system become more critical. This is especially true in a dual-labeling situation, in which long-pass filters must be applied to suppress the shorter wavelength in the "red channel." The cut-on wavelength must be well matched to the actual fluorescence spectrum of the dye to accomplish good imaging in the red channel.

### F. Effects of Spatial Sampling

All digital imaging systems are affected by the fact that they reproduce image information only in discrete points with discrete values. The conversion is done by sampling the intensity in the original continuous image in points laid out on a rectangular grid. This process may introduce some surprising artifacts if it is not performed properly, as demonstrated in Fig. 13. The problem encountered is that the sampling points are too sparse to represent the information in the original image properly. Although the illustration here appears to indicate that the problem is two dimensional, it affects confocal imaging in all three dimensions. Horizontal sampling artifacts are often easy to detect during data capture simply by comparing the optical image through the microscope binocular to the digital image. Artifacts due to vertical undersampling are much more difficult to see because no such direct comparison can be made.

Theoretical work (Shannon, 1948) shows that the minimum sampling distance that can be used without loss of information is half of the smallest feature in the input. In practice the rule of thumb is that the sampling rate should be about 2.3 times the largest spatial frequency in the input. Because the resolution of the optical system in the microscope sets the limit on information presented to the scanning system, the ultimate limit on pixel and section spacing is set by the point-spread function of the lens. The specimen itself may, however, allow a less strict condition depending on the size and spacing of the features present in the imaged area. If the sample is believed to be isotropic one should select the section-to-section distance equal to the horizontal pixel size to ensure that no vertical sampling artifacts are introduced. It is, however, never useful to scan sections that are closer together than the vertical resolution limit of the lens divided by 2.3.

### III. Conclusions

We have described artifacts that the interaction between the optics in the microscope and the specimen can cause. The most important is that the focal plane can move more or less than the microscope stage, depending on the index of refraction of the media above and below the coverslip. This effect can cause vertical distance errors in excess of 40%, when using a dry objective on a specimen in glycerol. It is therefore imperative that one either designs the experiment properly (e.g., a glycerol immersion objective could be used) or uses software that is cognizant of this phenomenon to collect and measure the data.

The lenses that are currently used for confocal microscopy are designed based on a set of optimization criteria that is not necessarily appropriate for confocal applications. We have shown that highly corrected lenses that theoretically ought to be ideal may behave erratically when used in confocal systems. It is also evident that spherical aberrations limit the performance of all microscope objectives when used for imaging deep below the coverslip.

## References

Carlsson, C. (1990). *Proc. Soc. Photo-Opt. Instrum. Eng.* **1245,** 68–80.

Carlsson, C., and Aslund, N. (1987). *Appl. Op.* **26,** 3232–3238.

Galbraith, W. Q. (1955). *Q. J. Microsc.* **96,** 285–289.

Keller, H. E. (1990). *In* "Handbook of Biological Confocal Microscopy" (J. B. Pawley, ed.), Rev. Ed., pp. 77–86. Plenum, New York.

Shannon, C. E. (1948). *Bell Syst. Tech. J.* **27,** 379–423; 623–656.

Taylor, D. L., and Salmon, E. D. (1989). *Methods Cell Biol.* **29,** 207–237.

**CHAPTER 4**

# Multicolor Laser Scanning Confocal Immunofluorescence Microscopy: Practical Application and Limitations

**T. Clark Brelje, Martin W. Wessendorf, and Robert L. Sorenson**

Department of Cell Biology and Neuroanatomy
University of Minnesota Medical School
Minneapolis, Minnesota 55455

# I. Introduction

Fluorescence is presently the most important imaging mode in biological confocal microscopy (Schotten, 1989; Tsien and Waggoner, 1990). In conventional microscopy, the illumination stimulates fluorescence throughout the entire depth of a specimen, rather than only in the focal plane. The contrast and resolution observed for structures within the focal plane can be severely reduced by the background fluorescence from out-of-focus structures. In contrast, confocal microscopy uses the combination of a focused illumination spot and a detection pinhole to restrict excitation and detection to a small, diffraction-limited volume within the focal plane (Brakenhoff *et al.*, 1979; Wilson and Sheppard, 1984). Out-of-focus structures do not contribute to the background because they receive little or no illumination, and any signal derived from them is rejected by the detector aperture. The illumination point can be scanned across the specimen to build an image of structures within the focal plane in which the out-of-focus background is virtually absent (White *et al.*, 1987; Amos, 1988; Carlsson, 1990). Over and above the improvement in image contrast and resolution, it is the capability to optically section intact or thick specimens that makes confocal microscopy extremely attractive for studies using fluorescent probes. Application of this optical sectioning capability has found widespread use within biology for the examination of the three-dimensional distribution of fluorescent probes within intact, fixed, or living specimens (Schotten, 1989; Paddock, 1991).

Because many biological problems cannot be unambiguously characterized by the examination of a single parameter, techniques for the independent detection of signals from multiple fluorescent probes are required. At present, this can most easily be done by using fluorescent probes that can be viewed selectively based on differences in their excitation and emission spectra. Until recently, the capacity of confocal microscopes to examine multiple fluorescent probes in a single specimen has been extremely limited compared to conventional fluorescence microscopy (DeBiasio *et al.*, 1987; Waggoner *et al.*, 1989; Wessendorf, 1990; Galbraith *et al.*, 1991) and flow cytometry (Hoffman, 1988; Shapiro, 1988; Lanier and Recktenwald, 1991).

Advances in fluorescent probe chemistry, economical laser availability, and confocal microscope instrumentation are making the enormous potential of multicolor laser scanning confocal microscopy (LSCM) available to a wider range of biologists. This article outlines the requirements for performing multicolor immunofluorescence studies with LSCM. First, the principles of immunofluorescence histochemistry necessary for the preparation of multilabeled specimens are summarized. Second, the technical aspects of confocal microscope instrumentation that affect its application to multicolor studies are examined. Third, the practical application and limitations of this technology are demonstrated for multicolor LSCM, using the inexpensive, air-cooled argon ion and krypton–argon ion lasers as light sources. Fourth, aspects of confocal microscopy that affect the comparison of images acquired with different excitation and/or emission wavelengths are examined. With this information, users should have a better understanding of the compromises needed to effect the accurate imaging of specimens stained with multiple fluorophores. Although this article concentrates on studies of fixed biological specimens, much of the information concerning the application and limitations of multicolor LSCM is applicable to the viewing of living specimens.

## II. Immunofluorescence Histochemistry

Immunofluorescence histochemistry involves the use of antibodies labeled with fluorophores to detect substances within a specimen. Several excellent discussions on various aspects of immunofluorescence histochemistry have been published (Pearse, 1980; Larsson, 1983; Sternberger, 1986; Wessendorf, 1990). Therefore this section focuses on issues of special concern in the use of multicolor immunofluorescence for the detection of multiple substances in a single specimen.

Immunofluorescence can be performed by either direct or indirect methods. Direct immunofluorescence involves the conjugation of the primary antibody with a fluorophore, such as fluorescein or rhodamine. For indirect immunofluorescence, the primary antibody is visualized by using a fluorophore-conjugated secondary antibody raised against the immunoglobulins of the species in which the primary antibody was raised. Indirect immunofluorescence is more commonly used because the labeling of each primary antibody is laborious and can decrease its affinity or specificity for its antigen. Moreover, direct methods may be less sensitive than indirect methods because theoretically more than one molecule of the secondary antibody can bind to a given molecule of the primary antibody. With the widespread use of indirect immunofluorescence for biological studies, a large number of secondary antibodies conjugated to various fluorophores have become commercially available.

Before accepting the localization of an antigen by indirect immunofluorescence, the specificity of the staining and visualization must be established. This characterization of a staining protocol is especially important for multicolor immunofluorescence because of the greatly expanded opportunities for cross-reactivity and artifactual staining.

### A. Fluorophores and Labeling Reagents

The most important factors in determining the limitations and capabilities of fluorescence microscopy are the physical characteristics of the fluorescent dyes used in biological studies (Tsien and Waggoner, 1990; Wells and Johnson, 1993). In particular, the extent to which a fluorophore absorbs light (i.e., the extinction coefficient) and the likelihood that an excited fluorophore will emit fluorescence (i.e., the quantum yield) or spontaneously decompose (i.e., photobleaching) imposes strict limits on this method (Wells *et al.,* 1990). Because specimens can be stained with a finite amount of fluorescent dye, it is important that the microscope efficiently excite and detect the limited number of photons emitted before its photodestruction. Although numerous fluorescent dyes exist, relatively few have been found suitable for immunofluorescence studies (Fig. 1). Because the selection of appropriate fluorophores is critical to the success of multicolor immunofluorescence studies, the important physical and spectral properties concerning their use will be briefly described.

The most important consideration in the selection of fluorescent dyes for the covalent labeling of antibodies, or other relevant biological molecules, is their intensity of fluorescence. This is particularly important for LSCM, in which exceedingly small quantities of fluorescent dyes must be detected over short intervals of time. With nonsaturating excitation rates, the relative brightness of a fluorescent dye is proportional to the product of its extinction coefficient at a given excitation wavelength and its quantum yield (Table I). Because both of these properties are sensitive to the local molecular environment (for example, pH of aqueous media, solvent polarity, and the proximity of quenching species), they must be determined for the actual conjugates of the fluorophores rather than for the unconjugated fluorescent dyes. For example, the high quantum yield for fluorescein in aqueous solution (~0.70) decreases to 0.20–0.35 when four fluorophores are bound to each antibody molecule (Tsien and Waggoner, 1990). This reduction in fluorescence on conjugation is due to the quenching by other bound dye molecules or through interactions with the labeled protein. Moreover, these interactions limit the increase in fluorescence intensity that can be obtained by conjugating higher numbers of fluorophores to each protein molecule. Besides these intrinsic properties of the conjugated fluorophore, their observed brightness is also directly influenced by the efficiency of excitation by the available light sources and detection by the commonly used detectors (such as the human eye, photographic film, or photomultiplier tubes).

Although the total fluorescence signal can be increased with higher illumination intensities or by integrating for a longer time, photochemical side effects such as photobleaching of the fluorophore or damage to the specimen limits the allowable light exposure. However, the high illumination intensities necessary for LSCM are already near the optical saturation limit of many fluorescent probes (Wells *et al.,* 1990; Wells and Johnson, 1993). Further increases in the illumination intensity will actually decrease the observed signal-to-background ratio because much higher levels of light are needed to saturate the background autofluorescence (Tsien and Waggoner, 1990). It is important to recognize that the average number of photons emitted by a fluorophore before photodestruction is determined by the ratio of the quantum yields for fluorescence and photobleaching (Mathies and Stryer, 1986). This suggests that longer observation times can be achieved only by increasing the concentration of the fluorophore, using lower illumination intensities to reduce the rate of fluorescence, or decreasing the rate of photobleaching. Therefore, the lowest illumination inten-

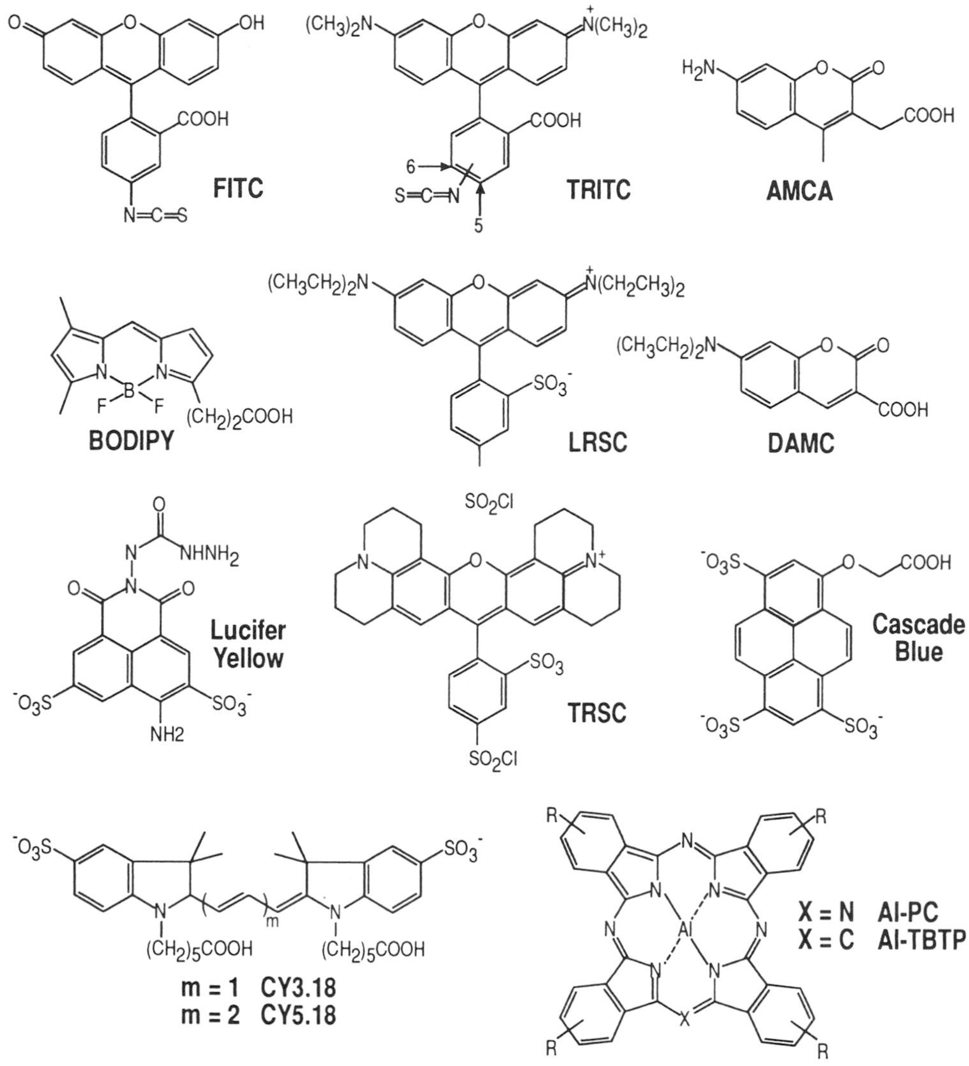

**Fig. 1** Chemical structures of common fluorophores for immunofluorescence studies. See Table I for the abbreviations used for each fluorophore and its spectral properties. Note that most commercial preparations of tetramethylrhodamine isothiocyanate (TRITC) are a mixture of the 5'- and 6'-isothiocyanate isomers.

sities that give images with an adequate signal to noise should be used for the collection of images by LSCM. The rate of photobleaching for some fluorophores can be reduced by the addition of chemical antioxidants, such as *p*-phenylenediamine (Johnson and de C. Nogueira Araujo, 1981; Johnson *et al.*, 1982) or *n*-propyl gallate (Giloh and Sedat, 1982), to the mounting media for fixed specimens. However, these antifade reagents are incompatible with living cells.

**Table I**
**Spectroscopic Properties of Common Probes for Immunofluorescence[a]**

| Fluorophore or labeling reagent | Abbreviation | Molecular weight | Excitation maximum (nm) | Emission maximum (nm) | Extinction coefficient ($\times 10^3\ M^{-1}cm^{-1}$) | Quantum yield | Reference |
|---|---|---|---|---|---|---|---|
| 7-Amino-4-methylcoumarin-3-acetic acid | AMCA | 233 | 347 | 445 | 15 | — | Khalfan et al. (1986); Wessendorf et al. (1990b,c) |
| Pyrenyloxytrisulfonic acid | Cascade Blue | 486 | 376, 399 | 423 | 23, 28 | — | Whitaker et al. (1991a); MP[b] |
| 7-Diethylaminocoumarin-3-carboxylic acid | DAMC | 261 | 391 | 474 | — | — | Staines et al. (1988) |
| Lucifer yellow | LY | 457 | 428 | 533 | 12 | — | MP |
| Fluorescein isothiocyanate | FITC | 389 | 496 | 518 | 67 | 0.20–0.35 | Waggoner et al. (1989) |
| 4,4-Difluoro-5,7-dimethyl-4-bora-3a,4a-diazaindacene 3-propionic acid | BODIPY | 292 | 503 | 511 | 80 | 0.40 | Haugland (1990); MP |
| Cyanine 3.18 | Cy3.18 | 718 | 554 | 565 | 150 | 0.15 | Mujumdar et al. (1993); BDS[c] |
| Tetramethylrhodamine isothiocyanate | TRITC | 444 | 554 | 576 | 67 | — | |
| Lissamine rhodamine sulfonyl chloride | LRSC | 577 | 572 | 590 | 83 | 0.04 | Chen (1969) |
| R-Phycoerythrin | R-PE | 240,000 | 480, 565 | 578 | 2,000 | 0.85 | Oi et al. (1982) |
| B-Phycoerythrin | B-PE | 240,000 | 546, 565 | 575 | 2,410 | 0.59 | Oi et al. (1982) |
| Texas Red sulfonyl chloride | TRSC | 625 | 592 | 610 | 87 | 0.01 | Titus et al. (1982) |
| Allophycocyanin | APC | 110,000 | 650 | 661 | 690 | 0.68 | Oi et al. (1982) |
| Cyanine 5.18 | Cy5.18 | 734 | 649 | 667 | 240 | 0.28 | Mujumdar et al. (1993); BDS |
| Aluminum tetrabenztriazaporphyrin | Al-TBTP | ~1,000 | 395, 656, 675 | 678 | 189 | 0.24 | Renzoni et al. (1992); BTG USA[d] |
| Aluminum phthalocyanine | Al-PC | 876 | 350, 675 | 680 | 160 | 0.50 | Renzoni et al. (1992) |
| Peridinin chlorophyll a-binding protein | PerCP | 35,000 | 470 | 680 | 380 | 1.00 | Recktenwald (1989) |

[a] These fluorescent probes are listed in order of increasing excitation and emission wavelengths. Except for LY and PerCP, all values are given for the individual fluorophores conjugated to IgG antibodies. All conjugates had dye/protein ratios of 2 to 4, except for the biological pigments (i.e., R-PE, B-PE, APC, and PerCP), which had dye/protein ratios of 1. The values for AMCA, Cy3.18, and Cy5.18 are for conjugates prepared from the corresponding succinimidyl esters. The extinction maxima for R-PE, B-PE, and APC are for the phycobiliproteins, which contain 34, 34, and 6 pigment molecules, respectively.

[b] MP, Molecular Probes, Inc. (Eugene, OR).

[c] BDS, Biological Detection Systems, Inc. (Pittsburgh, PA).

[d] BTG USA, British Technology Group USA, Inc. (Gulph Mills, PA).

Although the intensity of fluorescence is important, the utility of a fluorophore for the labeling of antibodies is determined by several additional properties. An important practical consideration is the availability of suitable labeling reagents for the preparation of conjugates with biological molecules (Haugland, 1983). Isothiocyanates are widely used to attach fluorescent dyes to neutral amino groups of proteins in buffers at pH 8.5–9.5. Other alternatives for the labeling of amino groups include succinimidyl esters, chlorotriazinyl groups, aziridines, and anhydrides. The fluorophore must not adversely affect the properties of the biological molecule after conjugation. For example, the fluorophore-to-protein ratio for antibodies must be carefully controlled to prevent their denaturation, precipitation, or loss of binding activity. Finally, the fluorophore should have low toxicity and biological activity so that studies with living tissue can be done.

## 1. Fluorescein

Fluorescein isothiocyanate (FITC) is the most widely used fluorescent probe for the preparation of conjugates with biological molecules (Hansen, 1967; Haugland, 1990). This xanthene dye (Fig. 1) is particularly useful for several reasons: conjugates are easily prepared because of the water solubility of FITC; it is brightly fluorescent because of its reasonably large extinction coefficients and high quantum yields after conjugation (Table I); and it has low nonspecific binding with most biological tissues. The preparation of fluorescein conjugates from the closely related (4,6-dichlorotriazinyl) aminofluorescein (DTAF) has been recommended because of its higher purity and stability (Blakeslee and Baines, 1976). Typically, three to five fluoresceins can be conjugated to each IgG antibody before self-quenching and altered binding affinities are observed. Fluorescein is maximally excited by blue light and emits primarily green to yellow fluorescence (Fig. 2). Although the excitation spectrum of fluorescein does not overlap with any of the intense emission peaks of mercury arc lamps (313, 334, 365, 405, 435, 546, and 578 nm), the output intensity in the range of 450 to 500 nm is sufficient for the excitation of fluorescein by conventional fluorescence microscopy. The 488-nm line of the argon ion laser used in flow cytometry and LSCM is ideally suited for near-maximal excitation of fluorescein.

In spite of its general usefulness, fluorescein does have several unfavorable properties. It is not particularly photostable, it is sensitive to changes in pH and solvent polarity, and its emission spectrum overlaps extensively with cellular autofluorescence. For fixed specimens, the photobleaching of fluorescein is effectively retarded by the addition of an antifade reagent to the mounting medium (see above). Structurally, the pH sensitivity of fluorescein is due to the presence of an ionizable carboxylate group conjugated to the $\pi$ electron system of the fluorophore, and has been employed in pH indicators such as 2′,7′-bis-(2-carboxyethyl)-5(and 6)-carboxyfluorescein (BCECF), seminaphthorhodafluors (SNARFs), and seminaphthofluoresceins (SNAFLs) (Whitaker et al., 1991b).

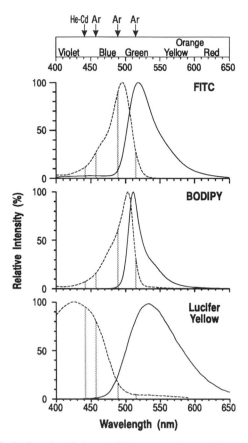

**Fig. 2** Excitation (dashed) and emission (solid) spectra of green fluorophores. *Top:* Fluorescein isothiocyanate (FITC)-conjugated donkey anti-mouse IgG (Jackson ImmunoResearch Laboratories, West Grove, PA). The excitation spectrum was scanned while measuring emission at 570 nm, and the emission spectrum was scanned while exciting at 370 nm. *Middle:* BODIPY-conjugated goat anti-mouse IgG (Molecular Probes, Eugene, OR). The excitation spectrum was scanned while measuring emission at 600 nm, and the emission spectrum was scanned while exciting at 370 nm. *Bottom:* Lucifer yellow (Sigma, St. Louis, MO). The excitation spectrum was scanned while measuring emission at 600 nm, and the emission spectrum was scanned while exciting at 370 nm. The emission lines for argon ion (Ar) and helium–cadmium (He–Cd) lasers are shown as vertical lines beneath the excitation spectra.

Therefore specimens stained with fluorescein should be mounted in aqueous media with a pH of at least 8 for the maximum intensity of fluorescence (Hiramoto *et al.*, 1964).

## 2. BODIPY

Boron dipyrromethene difluoride (BODIPY) has been proposed as a substitute for fluorescein (Worries *et al.*, 1985; Haugland, 1990). BODIPY conjugates are efficiently excited by blue light and emit primarily green fluorescence like fluorescein, but with a smaller Stokes shift and narrower excitation and emission peaks (Fig. 2). This characteristic usually requires the excitation or detection of BODIPY staining at suboptimal wavelengths. Major advantages of BODIPY compared to fluorescein include its insensitivity to changes in pH and solvent polarity. In addition, BODIPY has been reported to be more photostable than fluorescein conjugates (Haugland, 1990), but less photostable than the rhodamine Texas Red (Robitaille *et al.*, 1990). Unfortunately, at high concentrations of BODIPY the green fluorescence emission peak at ~515 nm decreases and a second peak of red fluorescence appears at ~620 nm (Pagano *et al.*, 1991; Haugland, 1992). Although this phenomenon probably requires interaction of multiple fluorophores, a similar relatively weak, red fluorescence can be observed from specimens brightly stained with BODIPY-conjugated secondary antibodies (T.C. Brelje, unpublished observations).

The development of additional BODIPY fluorophores with excitation and emission spectra shifted to longer wavelengths has been described by Molecular Probes (Eugene, OR) (Haugland, 1992). Unfortunately, the fluorescence from many of these derivatives is quenched upon conjugation to proteins. The development of red-shifted derivatives which are suitable for conjugation to proteins is being actively pursed and should be available in the near future (R. Haugland, personal communication).

## 3. Lucifer Yellow

Although infrequently used as a covalent label for biological molecules, Lucifer yellow is often used in immunofluorescence studies for the intracellular filling of cells (Stewart, 1978). It is intensely fluorescent, relatively photostable, and the presence of a free amino group makes it fixable in specimens. However, the extremely broad excitation and emission spectra of Lucifer yellow (Fig. 2) can complicate its independent detection in the presence of other fluorophores. In these cases, the use of alternate intracellular markers, such as biocytin (Horikawa and Armstrong, 1988) or *N*-(2-aminoethyl)biotinamide (Neurobiotin; Kita and Armstrong, 1991), that can be visualized with more specific fluorophores conjugated to avidin or anti-biotin antibodies is preferred.

## 4. Rhodamine Fluorophores

The rhodamines are xanthene derivatives structurally related to fluorescein, but with additional chemical substitutions that shift their excitation and emission spectra to longer wavelengths (Fig. 1). The most widely used rhodamines in order of increasing excitation and emission wavelengths are tetramethylrhodamine, Lissamine rhodamine, and Texas Red (Fig. 3). Although the lower quantum yields of rhodamine conjugates make them significantly dimmer than comparable fluorescein conjugates (Table I), they are generally more photostable and are pH insensitive (McKay *et al.*, 1981). Rhodamine conjugates must be

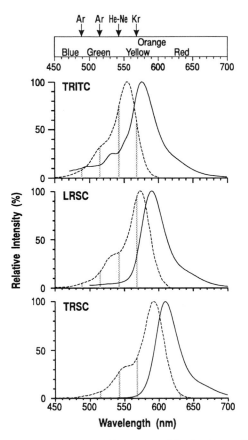

**Fig. 3** Excitation (dashed) and emission (solid) spectra of rhodamine-conjugated secondary antibodies (Jackson ImmunoResearch Laboratories). *Top:* Tetramethylrhodamine isothiocyanate (TRITC)-conjugated donkey anti-mouse IgG. The excitation spectrum was scanned while measuring emission at 610 nm, and the emission spectrum was scanned while exciting at 450 nm. *Middle:* Lissamine rhodamine sulfonyl chloride (LRSC)-conjugated donkey anti-mouse IgG. The excitation spectrum was scanned while measuring emission at 630 nm, and the emission spectrum was scanned while exciting at 480 nm. *Bottom:* Texas Red sulfonyl chloride (TRSC)-conjugated donkey anti-mouse IgG. The excitation spectrum was scanned while measuring emission at 650 nm, and the emission spectrum was scanned while exciting at 500 nm. The emission lines for argon ion (Ar), krypton ion (Kr), and helium–neon (He–Ne) lasers are shown as vertical lines beneath the excitation spectra.

carefully prepared because they are particularly susceptible to quenching when more than two or three dye molecules are covalently attached to each antibody molecule. Nonetheless, rhodamine staining can often appear quite bright by conventional fluorescence microscopy because their excitation spectra coincide with the strong 546-nm emission peak of mercury arc lamps. The hydrophobic nature of the rhodamines, especially for Texas Red and less so for tetramethylrhodamine, requires careful control of the number of fluorophores conjugated to each antibody. Higher fluorophore-to-protein ratios result in fluorescent quenching, denaturation and precipitation of the antibodies, and higher background staining. Although the excitation source available influences which rhodamine to use, the larger spectral overlap between fluorescein and tetramethylrhodamine has been observed to be a problem in the specific visualization of these fluorophores in multiple-labeled specimens (Wessendorf *et al.*, 1990a).

## 5. Phycobiliproteins

Phycobiliproteins are naturally occurring components of the light-collecting complexes of certain cyanobacteria and algae, and have considerable potential as fluorescent probes (Oi *et al.*, 1982; Kronick, 1986). These proteins have been engineered by natural selection for large extinction coefficients, high quantum yields, and to protect the covalently linked tetrapyrrole chromophores from quenching processes (Table I) (Glazer, 1989). Although designed to efficiently transfer energy from blue light to the chlorophyll photosynthetic system, the purified phycobiliproteins are highly fluorescent because the molecules no longer have any nearby acceptors to which to transfer the absorbed energy.

The most widely used phycobiliproteins for fluorescence studies are R-phycoerythrin, B-phycoerythrin, and allophycocyanin (Haugland, 1992). The phycoerythrins are efficiently excited by blue–green light and emit primarily yellow–orange fluorescence (Fig. 4). Because each contains a large number of chromophores, their fluorescence yield is equivalent to at least 30 fluorescein or 100 rhodamine fluorophores at comparable wavelengths (Oi *et al.*, 1982). The more efficient excitation of R-phycoerythrin by the 488-nm emission line of an argon ion laser has led to its widespread use with fluorescein for two-color studies using flow cytometry (Hoffman, 1988; Shapiro, 1988; Lanier and Recktenwald, 1991). The photostability of R-phycoerythrin is slightly less than that of fluorescein, whereas B-phycoerythrin is slightly more stable (White and Stryer, 1987). Although not as bright as the phycoerythrins, the longer wavelength allophycocyanin is efficiently excited by red light and emits far red fluorescence (Fig. 4).

Although these phycobiliproteins are brightly fluorescent, their unique properties must be considered when used as fluorescent labels. Their intensity of fluorescence is greatly reduced by denaturation of their protein component. R-Phycoerythrin fades rather rapidly with the high-intensity illumination used with LSCM (Schubert, 1991). Furthermore, the high molecular weights of the phycobiliproteins (Table I) restrict their penetration into the denser regions of fixed cells and thick specimens.

## 6. Cyanine Fluorophores

Cyanine 3.18 and 5.18 are sulfoindocyanine dyes from a family of fluorophores developed by A. Waggoner and colleagues at Carnegie-Mellon University (Southwick *et al.*, 1990; Mujumdar *et al.*, 1993). These sulfoindocyanine

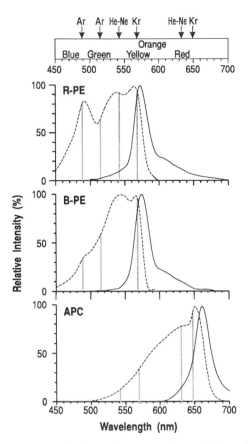

**Fig. 4** Excitation (dashed) and emission (solid) spectra of phycobiliprotein-conjugated secondary antibodies. *Top:* R-Phycoerythrin (R-PE)-conjugated goat anti-mouse IgG (Jackson Immuno-Research Laboratories). The excitation spectrum was scanned while measuring emission at 625 nm, and the emission spectrum was scanned while exciting at 475 nm. *Middle:* B-Phycoerythrin (B-PE)-conjugated goat anti-mouse IgG (Jackson ImmunoResearch Laboratories). The excitation spectrum was scanned while measuring emission at 625 nm, and the emission spectrum was scanned while exciting at 475 nm. *Bottom:* Allophycocyanin (APC)-conjugated goat anti-mouse IgG (Biomeda, Foster City, CA). The excitation spectrum was scanned while measuring emission at 710 nm, and the emission spectrum was scanned while exciting at 500 nm. The emission lines for argon ion (Ar), krypton ion (Kr), and helium–neon (He–Ne) lasers are shown as vertical lines beneath the excitation spectra.

dyes are highly water soluble, pH insensitive, and exhibit low nonspecific binding to biological specimens. Because of their large extinction coefficients and moderate quantum yields (Table I), their antibody conjugates are typically brighter and have greater photostability than those with fluorescein (Yu *et al.*, 1992; Mujumdar *et al.*, 1993). Because these cyanine fluorophores are as bright, if not brighter, in organic solvents, they are particularly useful with thick specimens that must be dehydrated and cleared before examination by LSCM (Mesce *et al.*, 1993).

With increasing length of the polymethine chain $[(-C=)_n]$ separating the indolenine nuclei (Fig. 1), the absorption and emission wavelengths of the cyanine chromophore shift to longer wavelengths (Southwick *et al.*, 1990). The excitation and emission spectra of cyanine 3.18 conjugates are similar to tetramethylrhodamine (Fig. 5). When used with conventional fluorescence microscopy and a mercury arc lamp, cyanine 3.18 has been found to give significantly brighter specific staining than either fluorescein or any of the rhodamines (Wessendorf and Brelje, 1992). The longer wavelength cyanine 5.18 is excited by red light and emits far red fluorescence, and can be used as a low molecular weight alternative to allophycocyanin (Fig. 5). Like other far red fluorophores, cyanine 5.18 is extremely difficult to observe by eye in conventional fluorescence microscopes because of the low sensitivity of the eye to red light above 650 nm.

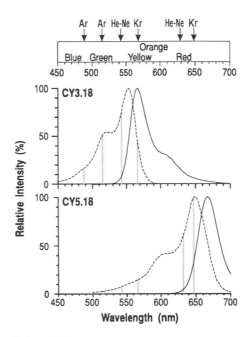

**Fig. 5** Excitation (dashed) and emission (solid) spectra of cyanine-conjugated secondary antibodies (Jackson ImmunoResearch Laboratories). *Top:* Cyanine 3.18 (CY3.18)-conjugated donkey anti-mouse IgGs. The excitation spectrum was scanned while measuring emission at 610 nm, and the emission spectrum was scanned while exciting at 490 nm. *Bottom:* Cyanine 5.18 (CY5.18)-conjugated donkey anti-mouse IgGs. The excitation spectrum was scanned while measuring emission at 710 nm, and the emission spectrum was scanned while exciting at 500 nm. The emission lines for argon ion (Ar), krypton ion (Kr), and helium–neon (He–Ne) lasers are shown as vertical lines beneath the excitation spectra.

## 7. Phthalocyanine Derivatives

Phthalocyanine derivatives suitable for conjugation to biological molecules were developed by Ultra Diagnostics Corp. (Schindele and Renzoni, 1990; Renzoni *et al.*, 1992) and licensed by British Technology Group USA (Gulph Mills, PA). Structurally related to the linking of tetrapyrroles by methine (—C=) groups in porphyrins, the phthalocyanines are composed of four iso-indole units linked by aza nitrogen atoms (—N=; Fig. 1). As with the porphyrins, metal atoms such as aluminum are usually inserted in the central ring of phthalocyanines. These metal-phthalocyanines are excited by both ultraviolet and far red light, and emit far red fluorescence (Fig. 6). Replacing one of the aza nitrogens by a methine carbon gives a tetrabenztriazaporphyrin that is similar to the corresponding phthalocyanine except that an additional red excitation peak occurs (Fig. 6). Although phthalocyanine conjugates are currently not commercially available, the increased use of far red fluorophores for all types of fluorescence studies should encourage their production.

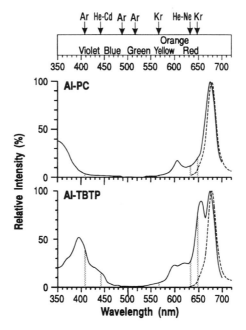

**Fig. 6** Excitation (dashed) and emission (solid) spectra of phthalocyanine derivatives conjugated to secondary antibodies (British Technology Group USA, Gulph Mills, PA). *Top:* Aluminum phthalocyanine (Al-PC)-conjugated goat anti-mouse IgG (Ultralight 680). *Bottom:* Aluminum tetra-benztriazaporphyrin (Al-TBTP)-conjugated goat anti-mouse IgG (Ultralight T680). The excitation spectra were scanned while measuring emission at 725 nm, and the emission spectra were scanned while exciting at 340 nm. The emission lines for argon ion (Ar), krypton ion (Kr), helium–cadmium (He-Cd), and helium–neon (He–Ne) lasers are shown as vertical lines beneath the excitation spectra.

## 8. Blue Fluorophores

Several ultraviolet-excitable, blue fluorophores have been used for immuno-fluorescence studies: 7-amino-4-methylcoumarin-3-acetic acid (AMCA; Khal-fan *et al.*, 1986; Wessendorf *et al.*, 1990a), diethylaminocoumarin (DAMC; Staines *et al.*, 1988), and Cascade Blue (pyrenyloxytrisulfonic acid; Whitaker *et al.*, 1991a; Fritschy *et al.*, 1992). All of these blue fluorophores are excited by ultraviolet light and emit blue fluorescence (Fig. 7). However, the greater over-lap between the emission spectra of DAMC and fluorescein makes it less attrac-tive for multicolor studies. AMCA is the most widely available of these blue fluorophores and has been successfully used for triple-labeling studies by con-ventional fluorescence microscopy (Wessendorf *et al.*, 1990a), flow cytometry (Delia *et al.*, 1991), and LSCM (Schubert, 1991; Ulfhake *et al.*, 1991).

### B. Immunofluorescence Staining Techniques

Staining methods using multicolor immunofluorescence techniques require careful characterization if the observed staining is to be validly interpreted. To prevent the occurrence of false positives (i.e., the appearance of staining in instances in which there is none), it is necessary to demonstrate for the staining protocol that (1) the fluorophores can be distinguished from each other by using the microscope filter sets, (2) the secondary antibodies specifically recognize only one of the primary antibodies, and (3) the primary antibodies are specific in their recognition of the substance against which they were raised (Fig. 8). This characterization can be most efficiently performed by addressing these issues sequentially. First, the specificity of visualization of the fluorophores is tested. Having established the specificity of the fluorophores, the specificity of the fluorophore-conjugated secondary antibodies can be tested. Once the specificity of the secondary antibodies is established, it is possible to use these reagents to examine the specificity of the primary antibodies. Although the tests for the occurrence of false positives will be addressed, it should also be noted that the combination of multiple detection schemes may obscure potential occurrences of multiple labeling and result in false negatives (Wessendorf, 1990; Wessendorf *et al.*, 1990a).

### 1. Visualization Specificity of Fluorophores

The choice of fluorophores used for immunofluorescence studies is critical. First, it is necessary to determine whether autofluorescence from substances intrinsic to the tissue can mimic the appearance of the fluorophores. This can be done by examining unstained specimens with the same set of excitation and emission filters intended for use with a fluorophore. If no fluorescence is de-tected, then no substances in the tissue would appear to mimic the emission of the fluorophore. Although the exact nature of the autofluorescent substances in biological tissues is unclear, it has been suggested that endogenous fluorophores

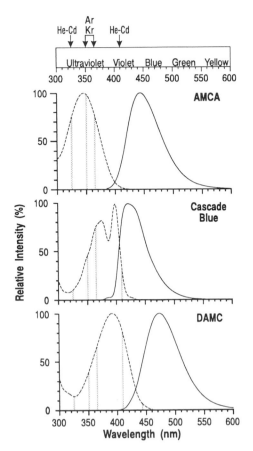

**Fig. 7** Excitation (dashed) and emission (solid) spectra of blue fluorophore-conjugated secondary antibodies. *Top:* 7-Amino-4-methylcoumarin-3-acetic acid (AMCA)-conjugated donkey anti-rabbit IgG (Jackson ImmunoResearch Laboratories). The excitation spectrum was scanned while measuring emission at 475 nm, and the emission spectrum was scanned while exciting at 370 nm. *Middle:* Pyrenyloxytrisulfonic acid (Cascade Blue)-conjugated goat anti-mouse IgG (Molecular Probes). The excitation spectrum was scanned while measuring emission at 500 nm, and the emission spectrum was scanned while exciting at 340 nm. *Bottom:* 7-Diethylaminocoumarin-3-carboxylic acid (DAMC)-conjugated avidin (Organon Teknika-Cappel, Durham, NC). The excitation spectrum was scanned while measuring emission at 530 nm, and the emission spectrum was scanned while exciting at 370 nm. The emission lines for argon ion (Ar), krypton ion (Kr), and helium–cadmium (He–Cd) lasers are shown as vertical lines beneath the excitation spectra.

include flavins, flavoproteins, reduced pyridine nucleotides, and lipofuscin pigments (Pearse, 1980; Lang *et al.*, 1991). Autofluorescence is usually the highest with excitation by violet–blue to blue light (400 to 450 nm) and decreases with increasing wavelength (Aubin, 1979; Benson *et al.*, 1979). However, cells containing significant amounts of porphyrins or chlorophyll will exhibit considerable far-red autofluorescence.

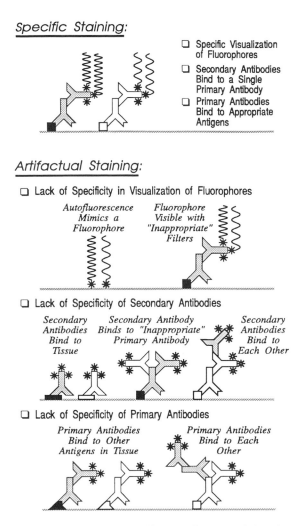

**Fig. 8** Diagrammatic representation of specific vs artifactual staining observed with two-color indirect immunofluorescence. The diagram of specific staining depicts the detection of individual antigens (solid and open squares) with separate combinations of primary and fluorophore-conjugated secondary antibodies (shaded and open). The visibility of fluorophores, using only the appropriate filters, is shown as the emission of a single wavelength of light from each secondary antibody. Other substances intrinsic to the tissue that may have an affinity for the primary or secondary antibodies is shown as rectangular and triangular binding sites.

When more than one fluorophore is used for the simultaneous detection of antibodies, it is also important to know whether one of the fluorophores can mimic the appearance of any other fluorophores used. The specificity of visualization of the fluorophores can be tested by staining individual specimens with one of the primary antibodies followed by the appropriate secondary antibody.

When these specimens are then examined by using the filter sets for each of the fluorophores, each specimen should be visible only with the appropriate filter set. Observation of staining with any of the other filter sets indicates that the protocol is not specific. This control should be performed in areas of brightest staining so as to maximize the likelihood of observing any lack of specificity.

## 2. Secondary Antibody Specificity

The simultaneous detection of more than one primary antibody depends on the availability of secondary antibodies that (1) do not cross-react with proteins intrinsic to the tissues being examined, (2) recognize only one of the primary antibodies, and (3) do not recognize each other. Without negative secondary antibody controls, reliable immunofluorescence is impossible. However, demonstrating secondary antibody specificity does not replace the need for primary antibody controls.

Whether the secondary antibody recognizes any substances intrinsic to a specimen can be examined by staining the specimen with only the secondary antibody in the absence of the primary antibody. The presence of staining could suggest that the secondary antibody is not specific. Although such staining may result from a specific interaction of the secondary antibody with an IgG-like epitope in the tissue, there may be other causes. These include the presence of naturally occurring antibodies in the serum against tissue epitopes, the presence of antibodies to contaminants in the immunizing antigen, and the presence of other serum proteins that can bind to constituents within the tissue. For this reason, the use of secondary antibodies that were affinity isolated before conjugation with the fluorophore may be beneficial. Although this should reduce the problem, it is not totally eliminated because the IgG coupled to the affinity column may also contain contaminants.

To prove that a secondary antibody recognizes only the primary antibody and not other constituents in the primary antibody solution is more difficult. First, it is necessary to demonstrate whether the secondary antibody is capable of staining the primary antibody. If staining results from sequential application of the primary and secondary antibodies, but not from the application of the secondary antibody alone, it would suggest that the secondary antibody recognizes something in the primary antibody solution that binds to the specimen. Second, it is necessary to demonstrate that the secondary antibody specifically recognizes the immunoglobulins of the primary antibody and not additional constituents in the antibody solution. This possibility can be tested by preincubating the primary antibody with the antigen against which it is directed. If this absorption control blocks all staining, it would appear that the staining is due to the secondary antibody recognizing the immunoglobulins of the primary antibody. If an absorption control is not possible, a similar control could be performed by examining the staining with preimmune serum from the same animal.

The simultaneous detection of more than one primary antibody with the corresponding secondary antibodies requires several more controls. It must be established that no secondary antibody has affinity for a primary antibody other than the one against which it is directed. This can be tested by staining specimens with only one of the primary antibodies and each of the secondary antibodies to be used. Assuming that the fluorophores can be specifically visualized, staining should be detected only with the filter set for the appropriate secondary antibody.

Once it is established that none of the secondary antibodies cross-react with the "inappropriate" primary antibodies, it is necessary to establish that no secondary antibody has an affinity for any of the other secondary antibodies being used. If multiple labeling is observed after incubating tissue with one primary antibody followed by all of the other secondary antibodies, this would suggest that one or more of the secondary antibodies have an affinity for another. This is most likely to occur when one of the secondary antibodies has been raised in the same or a closely related species to that in which one of the primary antibodies has been raised. Therefore it is essential to avoid using secondary antibodies raised in such species. The best choice is to use secondary antibodies raised in the same or similar species.

Secondary antibodies prepared specifically to avoid the above problems have become commercially available (e.g., Jackson ImmunoResearch Laboratories, West Grove, PA). These secondary antibodies are extensively adsorbed against solid phase-immobilized immunoglobulins and serum proteins of other species to minimize cross-reactivity with them. For example, the specific detection of mouse and rat monoclonal antibodies when used together is difficult because similar epitopes in both species will be recognized by most secondary antibodies to one of these species. However, these monoclonal antibodies can be distinguished by using fluorescein-conjugated donkey anti-mouse IgG that has been stripped of cross-reactivity to rat serum proteins, and rhodamine-conjugated donkey anti-rat IgG that has been stripped of cross-reactivity to mouse serum proteins. (It should be noted, however, that secondary antibodies adsorbed against closely related species should be used only when necessary because the IgG that is removed reduces epitope recognition of the "appropriate" IgG. As a result, the intensity of staining may suffer with some subclasses of IgGs.) An additional benefit in using reagents stripped of antibodies against serum proteins from the appropriate species is the reduction or elimination of cross-reactions to traces of these proteins present in normal tissues or absorbed from the culture medium by cells *in vitro* (Houser *et al.,* 1984).

Another issue to consider when using multiple secondary antibodies is whether the specimen is stained sequentially or simultaneously with each of the antibodies. The presence of small amounts of isoantibodies in serum from different individuals of the same species and/or heterophile antibodies in serum from different species may preclude the mixing of the sera into a single staining solution. If this occurs, the microprecipitates can frequently be observed on the surface of the specimen as small fluorescent particles. In this case, it would be best to stain the specimen by sequential application of the secondary antibodies.

## 3. Primary Antibody Specificity

Specific simultaneous detection of more than one substance depends on the availability of primary antibodies that (1) do not recognize other substances in the tissue being examined, (2) can be recognized specifically by secondary antibodies (see above), and (3) do not recognize each other. Even with well-characterized primary antibodies, it is important to demonstrate the specificity of staining with the primary antibodies whenever a new tissue is examined.

Before using a primary antibody for multicolor immunofluorescence studies, it is important to establish that each primary antibody recognizes the substance against which it was raised. This is typically done by testing whether staining can be blocked by absorption of the antibody with the relevant antigen. However, if the antiserum contains additional antibodies to contaminants in the antigen preparation, the absorption of the antiserum with an impure antigen may block staining but no distinction has been made between the desired and contaminating antibodies. In addition, testing whether staining can be blocked in an absorption control does not guarantee an antibody will recognize the substance as it occurs within the specimen, or after it has been altered by fixation. It is more difficult to test for cross-reactivity by a primary antibody with unknown substances in the specimen that contain epitopes similar to those against which the antibody had been raised. Because it is unclear how many tissue components are recognized by an antibody, it is preferable to refer to staining for a substance by immunocytochemistry as "immunoreactivity" in recognition of the shortcomings of the technique.

An additional concern with the simultaneous detection of more than one antigen is that the primary antibodies do not have an affinity for each other. This can be checked by simultaneously staining a region of a specimen known to contain immunoreactivity for only one of the antigens, using all of the primary and secondary antibodies for the multicolor immunofluorescence protocol. Assuming the secondary antibodies and fluorophores have been shown to be specific as described above, the presence of multiple labeling would strongly suggest that one of the other primary antibodies has affinity for the primary antibody being tested.

## 4. Background Staining

Because the detection of specific staining requires adequate contrast from the background staining, it is important to minimize the background observed when using immunofluorescent techniques. This is particularly important when image processing is employed (such as LSCM) because it is often possible to obtain acceptable images from the low-contrast background staining observed with control specimens. More important for LSCM is the effect of high background staining on the depth to which optical sections of acceptable quality can be acquired within thick specimens (see Section VI,A,4). There have been several suggestions to reduce the nonspecific staining observed with primary and secondary antibodies.

The presence of other antibodies in low amounts within the primary and secondary antisera can result in high background staining when the reagents are used at high concentrations. The first remedy for such "nonspecific staining" is to increase the dilution of the antisera. However, it can not easily be determined whether the lower background staining results from the decreased nonspecific or specific staining. For this reason, it might be expected that the greater capability of the microscope to visualize less intense staining would permit higher dilutions of the antisera to be used for increased specificity and low background staining.

Another widely used method to reduce background staining is to incubate the specimen with normal serum from the same species as the secondary antibody before applying the fluorophore-conjugated secondary antibody. The incubation with normal serum will presumably saturate nonspecific antibody-binding sites in the specimen. Although it may be possible to compete for the nonspecific binding by including normal serum in the dilution of the secondary antibody, in some cases the presence of small amounts of isoantibodies in serum from different individuals of the same species may result in the formation of micro-precipitates.

Nonspecific background staining may also be increased by the presence of overconjugated secondary antibodies, unconjugated fluorophore molecules, or impurities from the labeling reagent bound noncovalently to the secondary antibodies. These fluorescent compounds may then bind nonspecifically to tissue components when the secondary antibody is used. Early on, it was recognized that this type of background staining could be substantially reduced by absorption of conjugated antibodies with tissue powders (Coons and Kaplan, 1950). Today, this problem is reduced by using solid-phase adsorption with either hydrophobic beads (Spack et al., 1986) or normal serum from the same species as that of the specimen to be stained (Gailbraith et al., 1978). However, repeating this adsorption before use of the fluorophore-conjugated antibody can still be helpful to remove free dye released during storage. Similarly, we routinely reuse a secondary antibody solution because background staining appears to be reduced as the nonspecific staining is adsorbed with each use of the antibody. Typically, the reuse of antibody is limited only by its stability when stored in a diluted state.

Besides pretreating thick specimens with detergents to increase penetration into thick specimens, the addition of detergents to the various incubation solutions can help reduce background staining. Typically, we add Triton X-100 to the antisera (0.3%) and washing solutions (1%). At these concentrations, the Triton X-100 reduces nonspecific, low-affinity protein interactions with little or no affects on antigen–antibody binding. For especially thick specimens, relatively long wash times (24–48 hr) may be necessary to observe a reduction in background staining.

Although it is widely recognized that repeated freezing and thawing can affect the reactivity of antibodies, this is especially important for fluorophore-conjugated secondary antibodies. Besides altering the affinity of the secondary antibody, freezing and thawing of the conjugates may denature or aggregate the antibody molecules. These changes can make the conjugates more "sticky," with a marked increase in background staining. Therefore it may be preferable to store the antisera in an unfrozen state as a 50% glycerol solution in buffer at −20°C. Alternatively, the undiluted antisera can be stored for prolonged periods at 4°C if kept as sterile solutions.

## III. Instrumentation

The basic information describing the instrumentation necessary for fluorescence LSCM has been thoroughly presented in many excellent reviews and books (Wilson and Shepherd, 1984; Brakenhoff *et al.*, 1989b; Schotten, 1989; Pawley, 1990). In this section, only the aspects of confocal microscope design that are important for the adaptation of LSCM to multicolor immunofluorescence studies is examined. These issues include the ability to excite the common fluorophores with the widely available lasers, the selection of filters for the spectral isolation of individual fluorescence signals, and the limits imposed by the use of photomultiplier tubes as detectors.

### A. Laser Light Sources

Lasers have a number of unique properties, compared to other available light sources, that make them ideal for use with confocal microscopy (Gratton and van de Ven, 1990). Lasers have extremely high brightness, spatial coherence, low beam divergence, monochromatic output, low noise (i.e., beam intensity fluctuations), and can be focused into extremely small regions. Because the power requirements for fluorescence LSCM are minimal, usually only 1–3 m W (Gratton and van de Ven, 1990; Tsien and Waggoner, 1990; Wells *et al.*, 1990), most lasers with even minor emission lines in the ultraviolet and visible part of the light spectrum could potentially be used as light sources for LSCM. More important for biological applications is how efficiently the emission lines of a given laser can excite the fluorophores one wishes to use (Fig. 9). Unfortunately, the monochromatic output of lasers is also a weakness. None of the widely available air-cooled lasers can match the broad emission of the mercury or xenon arc lamps used with conventional fluorescence microscopy to excite fluorophores ranging from the ultraviolet to red regions of the light spectrum. The output of the laser must be more stable than the relative differences in the intensity of fluorescence to be detected during the acquisition of an image.

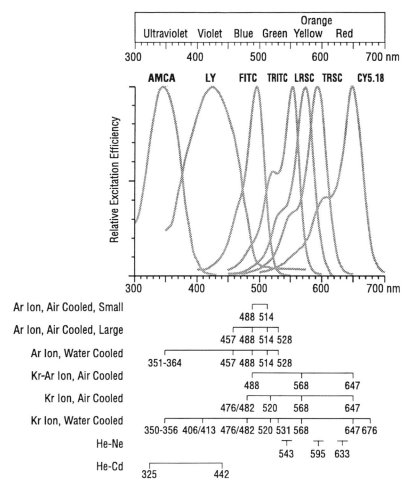

**Fig. 9** Comparison of the emission wavelengths from common lasers and the excitation spectra of fluorescent probes. The emission wavelength(s) available from various argon (Ar), krypton (Kr), krypton–argon (Kr–Ar), helium–neon (He–Ne), and helium–cadmium (He–Cd) lasers are shown. Note that the broad range of emission lines may not be simultaneously available from the larger, water-cooled ion lasers. The intense emission peaks from high-pressure mercury (Hg) arc lamps commonly used as a light source for conventional fluorescence microscopy are shown for comparison. The excitation spectra of representative fluorophores used in immunofluorescence studies are shown: 7-amino-methylcoumarin-3-acetic acid (AMCA), fluorescein (FITC), tetramethylrhodamine (TRITC), Lissamine rhodamine (LRSC), Texas Red (TRSC), and cyanine 5.18 (CY5.18). Lucifer yellow (LY) is commonly used as an intracellular label for microinjection experiments (Stewart, 1978).

Otherwise, differences in excitation intensity may be confused for actual variations in staining intensity. The output beam of the laser must be laterally stable, with the individual emission lines being colinear and parallel to lessen registration problems. Other important concerns regarding laser use with LSCM are cost, power requirements, method of waste heat removal, and reliability of operation.

## 1. Argon Ion Lasers

The most common type of laser for LSCM is a small, air-cooled argon ion laser with 25–50 mW of output power. This can be attributed to their low cost, stable output with low noise levels, minimal maintenance requirements, and long operational lifetimes (3000–5000 hr). These argon ion lasers have two major emission lines at 488 nm (blue) and 514 nm (green). The 488-nm line efficiently excites fluorescein (87% of its excitation maximum at 496 nm), but the 514-nm line is suboptimal for the various rhodamines (only 5 to 30% of their excitation maxima). Because 514-nm light also excites fluorescein (30% of its excitation maximum), other fluorophores (e.g., rhodamines) cannot be specifically excited in the presence of fluorescein with the 514-nm line. Typically, the larger, air-cooled argon ion lasers with 100–500 mW of output power are equipped with optics that allow a broader selection of emission lines ranging from 457 nm (violet–blue) to 528 nm (green). Lucifer yellow is more efficiently excited at 457 nm compared to 488 nm (81% vs 17% of its excitation maximum at 428 nm). Hence these larger lasers should be superior for the imaging of the small processes of Lucifer yellow-injected neurons (Mossberg and Ericsson, 1990). However, the increased autofluorescence observed with this shorter wavelength excitation line may be a problem with some specimens. The 528-nm line is the longest wavelength emission available from either air- or water-cooled argon ion lasers, but is infrequently used because it is difficult to maintain during the operational lifetimes of the laser. However, it does permit slightly more efficient (10–40% of their excitation maxima) excitation of the red fluorophores (Fox *et al.*, 1991).

The water-cooled argon ion lasers of 5–20 W of output power have also been used as a reliable source of ultraviolet emissions (35–363 nm) for LSCM (Amdt-Jovin *et al.*, 1990; Montag *et al.*, 1991; Schubert, 1991; Ulfhake *et al.*, 1991; Bliton *et al.*, 1993). Because of the higher ionization states of argon required for the stimulation of ultraviolet emissions, there are higher electrical and cooling requirements for these lasers. This reduces their operational lifetimes (1000 to 2000 hr) compared to the air-cooled argon ion lasers. Although water-cooled argon ion lasers have been used for live-cell imaging of ultraviolet excitable ion-sensitive probes (Lechleiter and Clapham, 1992), the high cost and maintenance requirements of these lasers have so far limited their use with LSCM. Nonetheless, the ultraviolet output of these lasers can also be used for immunofluorescence studies to efficiently excite blue fluorophores such as AMCA (Schubert, 1991; Ulfhake *et al.*, 1991). Unfortunately, the chromatic aberration present in most microscope lenses in the ultraviolet can severely compromise imaging (Ulfhake *et al.*, 1991; Bliton *et al.*, 1993). However, at least one commerical instrument has become available with the necessary optical modifications for ultraviolet confocal imaging (Bio-Rad Microscience, Cambridge, MA).

Although water-cooled argon ion lasers can be equipped with optics that permit simultaneous emission at both ultraviolet and visible wavelengths, emission of multiple lines makes it more difficult to stabilize the output power of these lasers when operating in a multiline mode. Typically, both air- and water-cooled ion lasers are operated in a light-control mode to minimize intensity fluctuations. The power supply output is regulated by a feedback circuit that samples the laser beam and adjusts the laser current to maintain constant light output. Although this works well for lasers emitting at a single wavelength, it is more difficult when the simultaneous emission from several lines occurs. For example, if the detector for the light control circuitry responds primarily to 488- and 514-nm light, there may be considerable fluctuations in the ultraviolet power output. In contrast, if the light control circuitry is used to stablize the ultraviolet emissions, large fluctuations in the power output at 488 nm may result. Therefore it may be preferable to use separate lasers as sources of ultraviolet and visible wavelengths to minimize intensity fluctuations.

## 2. Krypton and Krypton–Argon Ion Lasers

Although krypton ion lasers are similar in operation to argon ion lasers, the krypton ion has a wider range of visible emission wavelengths. The air-cooled krypton ion lasers of 15- to 200-mW output power have blue emission lines at 468, 476, and 482 nm, green lines at 520 and 531 nm, a yellow line at 568 nm, and red lines at 647 and 676 nm. This broad selection of wavelengths has the potential to efficiently excite most fluorophores requiring excitation by visible light (Fig. 9). Although this capability is enticing, krypton ion lasers are known for less reliable operation than similar argon ion lasers because of their lower output powers, higher noise levels, shorter operational lifetimes (<2000 hr), and greater sensitivity to changes in operation conditions (e.g., misaligned or dirty optics, gas pressure of the plasma tube, and power supply stability). Typically, these lasers have a limited lifetime due to depletion of the gas in their reservoirs that is used to replenish the plasma tube during aging. As if this were not bad enough, competition occurs between several of the krypton emission lines. This means that although the total output power of a krypton ion laser may stay constant when operating in a multiline mode, wide fluctuations in the intensity of the individual emission lines may occur. This excessive noise can make some of the wavelengths unusable for LSCM. Although it is less common, the use of the larger, water-cooled krypton ion lasers for LSCM has also been described (Brakenhoff et al., 1989a; Van Dekken et al., 1990).

Because of the promising characteristics of krypton–argon ion lasers, we attempted to address some of the shortcomings. We developed in collaboration with Bio-Rad Microscience and Ion Laser Technologies (Salt Lake City, UT) an air-cooled krypton–argon ion laser of 15-m W output power for use with LSCM. This laser operates in a multiline mode with a 4- to 5-m W output at 488 nm (blue), 568 nm (yellow), and 647 nm (red). To ensure the availability of more than enough light for the excitation of blue fluorophores such as fluorescein, a mixed gas krypton–argon ion laser was designed with the strong 488-nm emission of the argon ion instead of the weak blue emissions from the krypton ion. Similar to the argon ion lasers, the 488-nm line efficiently excites fluorescein, but the 568-nm krypton line is considerably more efficient than the 514-nm line for the excitation of the various rhodamines, especially Lissamine rhodamine (92% of its excitation maximum at 572 nm). In addition, the 647-nm line can efficiently excite far-red fluorophores such as cyanine 5.18 (98% of its excitation maximum at 649 nm).

## 3. Helium–Neon Lasers

As an alternative to krypton ion lasers for longer wavelength lines, helium–neon lasers are available with a 1- to 10-m W output at 543 nm (green), 595 nm (yellow), or 633 nm (red). These air-cooled lasers are inexpensive, have long lifetimes (~20,000 hr), and no adjustments of laser optics are needed because their emission wavelength cannot be changed. The 543-nm helium–neon laser can be used for more efficient excitation of rhodamines than is possible with an argon ion laser (Fig. 9) (Stelzer, 1990; Montag *et al.,* 1991; Schubert, 1991). As with the 647-nm line of the krypton ion lasers, the 633-nm helium–neon laser can be used for the excitation of far red fluorophores such as allophycocyanin or cyanine 5.18 (Fig. 9).

## 4. Helium–Cadmium Lasers

Helium–cadmium lasers can be used as an alternative ultraviolet light source instead of the water-cooled ion lasers. These lasers are air cooled and have 1–50 mW of output power at 325 nm (ultraviolet) or 442 nm (violet–blue). Because of their lower cost and operating requirements than the water-cooled argon lasers, helium–cadmium lasers have been used for many applications with flow cytometry that require ultraviolet excitation (Shapiro, 1988; Goller and Kubbies, 1992). A 442-nm helium–cadmium laser has been used in combination with an air-cooled argon ion laser for live-cell imaging by LSCM of changes in pH, using the ion-sensitive dye BCECF (Wang and Kurtz, 1990). Also, a true-color confocal reflection microscope with 442-nm helium–cadmium, 532-nm frequency-doubled neodymium–yttrium aluminum gamet (Nd-YAG), and 633-nm helium-neon lasers has been described (Cogswell *et al.,* 1992). The 325-nm line has less frequently been used for LSCM because it requires the use of special quartz optics (Brakenhoff *et al.,* 1979; Kuba *et al.,* 1991; Fricker and White, 1992).

## 5. Other Lasers

In addition to these lasers, a broad range of wavelengths is available from the use of tunable dye lasers and nonlinear wavelength expansion techniques (Gratton and van de Ven, 1990). The development of diode lasers emitting near 650 nm should also be excellent excitation sources for the excitation of far-red fluorophores. A particularly elegant application of high-power lasers is the two-photon excitation of ultraviolet-absorbing fluorophores by light with a wavelength twice that of the actual excitation wavelength (Denk *et al.,* 1990). However, these more exotic lasers are of limited availability to most biologists because of their high purchase and operating costs.

## B. Optical Filters

Regardless of whether conventional or confocal optics are used, the selection of appropriate optical filters is critical to the successful operation of any fluorescent microscope. Two types of optical filters are commonly used for fluorescence microscopy. Colored glass filters consist of dye molecules suspended in glass or plastic that absorbs some wavelengths of light and transmits other. Although these colored glass filters are highly efficient blockers of light, their optical properties will vary with the thickness of the filter, the dyes may themselves fluoresce, and conversion of absorbed high-intensity light to heat may change the special characteristics of the filter. In contrast, interference filters are made of multiple layers of reflective materials deposited on glass substrates. These thin layers of metals or dielectrics work by an additive process whereby the amplitudes of two or more overlapping waves are attenuated or reinforced. The major advantage of interference filters are their intrinsic non-fluorescence, negligible light scatter, and that they allow almost any desired spectral response to be obtained. These factors allow the design of complicated interference filters with multiple reflectance and transmittance bands (see Section IV,B,3 and 4). Because optical filters of all types are subject to damage and degradation, filter performance needs to be periodically monitored to verify continued performance at their design specifications.

Optical filters are characterized by their transmission and reflection properties and their intended use. Bandpass interference filters transmit one particular region of the light spectrum. Typically, they are specified according to their peak wavelength of transmission and the full bandwidth at half-maximal transmission. Shortpass and longpass filters are specified according to the wavelength at which half-maximal transmission occurs. Dichroic mirrors are typically long-pass filters designed to be utilized at an angle of incidence of 45° to the light path. As such, they reflect light of wavelengths shorter than the specified cut-off wavelength and transmit light of longer wavelengths. When used at other angles of incidence, the cut-off wavelength of the dichroic mirror will be shifted and the reflectance/transmittance boundary broadened.

## C. Detector Apertures

For multicolor LSCM with multiple detectors, it is beneficial to have separate, variable apertures for each detector. Although a single aperture could be positioned in the detection path before splitting the fluorescence into separate detectors, this configuration has several disadvantages. First, different aperture sizes are required to obtain the minimum depth of field for each fluorophore because the diameter of the Airy disk formed by their fluorescence is wavelength dependent (Brakenhoff *et al.*, 1990). Second, the use of separate, variable apertures provides the capability to balance the strength of the fluorescence signal against the rejection of the out-of-focus background fluorescence (*i.e.*, depth of field) for the optimum overall performance for each fluorophore (Wilson, 1989; Wells *et al.*, 1990). This is particularly important for biological specimens, in which considerable differences in the intensity of staining of each fluorophore in multiple-labeled specimens are frequently observed.

## D. Detectors

Although photomultiplier tubes (PMTs) are the most common detectors used in laser-scanning confocal microscopes (Art, 1990; Pawley, 1990), they are not necessarily the ideal detector. In an instrument with an efficient optical path, the detection of the fluorescence by the PMT can be the single least efficient step (Wells *et al.*, 1990). This is particularly important for multicolor LSCM because the response of PMTs is extremely sensitive to the wavelength of the detected photons. Although the quantum efficiency of the PMT may be as high as 25–30% for the detection of blue and green photons, this efficiency rapidly decreases as a nonlinear function with increasing wavelength. For example, the Bio-Rad MRC-600 uses PMTs with a prismatic S-20 photocathode surface (model 9828B; Thorn EMI, Rockaway, NJ) with a response typical of PMTs with extended red sensitivity. Nevertheless, the quantum efficiency for detection of photons decreases from ~11% at 500 nm, to ~5% at 600 nm, and <1% at 700 nm. Assuming the same fluorescence signal, this means that a fluorophore detected as red light will be detected with less than half of the efficiency of one detected as green light.

Several other issues must be considered when using PMTs with extended red sensitivity in confocal microscopes. Because the dark current of a PMT is primarily a function of the extent of red spectral response, the detection of weak fluorescence signals may be limited by their higher dark currents. In these red-sensitive PMTs, the lower work function of the photocathode results in more thermal events spontaneously ejecting electrons (Art, 1990). When imaging far red fluorophores, using the 647-nm line of a krypton–argon ion laser, we have observed a reduction in image contrast and increased dark current with prolonged use of the microscope. Presumably, this results from the heating of the PMTs by electrical components within the scan unit. Unfortunately, it is not possible to discriminate thermal events originating from the photocathode from photon-induced events. For optimal sensitivity it is necessary to use cooled PMTs to reduce the frequency of thermal events from the photocathode. Similarly, the higher dark current of PMTs induced by exposure to high light levels or room lighting can reduce the sensitivity of far red imaging for several hours to days.

## IV. Approaches to Multicolor Laser Scanning Confocal Microscopy

Examination of multiple fluorescent probes in a single specimen requires the independent detection of signals from each probe. This requires differences in their excitation and emission spectra. Two approaches have been used to spectrally isolate each fluorophore in a multiple-labeled specimen: (1) Use a single wavelength to simultaneously excite all fluorophores and separate their emissions in the detection path; and (2) use different excitation wavelengths and emission filters for the detection of each fluorophore. In both cases, the fluorophores and microscope filters must be carefully chosen to allow differences in their excitation and emission spectra to be exploited (Wessendorf, 1990; Galbraith *et al.*, 1989). Although not discussed here, separate detection by LSCM of fluorescent probes based on differences in fluorescence lifetimes is possible (Buurman *et al.*, 1992; Morgan *et al.*, 1992).

The advantages and disadvantages of these approaches for the spectral isolation of multiple fluorescence with LSCM will be examined below. Specific microscope configurations will be discussed to demonstrate the decisions and compromises necessary for the design of an instrument for multicolor LSCM. Because the use of lasers with ultraviolet emission lines with LSCM requires special optics and instrumentation, the following discussion will be limited to configurations with the widely available visible light lasers.

### A. Single-Wavelength Excitation of Multiple Fluorophores

The simultaneous excitation by a single wavelength of multiple fluorophores and separation of their emissions in the detection path places severe restrictions on the fluorophores to be examined. The excitation spectra of the fluorophores must partially overlap to permit excitation by a single wavelength of light. (However, for most combinations of fluorophores one will be excited much more efficiently than the others.) In contrast, their emission spectra should not overlap significantly so the signal from each fluorophore can be spectrally isolated with carefully chosen bandpass filters. In addition, the emission peaks of the shorter wavelength fluorophores should overlap minimally with the excitation peaks of the longer wavelength fluorophores to reduce the possibility of energy transfer between fluorophores (Chapple *et al.*, 1988). Because of these strict requirements, a considerable compromise in the efficiency of excitation and degree of spectral isolation of each signal is usually required for most combinations of fluorophores.

These factors have not prevented this approach from being extensively utilized for two-color immunofluorescence studies using flow cytometry with a single excitation beam (Loken *et al.*, 1977; Hoffman, 1988; Shapiro, 1988). Similar to LSCM, flow cytometry with laser light sources has relatively few wavelengths available for the excitation of fluorophores. However, a significant advantage for flow cytometry is that the sampling volume is a single cell, not the considerably smaller diffraction-limited volume of confocal microscopy. As a result, there is more latitude for balancing the efficiency of excitation, spectral isolation of the fluorescence signals, and sensitivity of detection. Nevertheless, it is usually impossible to achieve total spectral isolation of the fluorophores because their emission spectra always overlap to some extent. In these cases, the cross-talk between multiple detectors can usually be reduced by using electronic compensation to subtract a fraction of the signal detected in each spectral band from the others (Loken *et al.*, 1977). With this approach, double-labeling studies have become widespread, using the combination of fluorescein and R-phycoerythrin excited by the 488-nm line of argon ion lasers (Oi *et al.*, 1982). For this combination of fluorophores, fluorescein is measured as green fluorescence around 530 nm, whereas R-phycoerythrin is detected as orange–red fluorescence above 570 nm.

As for flow cytometry, this approach can be adapted to LSCM for multicolor studies using a single excitation wavelength. For single-detector instruments, the images of each spectral region must be collected after switching emission filters (Brodin *et al.*, 1988). However, fading or movement of the specimen during the sequential collection of the images complicates the comparison of the images. These problems are avoided by sampling simultaneously several spectral regions with multiple detectors (Amos, 1988; Carlsson, 1990). In this case, the corresponding pixels within the images will be in spatial and temporal registration because the same illumination point is the source of all fluorescence signals.

## 1. Two–Color Laser Scanning Confocal Microscopy with 514–nm Line of an Argon Ion Laser

The 514-nm line of the widely available air-cooled argon ion lasers has been successfully used for the imaging of specimens double labeled with fluorescein and one of the rhodamines (Brelje *et al.*, 1989; Fehon *et al.*, 1990; Schweitzer and Paddock, 1990; Stamatoglou *et al.*, 1990; Brelje and Sorenson, 1991; Vincent *et al.*, 1991; Wetmore and Elde, 1991). Although neither fluorophore is efficiently excited by the 514-nm line, sufficient light is absorbed by each to allow their fluorescence signals to be detected from brightly stained specimens. In this configuration (Fig. 10), the 514-nm line is selected with a narrow band-pass filter, reflected by a longpass dichroic mirror, and focused to a diffraction-limited volume within the specimen by the objective. The fluorescence signals are then transmitted by the same dichroic mirror into the detection path (Fig. 11). A second longpass dichroic mirror in the detection path reflects the shorter wavelength green fluorescence into one detector, and transmits the longer wavelength red fluorescence into another detector. The wavelength of light detected is further restricted by emission filters to 525–555 nm for the green fluorescence detector and longer than 600 nm for the red fluorescence detector. In addition, these filters must efficiently block the 514-nm light reflected by the specimen to prevent degradation of the observed signal-to-noise ratio.

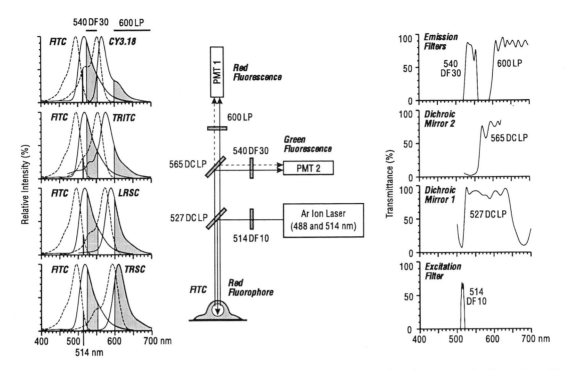

**Fig. 10** Filter configuration for simultaneous two-color imaging of specimens double labeled with fluorescein and a red fluorophore, using the 514-nm line of an argon laser. *Left:* The excitation (dashed) and emission (solid) spectra of various combinations of fluorescein and a red fluorophore, either cyanine 3.18 (CY3.18), tetramethylrhodamine (TRITC), Lissamine rhodamine (LRSC), or Texas Red (TRSC). The 514-nm line is shown as a vertical line beneath the excitation spectra. The wavelengths transmitted by the bandpass emission filters for detecting green and red fluorescence are shown as shaded regions on the emission spectra. Although a substantial region of each emission spectrum is sampled, the amount of cross-talk between the detectors cannot be determined from the normalized emission spectra shown, because the intensity of observed signals will depend on their relative concentrations within the specimen. *Center:* The filter configuration for simultaneous excitation of both fluorophores by 514-nm light. A second dichroic mirror is used to direct the green and red fluorescence into separate photomultiplier tubes (PMTs). *Right:* The transmittance spectra of the various excitation filters, dichroic mirrors, and emission filters are shown. Filter abbreviations: DF, bandpass filter with the specified center wavelength (nm) and full bandwidth at half-maximal transmission; DC, dichroic mirror with half-maximal transmission at the specified wavelength (nm) when at an angle of incidence of 45°; LP, longpass barrier filter with the specified cut-off wavelength (nm) between the shorter reflecting and long transmitting wavelengths.

From the emission spectra of fluorescein and the various rhodamines (Fig. 10), it appears that this configuration would require only minor corrections for the cross-talk between the green and red fluorescence detectors. Although excited less efficiently than tetramethylrhodamine, the longer wavelength Lissamine rhodamine and Texas Red should give better separation from the emission filter used for the green fluorescence detector. However, it should be noted that the emission spectra have been normalized as a percentage of the maximum

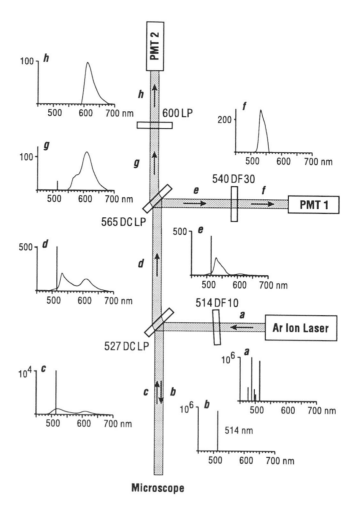

**Fig. 11** Explanation of how the filter configuration for two-color imaging with the 514-nm line of an argon ion laser separates the green and red fluorescence signals from a specimen double labeled with fluorescein and Texas Red. The argon (Ar) ion laser operates in a multiline mode with output at several wavelengths (a). A narrow bandpass filter (514 DF 10) selects the 514-nm line (b), reflected by a longpass dichroic mirror (527 DC LP), and directed into the microscope. The fluorescence signals and a significant fraction of the excitation light return from the microscope (c), and are passed by the dichroic mirror (d). A second longpass dichroic mirror (565 DC LP) in the detection path reflects the shorter wavelength green fluorescence into one detector (e), and transmits the longer wavelength red fluorescence into another detector (g). Two emission filters (540 DF 30 and 600 LP) are used to restrict the detection to the regions of maximum separation of the fluorescence signals and to block the remaining reflected 514-nm light (f and h). Note that the spectra are shown so the total signal detected in both detectors will be approximately equal.

fluorescence signal observed for each fluorophore. This comparison does not consider the differences in the efficiency of excitation and quantum yield of the fluorophores, the fluorophore/protein ratios of the secondary antibodies, and the relative intensity of the staining within a specimen. To demonstrate the magnitude of these issues, solutions of fluorescein and Texas Red conjugated to secondary antibodies were examined by spectrofluorometry (Fig. 12). When this is done, the previously small contribution of fluorescein to the red

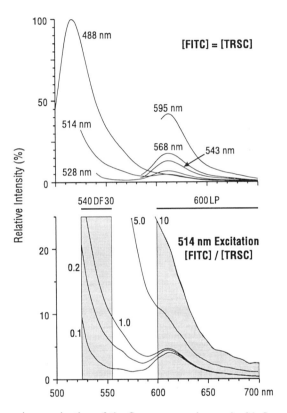

**Fig. 12** Spectroscopic examination of the fluorescence observed with fluorescein (FITC)- and Texas Red (TRSC)-conjugated IgGs. *Top:* The emission spectra of an equimolar solution of the fluorophore-conjugated goat anti-mouse IgGs at the indicated excitation wavelengths. (Note that the concentrations are based on the fluorophore instead of protein because of the slight differences in the fluorophore/protein ratios of the conjugates.) For excitation by 514-nm light, the amount of red fluorescence observed at wavelengths longer than 600 nm is barely detectable in the presence of the longer wavelength fluorescence from FITC. Although more red fluorescence from TRSC is observed with increasing excitation wavelength, its relative intensity compared to that from FITC with 488-nm excitation is considerably less. *Bottom:* The red fluorescence from FITC increases as its relative concentration increases in comparison to TRSC. Even for an equimolar solution, the longer wavelength emissions from FITC still contribute one-third of the total red fluorescence signal observed at wavelengths longer than 600 nm.

fluorescence signal detected at wavelengths longer than 600 nm is now as much as, if not more than, that from Texas Red. This is partially the result of the more efficient excitation of FITC by 514-nm light, but may also reflect the lower quantum yields of Texas Red conjugates (Table I). As a result, staining with the rhodamine will have to be especially bright and cross-talk compensation may still be necessary to remove the fluorescein signal observed in the red fluorescence detector (see Section V,A,3).

## 2. Cross–Talk Compensation

As routinely done for two-color studies with flow cytometry, the cross-talk between detectors in two-color LSCM with a single excitation wavelength can be reduced by subtracting a fraction of each signal from the others (Mossberg and Ericsson, 1990; Vassy *et al.,* 1990; Brelje and Sorenson, 1991; Lynch *et al.,* 1991; Carlsson and Mossberg, 1992). This cross-talk compensation is typically done after collection of the individual images by using linear image processing operations to subtract, with an appropriate coefficient, the image observed in one detector from the other image. The magnitude of this cross-talk correction can be estimated by imaging single-labeled specimens with the "inappropriate" detector(s), using the identical instrument configuration (*i.e.,* intensity of excitation light, pinhole sizes, gain and black level of the photomultiplier tubes, and objective). Alternately, if the images contain spatially distinct structures stained only with one of the fluorophores, the correction factor can be estimated from the ratio between intensities of respective pixels in each image.

This approach to cross-talk compensation requires that the relationship between fluorophore concentration and the intensity of fluorescence be constant for all pixels within the images. Because photomultiplier tubes are normally used as detectors for LSCM, good linearity between the observed intensity of fluorescence and the measured signal is expected. More important is the influence of the local environment on the fluorophore and fading of the fluorescence from the region of the specimen being examined. If these effects only alter the observed intensity of fluorescence, the relative contribution of fluorescence signals collected in different spectral regions will not be altered. However, any shifts in the emission spectra of the fluorophores will affect the relative distribution of their fluorescence signals between the detectors. Although large changes in the emission spectra are unlikely for the widely used fluorophores, the occurrence of small shifts with the intense illumination conditions used for LSCM cannot be dismissed. A comparatively large change in the measured signals may be observed because of this shift due to the highly nonlinear relationship between quantum efficiency and wavelength of detected light for the photomultiplier tubes typically used as detectors (see Section III,D). For example, shifts in the emission spectra of fluorescein and tetramethylrhodamine at different concentrations have been observed with excitation intensities similar to those used with LSCM (Carlsson and Mossberg, 1992). Because of these difficulties, the relative relationship between the fluorescence signals observed in different spectral regions will not be constant over the region of the specimen examined.

Unlike flow cytometry, the additional demands imposed by the requirements of confocal imaging can further reduce the effectiveness of this cross-talk compensation technique. In particular, the wavelength-dependent imaging properties can alter the detection efficiency and the region of the specimen sampled for each pixel in images acquired in different spectral regions. Axial chromatic aberration within the optical components of the microscope will result in a noticeable shift in the focal plane at the different wavelengths (Fricker and White, 1992). Lateral chromatic aberration can also vary the off-axis collection efficiencies for light of different wavelengths (Wells *et al.*, 1990). Similarly, a small amount of spherical aberration is sufficient to cause severe reduction in collection efficiency and resolution as the focal plane is moved deeper within a specimen (Sheppard and Gu, 1991; see also Section VI,A,2). Even if these aberrations can be reduced or avoided, differences in resolution will alter the diffraction-limited volume of the specimen sampled for the same pixel in images acquired in different spectral regions (Table II). As the difference between the excitation and detection wavelengths for a fluorophore increases, the images will be of lower resolution and have less rejection of out-of-focus fluorescence (*i.e.*, thicker optical sections; Wilson, 1989). However, this loss in resolution will be less than that observed with conventional microscopy because resolution is dependent on both the excitation and emission wavelengths for fluorescence confocal microscopy. As a result of these wavelength dependencies of imaging, the contribution of a stained structure to the same pixel will not be identical in images acquired in different spectral regions.

The difficulties in using this compensation technique for the correction of cross-talk between images acquired in different spectral regions can be easily demonstrated by examining specimens stained only with fluorescein. Using the previously discussed configuration (Fig. 10), images of a fluorescein-stained specimen were acquired in both the green and red fluorescence detectors (Fig. 13A and B, respectively). Although the images appear similar, the lower signals observed in the red fluorescence detector result in a lower signal-to-background ratio (*i.e.*, higher background staining) and a loss of detail. Because both images were acquired with an identical peak pixel value, the red/green fluorescence ratio image should have a value of 1.0 for all pixels. Acutally, a range of values from 0.8 to 6.0 is observed in the ratio image (Fig. 13C). The low-intensity background pixels apparently skew the histogram to larger ratio values (Fig. 14A). If pixels having an intensity below 10% of the maximum value are ignored in calculating the ratio image (Fig. 13D), a narrower range of ratio values centered on a peak value of 1.0 is observed (Fig. 14, *top*). However, this peak still represents a rather large range of ratio values (0.8 to 1.2). If the pixel value of the red fluorescence image is graphed against its ratio value, a relatively constant ratio (1.00 ± 0.2) is observed for the brighter pixels (Fig. 14, *bottom*). The use of a nonlinear function for the correction factor should give better results than choosing a single value based only on the brightest pixels. However,

**Table II**
**Theoretical Microscope Resolutions**[a]

| Wavelength (nm) | Lateral resolution ($\mu$m) | | | Axial resolution ($\mu$m) | | |
|---|---|---|---|---|---|---|
| | ×10 NA 0.40 $n = 1.0$ | ×40 NA 0.85 $n = 1.0$ | ×60 NA 1.40 $n = 1.516$ | ×10 NA 0.40 $n = 1.0$ | ×40 NA 0.85 $n = 1.0$ | ×60 NA 1.40 $n = 1.516$ |
| **Confocal fluorescence microscope** | | | | | | |
| 351/450 | 0.43 | 0.20 | 0.12 | 3.48 | 0.78 | 0.45 |
| 488/518 | 0.55 | 0.26 | 0.16 | 4.50 | 0.99 | 0.56 |
| 514/540 | 0.58 | 0.27 | 0.17 | 4.70 | 1.03 | 0.58 |
| 514/610 | 0.61 | 0.29 | 0.18 | 4.95 | 1.09 | 0.58 |
| 514/680 | 0.64 | 0.30 | 0.18 | 5.20 | 1.10 | 0.64 |
| 568/590 | 0.64 | 0.30 | 0.18 | 5.17 | 1.09 | 0.64 |
| 647/680 | 0.72 | 0.34 | 0.21 | 5.88 | 1.28 | 0.72 |
| **Confocal reflection microscope** | | | | | | |
| 351 | 0.39 | 0.18 | 0.11 | 3.12 | 0.70 | 0.39 |
| 488 | 0.54 | 0.25 | 0.15 | 4.45 | 0.97 | 0.54 |
| 514 | 0.56 | 0.27 | 0.16 | 4.58 | 1.01 | 0.57 |
| 568 | 0.63 | 0.29 | 0.18 | 5.05 | 1.12 | 0.62 |
| 647 | 0.71 | 0.34 | 0.21 | 5.76 | 1.27 | 0.71 |
| **Conventional microscope** | | | | | | |
| 351 | 0.54 | 0.25 | 0.17 | 4.39 | 0.97 | 0.63 |
| 450 | 0.69 | 0.32 | 0.21 | 5.63 | 1.25 | 0.81 |
| 488 | 0.74 | 0.35 | 0.23 | 6.10 | 1.35 | 0.88 |
| 518 | 0.79 | 0.37 | 0.24 | 6.48 | 1.43 | 0.93 |
| 568 | 0.87 | 0.41 | 0.27 | 7.10 | 1.57 | 1.02 |
| 590 | 0.90 | 0.42 | 0.28 | 7.38 | 1.63 | 1.06 |
| 647 | 0.99 | 0.46 | 0.30 | 8.09 | 1.79 | 1.16 |
| 680 | 1.04 | 0.49 | 0.32 | 8.50 | 1.88 | 1.22 |

[a] The conventional microscope resolutions were calculated with Eq. (1) for the lateral and Eq. (2) for the axial directions:

$$\Delta r = 0.61 \, \lambda/\eta \sin \alpha \tag{1}$$
$$\Delta z = 2 \, \lambda/\eta \sin^2 \alpha \tag{2}$$

where $\lambda$ is the wavelength of light, $\eta \sin \alpha$ is the numerical aperture (NA) of the objective, and $\eta$ is the refractive index of the immersion medium. A decrease in light intensity of ~27.7% laterally and ~19.3% axially is detectable between two point light sources placed this distance apart (Bliton *et al.*, 1993). The confocal resolutions are given as the distance between the peaks of two confocal point spread functions (PSFs) required to give a summed profile with the appropriate intensity decrease between the peaks. The confocal PSFs were calculated by multiplying together the PSF intensity profiles for the excitation and emission wavelengths as described by Eq. (3) in the lateral and Eq. (4) in the axial directions (Brakenhoff *et al.*, 1989):

$$I_{\text{lateral}}(v) = \text{const}[J_1(v)/v]^2 \quad \text{with } v = 2\pi r \eta \sin \alpha \tag{3}$$
$$I_{\text{axial}}(\omega) = \text{const}[\sin(\omega/4)]^2/(\omega/4)^2 \quad \text{with } \omega = 2\pi z \eta \sin^2\alpha/\lambda \tag{4}$$

where $J_1(v)$ is the first-order Bessel function.

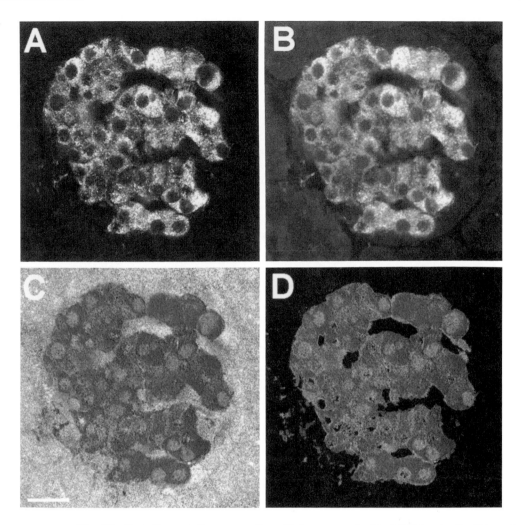

**Fig. 13** Test of cross-talk compensation with images acquired by LSCM, using the 514-nm line of an argon ion laser for two-color imaging (Fig. 10). (A) Image acquired in the green fluorescence detector and (B) image acquired in the red fluorescence detector. Each image was collected with a similar peak pixel value of white (i.e., 255). (C) The ratio image obtained by dividing the red by the green fluorescence image. The ratio values are displayed so a value of 4.0 or greater is shown as white and a value of 1.0 is dark gray (i.e., 64). (D) The ratio image obtained by considering pixels having an intensity below 10% of the maximum value (i.e., 25) as background; these pixels are displayed in black. Scale bar = 25 $\mu$m. Nikon ×40, NA 0.85.

the large range of ratio values for pixels of the same intensity (note the large error bars in Fig. 14B) suggests the local environment within the specimen affected the relative distribution of the fluorescence signal between the detectors. This means that even pixels of identical intensity cannot be corrected to the

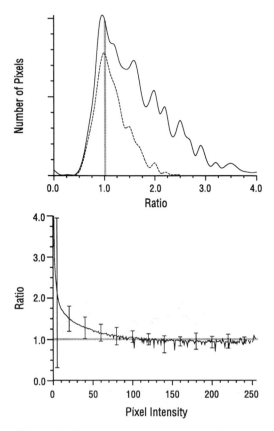

**Fig. 14** Estimation of the ratio value necessary to compensate the cross-talk of the fluorescein signal into the red fluorescence detector. *Top:* Histogram of the ratio values observed for Fig. 13C (solid) and Fig. 13D (dashed). Even when the background pixels are ignored, a broad peak centered at 1.0 is still observed. *Bottom:* A graph of the observed ratio value (average ± SEM) vs pixel intensity of the red fluorescence image. Although a relatively constant ratio is observed for the brighter pixels, note the large error bars indicating a large range of values for pixels of the same intensity.

same extent. Therefore it is impossible to avoid having pixels within the image that either under- or overcompensated irregardless of the correction factor used. The extent to which this increases the uncertainty in the corrected intensity values will have to be determined for each type of preparation because of the large number of factors involved.

Therefore this cross-talk compensation technique is only partially effective for images acquired in different spectral regions by LSCM. Unfortunately, this approach can only improve the separation of the fluorescence signals from brightly stained, double-labeled specimens. It does improve the efficiency of excitation or detection of the fluorophores. This makes it especially difficult, if not impossible, to determine if a structure is lightly stained with one fluorophore when substantial "bleed-through" from the other fluorophore occurs. Therefore this compensation technique is best suited for the correction of crosstalk between images in which each fluorophore stains spatially distinct structures.

## B. Multiple-Wavelength Excitation of Multiple Fluorophores

The most powerful approach for the spectral isolation of multiple fluorophores is to use different excitation wavelengths and emission filters for the detection of each fluorophore. The preferential excitation of each fluorophore is possible because for every fluorophore, at some wavelength longer than its excitation maximum, the photons will not be sufficiently energic to stimulate the electrons of the fluorophore into the excited states from which fluorescent emissions occur. However, an emission filter is necessary to block the small amount of fluorescence inefficiently excited from any longer wavelength fluorophores also present in the specimen. Thus, the use of separate filter sets to image each fluorophore provides the requisite degrees of freedom necessary for the optimal excitation of each fluorophore and the spectral isolation of its fluorescence emission. Although this approach is widely used for conventional fluorescence microscopy (DeBiasio et al., 1987; Waggoner et al., 1989; Wessendorf, 1990), its application for multicolor LSCM has been limited by the lack of economical lasers with broadly spaced emission lines.

Besides the availability of appropriate lasers, a major difficulty in using multiple excitation wavelengths with LSCM is the need to use separate filter sets to obtain images of each fluorophore. When a set of images is taken of the same field of the microscope, in general the images are not accurately superimposable. For example, we frequently observed lateral shifts of at least 0.5–1.0 $\mu$m when changing filter sets and using a ×60 objective. More important is the misalignment between the illumination beam and the detector apertures required for optimal confocal imaging. Practically, this means that the microscope must be realigned after changing filter sets to ensure that the illumination source and detector aperture overlap in the focal plane (Stelzer, 1990).

Even minor changes in the orientation, thickness, or surface characteristics of filters in the illumination path can shift the images or require realignment of the confocal apertures when using separate filter sets. This is mostly due to differences in the dichroic mirror. Therefore the use of filter configurations in which images of each fluorophore are acquired with the same dichroic mirror is preferred. In this case, the images will be within registration to the maximum extent possible with the objective lens being used. The following configurations will illustrate several ways to use the optimal excitation and emission filters for each fluorophore without having to use separate dichroic mirrors.

### 1. Two-Color Laser Scanning Confocal Microscopy with 488/514-nm Lines of an Argon Ion Laser

A simple application of using multiple excitation wavelengths with LSCM is to use two of the emission lines from an air-cooled argon ion laser to improve the imaging of specimens double labeled with fluorescein and rhodamine (Mossberg and Ericsson, 1990; Akner *et al.*, 1991). Although the imaging of the rhodamine is not improved, the 488-nm line excites fluorescein much more efficiently than the 514-nm line (Fig. 15). Similarly, the emission filter for the detection of the green fluorescence can be shifted to shorter wavelengths centered on the emission peak of fluorescein at 518 nm. Unlike the configuration using simultaneous 514-nm excitation, this filter set allows the imaging of fluorescein almost as

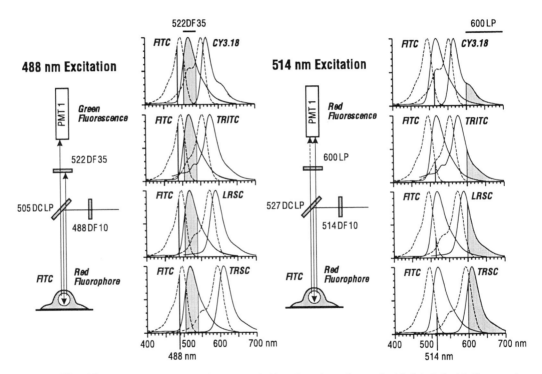

**Fig. 15** Filter configurations for sequential imaging of specimens double labeled with fluorescein and a red fluorophore, using the 488- and 514-nm lines of an argon ion laser. *Left:* The filter set for detection of green fluorescence, using 488-nm excitation. *Right:* The filter set for detection of red fluorescence, using 514-nm excitation. The separate filter sets must be changed to allow sequential imaging of the green and red fluorescence from the specimen. The excitation (dashed) and emission (solid) spectra of various combinations of fluorescein and a red fluorophore, either cyanine 3.18 (CY3.18), tetramethylrhodamine (TRITC), Lissamine rhodamine (LRSC), or Texas Red (TRSC), are also shown. The excitation wavelength (solid line) and regions of the emission spectra transmitted by the bandpass emission filters (shaded regions) are also indicated. See Fig. 10 for filter abbreviations.

efficiently as in single-labeled specimens. It will also reduce the amount of fluorescence from tetramethylrhodamine observed in the green fluorescence image. With a second filter set, the rhodamine is imaged as before, using the 514-nm line and the same red fluorescence emission filter. If the 528-nm line is available from the argon ion laser, it can be used to more efficiently excite the rhodamine and reduce cross-talk because fluorescein is only weakly excited by this wavelength (5% of its excitation maximum).

Unfortunately, these advantages for imaging of double-labeled specimens are partially offset by the use of separate filter sets for each excitation wavelength. The nonoverlapping images and misalignment of the microscope could be avoided if the filter configuration for simultaneous excitation of both fluorophores with the 514-nm line (Fig. 10) could be modified for use with both the 488- and 514-nm lines. One approach is to use the same filter configuration and use multiple excitation filters to select either the 488- or 514-nm line. This is possible because the longpass dichroic mirror will also reflect the shorter wavelength 488-nm light onto the specimen. If both excitation lines are used for simultaneous imaging, the more efficient excitation of fluorescein by the 488-nm line will increase the breakthrough of fluorescein into the red fluorescence detector. Another approach is to use a partially reflecting mirror (for example, a 10% reflectance/90% transmittance mirror) instead of a longpass dichroic mirror to reflect the illumination beam onto the specimen (Fig. 16). This permits the use of either excitation wavelength and the more efficient emission filter for the detection of fluorescein previously used with the separate filter sets (Fig. 15). When this shorter wavelength emission filter is used, the simultaneous imaging of both fluorophores is no longer possible because the reflected 514-nm light will be observed in the green fluorescence detector. The disadvantage of this mirror is that it requires higher output powers because only 10% of the available light is actually reflected on the specimen. In addition, the other emission lines (*i.e.*, 457 or 528 nm) available from argon ion lasers could be used with this configuration (Mossberg and Ericsson, 1990), but their lower output powers may be a problem.

## 2. Two-Color Laser Scanning Confocal Microscopy with Argon Ion and Helium–Neon Lasers

Although use of the various emission lines from the air-cooled argon ion lasers extends the capability to image double-labeled specimens, what is actually needed is additional excitation wavelengths that do not significantly excite fluorescein (i.e., >540 nm) and more efficiently excite the rhodamines. One approach is to use instruments with multiple lasers. Typically, an inexpensive helium–neon laser with an emission line at 543 or 633 nm has been used in combination with an argon ion laser (Stelzer, 1990; Montag *et al.*, 1991; Schubert, 1991; Fricker and White, 1992; Szarowski *et al.*, 1992). The 543-nm line can efficiently excite tetramethylrhodamine (76% of its excitation maximum

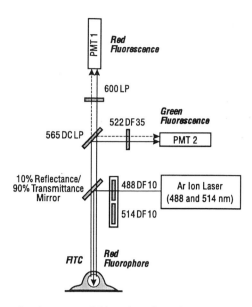

**Fig. 16** Filter configuration for sequential imaging of specimens double labeled with fluorescein and a red fluorophore using the 488- and 514-nm lines of an argon ion laser with a single filter set. This filter set is identical to that shown for simultaneous excitation by 514-nm light (Fig. 10), except that a 10% reflectance/90% transmittance mirror is used instead of a dichroic mirror. In this case, 10% of the laser light will be reflected onto the specimen, and 90% of the emitted fluorescence transmitted into the detection path. Selection of the various laser wavelengths is done by positioning the appropriate excitation filter in the illumination path. See Fig. 10 for filter abbreviations.

at 554 nm), but is still suboptimal for the longer wavelength Lissamine rhodamine and Texas Red (only 29–35% of their excitation maximums). Although most studies have used separate filter sets with these instruments, the filter configuration using 488/514-nm excitation with a 10% reflection/90% transmittance mirror (Fig. 16) can be easily modified for use with the 543-nm line. Because the 543-nm line does not significantly excite fluorescein, the red fluorescence detector can be used with an emission filter that transmits from 570 nm and above. However, with only 10% of the excitation light being reflected on the specimen, insufficient intensity may be available for the optimal excitation of the fluorophores with the lower power helium–neon lasers. Alternatively, use of a helium–neon laser with a 633-nm emission line allows the efficient excitation of a far red fluorophore such as allophycocyanin or cyanine 5.18 (60–83% of their excitation maximums).

Unfortunately, the expanded capabilities of these multiple laser instruments are offset by an increase in complexity. Beyond the requirement to keep multiple lasers in proper operation, additional optics are necessary to merge the output of the lasers into a single illumination beam. For correct operation of the confocal imaging system, the focused spot formed from the illumination sources by the objective lens must coincide both axially and transversely. If the filter configuration discussed above is used, the output of each laser must be superimposed and enter the microscope as coincidental, parallel beams to prevent misalignment of the regions scanned by the individual beams. The individual laser beams can be combined with a series of beam steering and dichroic mirrors or by passing each through the same fiber optic cable. If separate filter sets are used, this alignment is not as critical because the images will be misaligned by the switching of the dichroic mirrors.

## 3. Two-Color Laser Scanning Confocal Microscopy with Krypton–Argon Ion Laser

As an alternative to multiple laser instruments for the imaging of double-labeled specimens, the use of the 488- and 568-nm lines of a single, krypton–argon ion laser is especially attractive (Brelje and Sorenson, 1992). As before, a filter configuration that allows the use of either excitation wavelength with the same dichroic mirror is required to avoid needing to realign the microscope when changing filter sets (Fig. 17). This is possible with a dual-dichroic mirror with two reflection bands centered on the laser lines and that transmits at all other wavelengths. Although a 10% reflectance/90% transmittance mirror could be used instead, the higher efficiency reflection of each excitation wavelength onto the specimen by the dual-dichroic mirror allows the laser to be operated at lower output powers. The lower operating current should lengthen the useful life of the laser by reducing the effect of degrading mechanisms within the plasma tube. As with the previous filter configurations, a longpass dichroic mirror placed in the detection path is used to direct the green and red fluorescence into separate detectors. The excitation filters should be slightly tilted ($<2°$) to avoid interference effects caused by specular reflections and to prevent reflection of the other laser lines back into the plasma tube. If this occurs, the operating current and noise characteristics of the laser may be substantially altered.

Using this configuration, the fluorescence signals from the fluorophores can be collected by sequential or simultaneous excitation with the 488- and 568-nm lines. Although sequential excitation improves the spectral isolation of the fluorophores, simultaneous excitation is useful for the rapid surveying of specimens to select regions for further examination. Subsequently, the identified regions of the specimen can be examined with a single excitation wavelength to verify the presence of double labeling. For simultaneous imaging, it is preferable to have emission lines of similar output powers to allow relatively equal excitation of both fluorophores.

The krypton–argon ion laser has already been successfully used in several biological studies to image specimens double labeled with fluorescein and cyanine 3.18 (Elde *et al.,* 1991; Sorenson *et al.,* 1991).

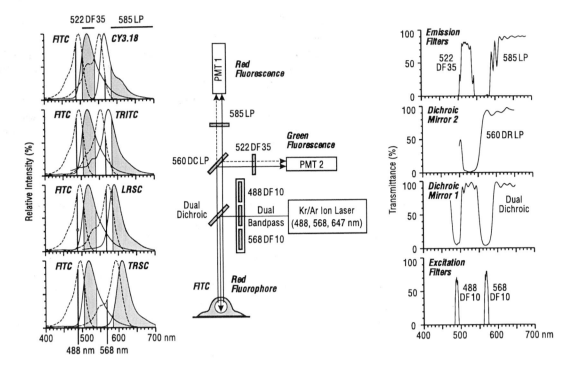

**Fig. 17**  Filter configuration for imaging of specimens double labeled with fluorescein and a red fluorophore, using the 488- and 568-nm lines of a krypton–argon ion laser. *Left:* The excitation (dashed) and emission (solid) spectra of various combinations of fluorescein and a red fluorophore, either cyanine 3.18 (CY3.18), tetramethylrhodamine (TRITC), Lissamine rhodamine (LRSC), or Texas Red (TRSC). The 488- and 568-nm lines are shown as vertical lines beneath the excitation spectra. The wavelengths transmitted by the bandpass emission filters for detecting green and red fluorescence are shown as shaded regions on the emission spectra. *Center:* The filter configuration for sequential or simultaneous excitation of the fluorophores by 488- and 568-nm light. Selection of the various laser wavelengths is done by positioning the appropriate excitation filter in the illumination path. The transmittance spectra for the dual-bandpass excitation filter is not shown because it is almost identical to the combination of the individual 488- and 568-nm excitation filters. *Right:* The transmittance spectra of the various excitation filters, dichroic mirrors, and emission filters are shown. See Fig. 10 for filter abbreviations.

## 4. Three-Color Laser Scanning Confocal Microscopy with Krypton–Argon Ion Laser

The filter configuration for two-color imaging with the krypton–argon ion laser can be easily modified to also allow the use of the 647-nm line for imaging (Fig. 18). This extends the usable spectral range into the far-red region of the light spectrum and permits the imaging of specimens triple labeled with fluorescein, rhodamine, and a far red fluorophore such as cyanine 5.18 or allophycocyanin (Brelje and Sorenson, 1992). The efficient excitation of each fluorophore

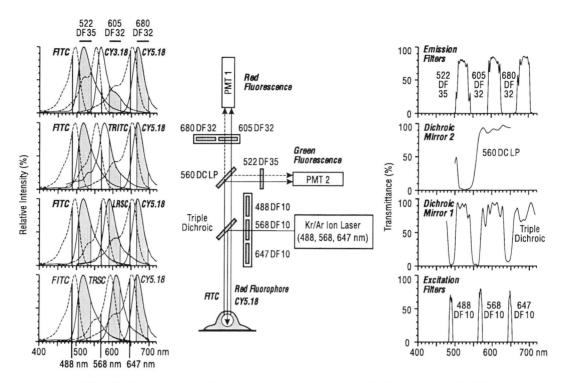

**Fig. 18** Filter configuration for imaging of specimens triple labeled, using the 488-, 568-, and 647-nm lines of a krypton–argon ion laser. *Left:* The excitation (dashed) and emission (solid) spectra of various combinations of fluorescein (FITC), a red fluorophore, and cyanine 5.18. The following red fluorophores are shown: cyanine 3.18 (CY3.18), tetramethylrhodamine (TRITC), Lissamine rhodamine (LRSC), and Texas Red (TRSC). The laser lines are shown as vertical lines beneath the excitation spectra. The wavelengths transmitted by the bandpass emission filters for detecting the fluorophores are shown as shaded regions on the emission spectra. *Center:* The filter configuration for imaging of triple-labeled specimens. The triple-dichroic mirror allows the reflection of each excitation wavelength onto the specimen and the transmittance of the fluorescence from the various fluorophores with the same dichroic mirror. Because the Bio-Rad MRC-600 has only two detectors, the emission filter for one photomultiplier (PMT 1) must be switched in addition to the excitation filters for the red fluorophore and CY5.18. *Right:* The transmittance spectra of the various excitation filters, dichroic mirrors, and emission filters are shown. See Fig. 10 for filter abbreviations.

by only one of these wavelengths and their well-separated emission peaks should allow the independent detection of fluorescence signals from each in the presence of the others. The only changes required for adapting the dual-excitation wavelength filter configuration is the replacement of the dual-dichroic mirror by a triple-dichroic mirror, and the ability to switch emission filters for the red fluorescence detector. Because the instrument we use has only two detectors (the Bio-Rad MRC-600), the appropriate excitation and emission filters must be selected to allowing imaging with either the 568- and 647-nm lines.

If these emission filters are positioned between the detector aperture and the photomultiplier tube, no realignment of the detector aperture is required when switching between the emission filter.

Unfortunately, this use of two detectors restricts simultaneous imaging to only two of the three fluorophores. With the filter configuration shown in Fig. 18, only fluorescein and either rhodamine or cyanine 5.18 can be simultaneously imaged. If the second dichroic mirror is replaced by a longpass dichroic mirror centered on 640 nm, the simultaneous imaging of the green fluorescence from fluorescein or the red fluorescence from a rhodamine in one detector, and the far-red fluorescence from cyanine 5.18 in the other, is possible. Because this dichroic mirror is in the detection path, and not in the illumination path from the laser to the specimen, it can be exchanged with the previous dichroic mirror without shifting the region of the specimen scanned, but realignment of the detector apertures will be necessary.

The advantage of an instrument with three detectors is it would allow the simultaneous imaging with any combination of two or all three of the emission lines available from the krypton–argon ion laser. An additional dichroic mirror can be used to separate the red and far red fluorescence into separate detectors. This capability would be particularly useful for the surveying of specimens for regions with a particular staining pattern or for time-resolved imaging of living specimens.

## V. Practical Aspects of Multicolor Laser Scanning Confocal Microscopy

In discussing the practical application of LSCM for multicolor immunofluorescence studies, the use of the inexpensive, air-cooled argon ion and krypton–argon ion lasers as light sources will be compared. The implications of using the limited number of excitation wavelengths available from these lasers for the detection and spectral isolation of fluorophores in single- and multilabeled specimens is demonstrated. Finally, several examples of the advantages of specific visualization of fluorophores with a krypton–argon ion laser are shown.

### A. Multicolor Laser Scanning Confocal Microscopy with Air-Cooled Argon Ion Laser

Although a restricted range of emission lines is available from an air-cooled argon ion laser, it has been successfully used for multicolor LSCM with fluorescein and a rhodamine (Brelje *et al.*, 1989; Fehon *et al.*, 1990; Mossberg and Ericsson, 1990; Mossberg *et al.*, 1990; Schweitzer and Paddock, 1990; Stamatoglou *et al.*, 1990; Brelje and Sorenson, 1991; Vincent *et al.*, 1991; Wetmore and Elde, 1991). As will be shown below, the inefficient visualization of one or both fluorophores with this configuration limits its use to the imaging of brightly stained specimens in which the relative intensity of the staining of the fluorophores can be carefully controlled to balance their detection and the cross-talk between the detectors. However, it is difficult to specifically visualize each fluorophore. Thus it is difficult to determine whether a structure is double labeled. As a result, this approach is best used when the individual fluorophores label structures that are spatially separated (i.e., single objects are not expected to be double labeled).

## 1. Visualization Specificity of Fluorophores with Argon Ion Laser

The specificity of the fluorophores with respect to the microscope filters was examined by attempting to visualize each fluorophore individually with the filter configurations used for the imaging of specimens double labeled with fluorescein and a red fluorophore (Figs. 10 and 15). To provide specimens with strong fluorescent signal with a minimum of background, spinal cord sections were stained for the presynaptic marker synaptophysin with the various fluorophore-conjugated secondary antibodies. Synaptophysin is a calcium-binding glycoprotein located in the membrane of synaptic vesicles (Jahn *et al.*, 1985; Wiedenmann and Franke, 1985). Because the intracellular injection of cells is frequently used in combination with immunofluorescence, the specificity of Lucifer yellow was also examined with these filters. A Lucifer yellow-injected neuron in the sacral parasympathetic nucleus of the spinal cord was employed for that purpose. With these intensely stained specimens, the chance of observing each fluorophore with the inappropriate filters is maximized.

When using the filter configuration for simultaneous excitation by the 514-nm line of an argon ion laser (Fig. 10), the green fluorophores could be observed in both the green and red fluorescence detectors (Fig. 19). In these green fluorescence images, the numerous varicosities containing synaptophysin-like immunoreactivity on the cell bodies and processes of the large motor neurons in the dorsal horn of the spinal cord are easily appreciated for both the fluorescein- and BODIPY-stained specimens. Although less than 5% of the fluorescein and 1% of the BODIPY emission spectra overlap with the transmittance region of the 600-nm longpass filter (Fig. 10), both fluorophores could also be observed in the red fluorescence detector with the same intensity of laser illumination. Although the fluorescence signal was weaker than that observed in the green fluorescence detector, both fluorophores could be easily imaged by increasing the gain of the photomultiplier tube used as the red fluorescence detector. Because of the narrow emission peak of BODIPY, its relative intensity observed between the red and green fluorescence detectors was half of that observed for fluorescein. In contrast, the extremely broad emission spectra of Lucifer yellow allowed its detection with almost equal efficiency in both the green and red fluorescence detectors of an intracellular-labeled neuron. This suggests that the cross-talk of fluorescence from the green fluorophore into the red fluorescence detector will be a problem for double-labeled specimens.

When using the filter configuration for sequential excitation by the 488- and

## 514 nm Excitation

| Green Fluorescence (540 DF 30) | Red Fluorescence (600 LP) | 488 nm Excitation Green Fluorescence (522 DF 35) |

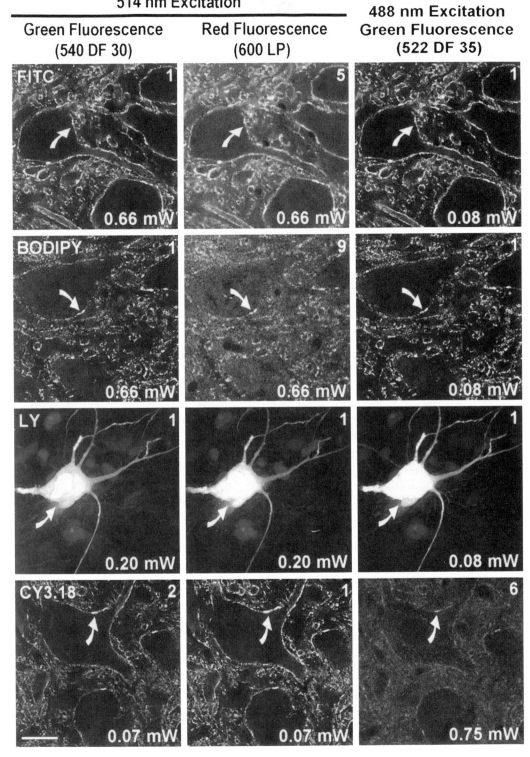

514-nm lines of an argon ion laser (Fig. 15), the more efficient excitation of the green fluorophores by the 488-nm light allowed comparable green fluorescence images to be obtained with only one-eighth of the illumination intensity required with 514-nm light (0.08 vs 0.66 mW). As expected, the use of a separate filter set for the detection of the red fluorescence with 514-nm excitation did not alter the visibility of these fluorophores (data not shown).

Similar to the lack of specificity in visualization of the green fluorophores, most of the red fluorophores could be observed in both the green and red fluorescence detectors when using the filter configuration for simultaneous excitation by the 514-nm line of an argon ion laser (Figs. 19 and 20). Because of the large overlap between the emission spectra of the shorter wavelength red fluorophores and the green fluorescence emission filter (Fig. 10), cyanine 3.18, tetramethylrhodamine, and R-phycoerythrin were easily observed with the green fluorescence detector. In addition, the R-phycoerythrin was difficult to image because of its rapid fading with repeated scanning. The longer wavelength Lissamine rhodamine was slightly less visible, and Texas Red was undetectable in the green fluorescence detector (Fig. 20). Although the increased specificity of visualization with Texas Red is desirable, it should be noted that the inefficient excitation of Texas Red by 514-nm light (<7% of its excitation maximum at 592 nm) substantially reduces the sensitivity of detection in weakly stained specimens. For more efficient detection of fluorescence from a red fluorophore, the shorter wavelength fluorophores would be preferred if the cross-talk into the green fluorescence detector could be reduced.

As previously suggested (see Section IV,B,1), using the filter configuration for sequential excitation by the 488- and 514-nm lines of an argon ion laser should reduce the cross-talk of the red fluorophores into the green fluorescence detector (Figs. 19 and 20). Nonetheless, the presence of significant green fluorescence from tetramethylrhodamine and R-phycoerythrin still resulted in their being observed in the green fluorescence detector. This suggests that the more efficiently excited cyanine 3.18 and Lissamine rhodamine would be preferable with this configuration. However, even though the overlap between the emission spectra of cyanine 3.18 and the green fluorescence emission filter is quite small (Fig. 10), the superior brightness of this fluorophore makes even this small amount significant for brightly stained specimens.

---

**Fig. 19** Specificity of visualization of fluorophores, using the microscope filters for two-color imaging with the 514-nm line of an argon ion laser. Rat spinal cord sections were stained with a mouse monoclonal antibody against synaptophysin and either fluorescein (FITC)-conjugated donkey anti-mouse IgG, BODIPY-conjugated goat anti-mouse IgG, or cyanine 3.18 (CY3.18)-conjugated donkey anti-mouse IgG. Single optical sections of a region within the ventral horn are shown for each of these fluorophores. For Lucifer yellow (LY), projections of 20 images acquired at 1.0-$\mu$m intervals through an intracellularly injected neuron within the superior cervical ganglion are shown. The intensity of laser illumination used to acquire the images is given in milliwatts (mW). The relative increase in photomultiplier gain and contrast for the images of each fluorophore is indicated in the upper right of each image. Scale bar = 25 mm. Nikon ×60 NA 1.4.

| Green Fluorescence (540 DF 30) | Red Fluorescence (600 LP) | 488 nm Excitation Green Fluorescence (522 DF 35) |

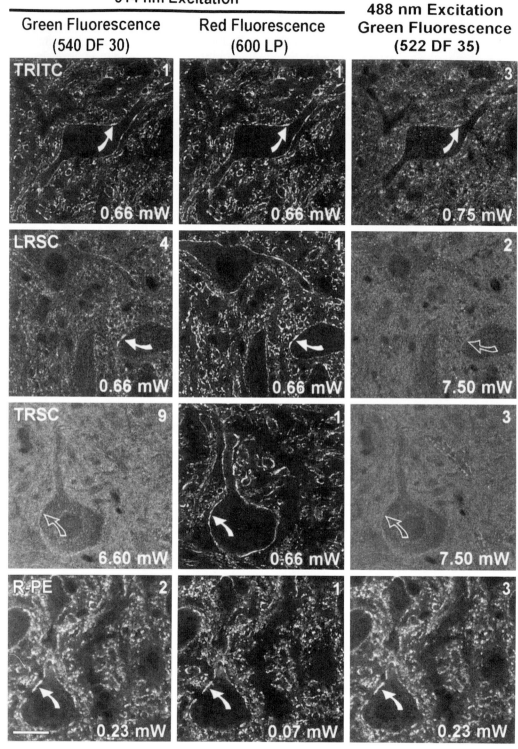

In summary, it was not possible to specifically visualize most of the fluorophores examined, using the 488- and/or 514-nm lines of an argon ion laser. This suggests that relative staining intensity of the green and red fluorophores in the double-labeled specimens must be carefully controlled to balance their detection and cross-talk between the detectors. In addition, the detection of the specific double labeling of structures will be hindered by the likely presence of artifactual double labeling resulting from structures intensely stained with a single fluorophore.

## 2. Observations on Two–Color Laser Scanning Confocal Microscopy with Argon Ion Laser

To demonstrate the difficulty in imaging double-labeled specimens with an argon ion laser, spinal cord sections were stained for the neurotransmitters serotonin and substance P. In the superficial dorsal horn, a smaller number of serotonin-immunoreactive nerve fibers occurs interspersed among the large number of intensely stained substance P-immunoreactive nerve fibers. Previous studies have demonstrated that these neurotransmitters exist in separate populations of fibers in the superficial dorsal horn (Wessendorf and Elde, 1985). This provides an excellent test specimen for examining, using an argon ion laser, the detection of the fluorophores in a double-labeled specimen.

As expected, separate populations of fibers were observed when stained for serotonin with a fluorescein-conjugated secondary antibody and when stained for substance P with a Lissamine rhodamine-conjugated secondary antibody (Color Plate 7). In this case, the intense staining of substance P allows its imaging with minimal cross-talk of the weaker fluorescein staining of serotonin. The few instances of apparent coexistence result from the superimposition of individual fibers separated in different optical sections during the formation of the projection image.

In contrast, a markedly different distribution of staining was observed with similar sections stained for serotonin with a Lissamine rhodamine-conjugated secondary antibody and for substance P with a fluorescein-conjugated secondary antibody (Color Plate 7). In this case, it appears that most of the observed fibers are double labeled for both neurotransmitters. The total absence of fibers stained only with fluorescein and the infrequent fibers stained only with

**Fig. 20** Specificity of visualization of fluorophores, using the microscope filters for two-color imaging with the 514-nm line of an argon ion laser. Rat spinal cord sections were stained with a mouse monoclonal antibody against synaptophysin and then with tetramethylrhodamine (TRITC)-, Lissamine rhodamine (LRSC)-, Texas Red (TRSC)-, or R-phycoerythrin (R-PE)-conjugated donkey anti-mouse IgGs. Single optical sections of a region within the ventral horn are shown for each of these fluorophores. The intensity of laser illumination used to acquire the images is given in milliwatts (mW). The relative increase in photomultiplier gain and contrast for the images of each fluorophore is indicated in the upper right of each image. Scale bar = 25 mm. Nikon ×60 NA 1.4.

## 514 nm Excitation

| Green Fluorescence (540 DF 30) | Red Fluorescence (600 LP) | "Corrected" Red Fluorescence |
|---|---|---|

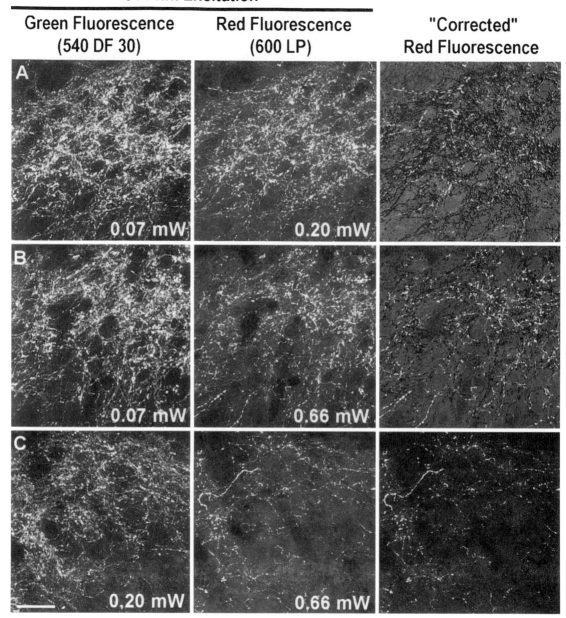

**Fig. 21** Cross-talk of FITC fluorescence into the red fluorescence detector, using the 514-nm line of an argon ion laser for two-color imaging (Fig. 10). Rat spinal cord sections were stained with goat anti-serotonin and rabbit anti-substance P antisera. A 1:100 dilution of the Lissamine rhodamine-conjugated donkey anti-goat IgG was used with 1:100 (A), 1:500 (B), and 1:1000 (C) dilutions of the fluorescein-conjugated donkey anti-rabbit IgG. In this region of the spinal cord, the superficial dorsal horn, coexistence would not be expected. A corresponding decrease in the amount of fluorescein fluorescence was observed in the red fluorescence image with the increasing dilution of the fluorescein-conjugated secondary antibody. The rhodamine fluorescence was estimated by

Lissamine rhodamine suggests that cross-talk of fluorescein into the red detector occurred. This occurred because the intense staining of substance P was visualized with fluorescein, and the weaker serotonin staining was visualized with the less bright fluorophore, Lissamine rhodamine. Therefore the amount of red fluorescence from the strongly stained fluorescein fibers is the same, if not more than, the amount of red fluorescence from the Lissamine rhodamine fibers. In this case, compensation for "bleed-through" of the fluorescein signal into the red fluorescence image is not possible because the Lissamine rhodamine-stained fibers are so inefficiently imaged. This demonstrates how the inability to specifically visualize the fluorophores with an argon ion laser can alter the apparent distribution of staining. This dramatically limits the use of this approach with specimens that have relatively weak or unknown staining patterns.

## 3. Cross-Talk between Detectors with Double-Labeled Specimens

Because it is not possible to specifically visualize both fluorophores in double-labeled specimens with an argon ion laser, it is important that the relative staining intensity of the green and red fluorophores be carefully controlled to balance their detection and cross-talk between the detectors. To demonstrate the consequences of these adjustments, further attempts were made to specifically visualize both fluorophores when observing spinal cord sections stained for the neurotransmitters serotonin and substance P.

Because of the inefficient excitation of the red fluorophore by 514-nm light, the cross-talk of the fluorescein into the red fluorescence detector can be a problem for specimens with intense fluorescein staining. As previously shown (Color Plate 7), considerable cross-talk of the fluorescein signal into the red fluorescence detector is observed when substance P is stained with a fluorescein-conjugated secondary antibody and when serotonin is stained with a Lissamine rhodamine-conjugated secondary antibody. When these fluorophore-conjugated secondary antibodies are used at similar dilutions, the cross-talk of fluorescein into the red fluorescence detector is more than the signal from the Lissamine rhodamine (Fig. 21A). Although this cross-talk can be compensated by subtracting a fraction of the green fluorescence image from the red fluorescence image, the ability to detect serotonin fibers lightly stained with Lissamine rhodamine in the "corrected" red fluorescence image is greatly reduced (Fig. 21A). To reduce the cross-talk of fluorescein into the red fluorescence detector, the intensity of the fluorescein staining can be reduced by

---

subtracting a fraction [100% for (A), 75% for (B), and 15% for (C)] of the corresponding green fluorescence image from the observed red fluorescence images. With the reduction in fluorescein staining, a corresponding increase in the number of fibers in these "corrected" red fluorescence images is observed. This reflects the difficulty in detecting the red fluorescence from Lissamine rhodamine when fluorescein contributes the majority of the signal to the red fluorescence image. Each image is a projection of 16 optical sections acquired at 1.0-$\mu$m intervals. Scale bar = 25 $\mu$m. Nikon ×60, NA 1.4.

using higher dilutions of the fluorescein-conjugated secondary antibody (Fig. 21B and C). In these cases, the reduction in cross-talk from fluorescein is easily appreciated by the higher illumination intensity (0.66 vs 0.20 mW) necessary to obtain an image in the red fluorescence detector. Because of the improved separation of the signals from the fluorophores into the green and red fluorescence detectors, a large number of serotonin fibers in the "corrected" red fluorescence images can be observed after cross-talk compensation (Fig. 21B and C). Although this approach improved the detection of the rhodamine staining and reduced cross-talk from fluorescein into the red fluorescence image, it is probably preferable to switch the secondary antibodies so fluorescein is used to visualize the more difficult-to-detect serotonin fibers.

On the other hand, a similar cross-talk problem can occur with the red fluorophore into the green fluorescence detector when double-labeled specimens are intensely stained with a red fluorophore. Although this cross-talk could also be reduced by staining substance P less intensely with the red fluorophore, this is not really practical because intense staining of the red fluorophore is required to compensate for its inefficient excitation by 514-nm light. A better approach is to use red fluorophores with emission spectra that are shifted to longer wavelengths that have less overlap with the green fluorescence emission filters (Fig. 22). When using the filter configuration for sequential excitation by the 488- and 514-nm lines of an argon ion laser (Fig. 10), the cross-talk of cyanine 3.18 and tetramethylrhodamine into the green fluorescence detector is similar in intensity to the fluorescein signal (Fig. 23). In contrast, no cross-talk of the longer wavelength Lissamine rhodamine and Texas Red into the green fluorescence detector was observed. Because the green fluorescence emission filter is at shorter wavelengths with the filter configuration for sequential excitation by the 488- and 514-nm lines of an argon ion laser (Fig. 15), this configuration dramatically reduced the cross-talk of the red fluorophores into the green fluorescence detector (Fig. 23). In addition, it should be noted that cyanine 3.18 required a lower illumination intensity than the rhodamines (0.07 vs 0.66 mW) to obtain a red fluorescence image of the substance P staining.

As demonstrated by these specimens, two-color imaging with an argon ion laser is practical only for some combinations of fluorophores when their relative staining intensity can be carefully controlled. Usually, the less efficient imaging of the red fluorophore requires that it be used to visualize the more strongly staining antigen. However, if both substances of interest can only be weakly stained, two-color imaging with an argon ion laser of these specimens may not be possible.

## 4. Is Three-Color Laser Scanning Confocal Microscopy with an Argon Ion Laser Possible?

Although three-color fluorescence detection with a single excitation wavelength from an argon ion laser has been reported for flow cytometry (Festin *et al.*, 1990; Afar *et al.*, 1991; Lansdorp *et al.*, 1991), it is unclear whether

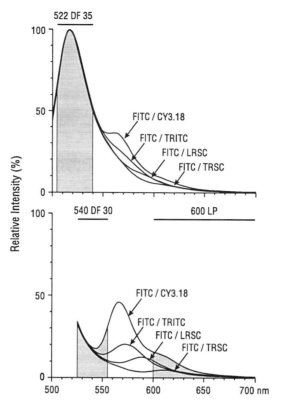

**Fig. 22** Spectroscopic examination of the fluorescence observed from an equimolar solution of fluorescein (FITC)- and various red fluorophore-conjugated IgGs. (Note that the concentrations are for the fluorophores instead of the protein because of the slight differences in the fluorophore/ protein ratios of the conjugates.) The following red fluorophores were used in combination with fluorescein-conjugated goat anti-mouse IgG: cyanine 3.18 (CY3.18)-, tetramethylrhodamine (TRITC)-, Lissamine rhodamine (LRSC)-, or Texas Red (TRSC)-conjugated goat anti-mouse IgGs. The emission spectra of the various combinations of fluorophores in response to excitation by 488-nm light (*top*) or 514-nm light (*bottom*) are shown. The regions of the emission spectra that are transmitted by the bandpass emission filters are also shown (shaded regions). Note the increased contribution of the shorter wavelength red fluorophores to the emission that would be observed through the green fluorescence emission filter used with 514-nm excitation (*bottom*).

this approach can be successfully applied to multicolor LSCM. Three-color flow cytometry with a single excitation wavelength is usually done with 488-nm excitation of fluorescein (peak emission wavelength of 520 nm), R-phycoerythrin (peak emission wavelength of 575 nm), and one of the phyco-biliprotein tandem conjugates (peak emission wavelengths of 610–670 nm; Fig. 24). These tandem conjugates have extremely large Stokes shifts and include R-phycoerythrin/allophycocyanin (Glazer and Stryer, 1983), R-phycoerythrin/ Texas Red (Festin *et al.*, 1990), R-phycoerythrin/cyanine 5.18 (Lansdorp *et al.*, 1991), or the photosynthetic pigment from dinoflagellates, peridinin chlorophyll

514 nm Excitation

| Green Fluorescence (540 DF 30) | Red Fluorescence (600 LP) | 488 nm Excitation Green Fluorescence (522 DF 35) |
|---|---|---|

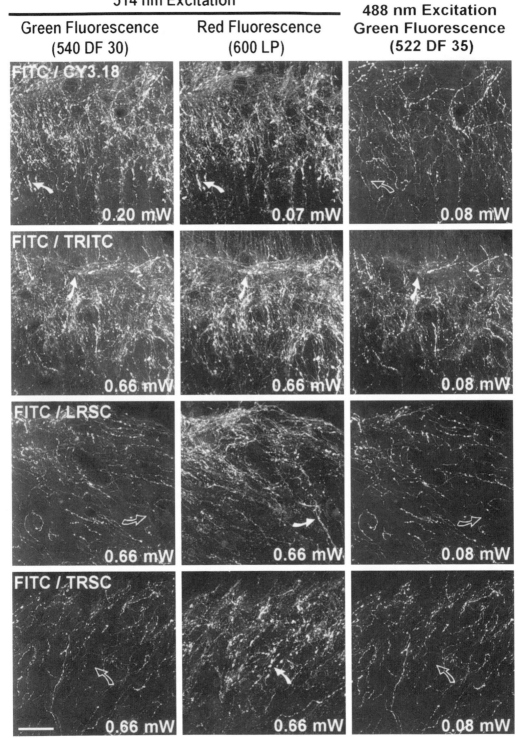

FITC / CY3.18 — 0.20 mW | 0.07 mW | 0.08 mW

FITC / TRITC — 0.66 mW | 0.66 mW | 0.08 mW

FITC / LRSC — 0.66 mW | 0.66 mW | 0.08 mW

FITC / TRSC — 0.66 mW | 0.66 mW | 0.08 mW

*a* binding protein (Recktenwald, 1989; Afar *et al.*, 1991). Because the correction of the cross-talk between images becomes more difficult as the difference between the excitation and emission wavelengths increases (see Section IV,A,2), this approach should be less successful than that observed for two-color LSCM with a single excitation wavelength.

To test this possibility, rat pancreatic islets of Langerhans were stained for the major islet hormones. This specimen was chosen because the major islet hormones (insulin, glucagon, and somatostatin) are easily stained and are synthesized within distinct cell types within the islet (β, α, and δ cells, respectively). The combination of fluorescein, cyanine 3.18, and the tandem conjugate of R-phycoerythrin/cyanine 5.18 (R-PE–CY5.18) was chosen because of the exceptional brightness of the cyanine fluorophores. After several trials examining the relative staining intensity of these fluorophores, it was determined that it was necessary in this case to reduce the intensity of the fluorescein and cyanine 3.18 staining to reduce cross-talk into the far-red fluorescence image of the R-PE–CY5.18 staining. Therefore dilutions of 1 : 500, 1 : 200, and 1 : 50 for fluorescein-, cyanine 3.18-, and R-PE–CY5.18-conjugated secondary antibodies, respectively, were used for the triple labeling of islets.

Although the use of either 488- or 514-nm excitation for imaging of all three fluorophores was possible, sequential excitation with the 488-nm line for fluorescein and the 514-nm line for cyanine 3.18 and R-PE–CY5.18 was used to increase the spectral isolation of fluorescein from the red fluorophores (Fig. 25). However, it can be seen that the greater difference between the excitation and observation wavelengths leads to a substantial decrease in the apparent "confocality" of the R-PE–CY5.18 image. In addition, the use of 488-nm excitation allowed imaging of the weak fluorescein staining required to reduce cross-talk into the images of the other two fluorophores (Fig. 26). To obtain an image of the cyanine 3.18 staining, it was still necessary to compensate for the cross-talk of fluorescein into the red fluorescence image by subtracting 40% of the green fluorescence image from the red fluorescence image. Similarly, an image of the

---

**Fig. 23**  Cross-talk of the red fluorophore into the green fluorescence detector, using an argon ion laser for two-color imaging. Rat spinal cord sections were stained with goat anti-serotonin and rabbit anti-substance P antisera. Fluorescein (FITC)-conjugated donkey anti-goat IgG was used in combination with either cyanine 3.18 (CY3.18)-, tetramethylrhodamine (TRITC)-, Lissamine rhodamine (LRSC)-, or Texas Red (TRSC)-conjugated donkey anti-rabbit IgGs. All secondary antibodies were used as 1:100 dilutions. In this region of the spinal cord, the superficial dorsal horn, coexistence would not be expected. The shorter wavelength red fluorophores, both cyanine 3.18 and tetramethylrhodamine, are visible in the green fluorescence images collected with 514-nm excitation (Fig. 10). However, the more optimal filter set using 488-nm excitation (Fig. 15) allows a more specific detection of the green fluorescence from fluorescein for these red fluorophores. Also, note the lower illumination intensity needed to acquire the image of the cyanine 3.18 staining compared to the rhodamines. Each image is a projection of 16 optical sections acquired at 1.0-μm intervals through the superficial dorsal horn. Scale bar = 25 μm. Nikon ×60 NA 1.4.

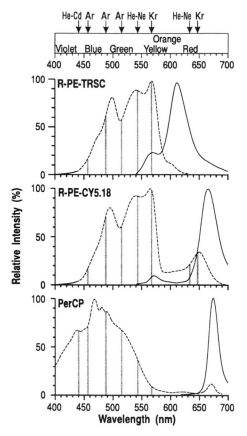

**Fig. 24** Excitation (dashed) and emission (solid) spectra of large Stokes shift fluorophores derived from photosynthetic pigments. *Top:* The tandem conjugate of R-phycoerythrin and Texas Red with streptavidin (R-PE–TRSC; Gibco Life Technologies, Grand Island, NY). The excitation spectrum was scanned while measuring emission at 650 nm, and the emission spectrum was scanned while exciting at 490 nm. *Middle:* The tandem conjugate of R-phycoerythrin and cyanine 5.18 (R-PE–CY5.18) with goat anti-mouse IgG (Jackson ImmunoResearch Laboratories). The excitation spectrum was scanned while measuring emission at 710 nm, and the emission spectrum was scanned while exciting at 490 nm. *Bottom:* Peridinin chlorophyll *a*-binding protein (PerCP; provided by Diether Recktenwald of Becton Dickinson, San Jose, CA). The excitation spectrum was scanned while measuring emission at 710 nm, and the emission spectrum was scanned while exciting at 390 nm. The emission lines for argon ion (Ar), krypton ion (Kr), helium–cadmium (He–Cd), and helium–neon (He–Ne) lasers are shown as vertical lines beneath the excitation spectra.

R-PE–CY5.18 staining was obtained from the far-red fluorescence image by subtracting 20% of the fluorescein and 50% of the cyanine 3.18 images.

These images of a triple-labeled islet can be merged to form a color image that allows the distribution of the islet hormones to be examined. Because individual islet cells synthesize only a single hormone, the occurrence of double- and

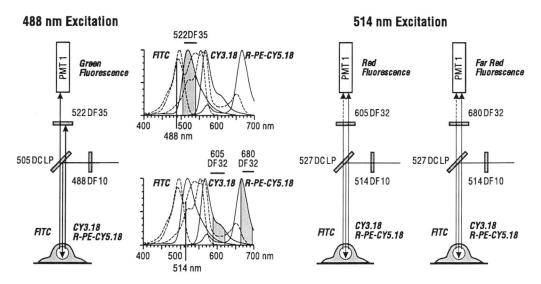

**Fig. 25** Filter configurations for sequential imaging of triple-labeled specimens, using an argon ion laser. *Left:* The filter set for the detection of green fluorescence, using 488-nm excitation. *Right:* The filter sets for the detection of red and far red fluorescence, using 514-nm excitation. The excitation (dashed) and emission (solid) spectra of the fluorescein (FITC), cyanine 3.18 (CY3.18), and tandem conjugate of R-phycoerythrin/cyanine 5.18 (R-PE–CY5.18) are shown in the middle. The excitation wavelength (solid line) and regions of the emission spectra transmitted by the bandpass emission filters (shaded regions) are also shown. See Fig. 10 for filter abbreviations.

triple-labeled cells in the images as collected is artifactual (Color Plate 8A). Although compensation of the cross-talk between the images dramatically improves the separation of the fluorescence signals (Color Plate 8B), several cells still appear to be double labeled for insulin and glucagon in the "corrected" images. This is not surprising considering that the loss of resolution in the far red fluorescence image will hinder the compensation of cross-talk and determination of which cells were actually stained for glucagon. This difficulty in cross-talk compensation and the need to carefully adjust the relative staining intensity of the fluorophores demonstrates the difficulty of this approach and its susceptibility to artifactual multiple labeling.

## B. Multicolor Laser Scanning Confocal Microscopy with Air-Cooled Krypton–Argon Ion Laser

The broad range of emission wavelengths available from an air-cooled krypton–argon ion laser allows the use of different excitation wavelengths and emission filters for the detection of specific fluorophores. For appropriate combinations of fluorescent dyes, this approach allows the more efficient and independent detection of more than one fluorophore in a single specimen by LSCM.

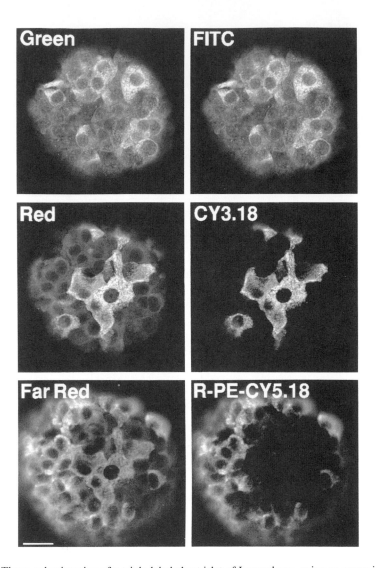

**Fig. 26** Three-color imaging of a triple-labeled rat islet of Langerhans, using an argon ion laser. The major islet cell types were stained with guinea pig anti-insulin serum, rabbit anti-somatostatin serum, and a mouse anti-glucagon monoclonal antibody. The following secondary antibodies were used: fluorescein-conjugated donkey anti-guinea pig IgG, cyanine 3.18 (CY3.18)-conjugated donkey anti-rabbit IgG, and a tandem conjugate of cyanine 5.18 and R-phycoerythrin (R-PE–CY5.18) with donkey anti-mouse IgG. *Left:* Projections of six optical images acquired at 1.0-$\mu$m intervals, using the filter configurations shown in Fig. 25. Because individual islet cells produce a single hormone, the occurrence of stained cells in more than one of the images indicates the failure to spectrally isolate the fluorophores completely. *Right:* The distribution of staining after compensation for cross-talk between the observed images. FITC staining was assumed to be represented by the green fluorescence image. CY3.18 staining was estimated by subtracting 40% of the green fluorescence image from the red fluorescence image. Similarly, R-PE–CY5.18 staining was estimated by subtracting 20% of the green fluorescence image and 50% of the "CY3.18" image from the red fluorescence image. Scale bar = 25 $\mu$m. Olympus ×40  NA 0.85.

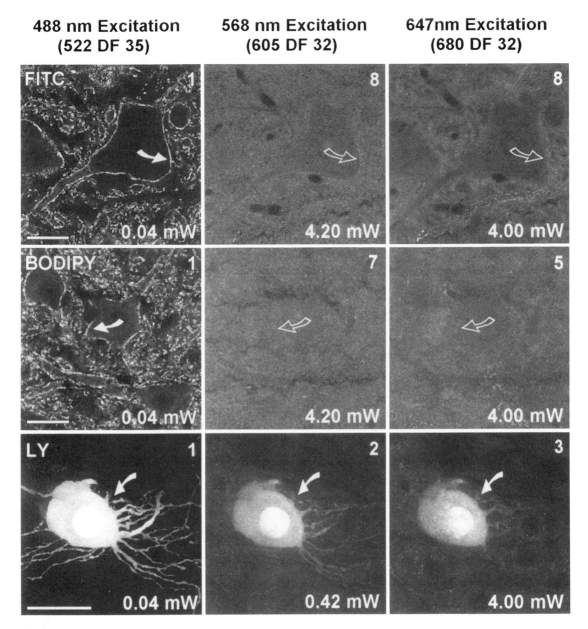

**488 nm Excitation (522 DF 35)** | **568 nm Excitation (605 DF 32)** | **647nm Excitation (680 DF 32)**

**Fig. 27** Specificity of visualization of green fluorophores, using the microscope filters for three-color imaging with a krypton–argon ion laser. Rat spinal cord sections were stained with a mouse monoclonal antibody against synaptophysin and either fluorescein (FITC)-conjugated donkey anti-mouse IgG or BODIPY-conjugated goat anti-mouse IgG. Single optical sections are shown for each of these fluorophores. For Lucifer yellow (LY), projections are shown of 20 images acquired at 1.0-$\mu$m intervals through an intracellularly injected neuron within the parasympathetic nucleus. The intensity of laser illumination used to acquire the images is given in milliwatts (mW). The relative increase in photomultiplier gain and contrast for the images of each fluorophore is indicated in the upper right of each image. Scale bars = 25 mm. Nikon ×60 NA 1.4.

In addition, the specific visualization of each fluorophore permits the investigation of specimens with staining for the coexistence substances.

## 1. Visualization Specificity of Fluorophores with Krypton–Argon Ion Laser

The specificity of the fluorophores with respect to the microscope filters was investigated by attempting to visualize each fluorophore with the filter configuration for the imaging of triple-labeled specimens and a krypton–argon ion laser (Fig. 18). In addition, as done for our studies on the argon ion laser (see Section V,A,1), specimens stained for synaptophysin with the various fluorophore-conjugated secondary antibodies and a Lucifer yellow-injected neuron were examined.

Unlike the argon ion laser (Fig. 19), the filter configurations for three-color imaging with a krypton–argon ion laser could be used to specifically visualize the green fluorophores, except for Lucifer yellow (Fig. 27). With the filters for 488-nm excitation, the distribution of numerous varicosities containing synaptophysin-like immunoreactivity on the cell bodies and processes of neurons is easily appreciated for both the fluorescein- and BODIPY-stained specimens. Even when the intensity of laser illumination was increased 100-fold and photon counting was used, no staining whatsoever beyond autofluorescence was observed in the red and far red fluorescence images obtained with the filters for 568- or 647-nm excitation. Unlike the 514-nm excitation used with an argon ion laser, these longer excitation wavelengths from a krypton–argon ion laser are well past the excitation maximums of these green fluorophores. In contrast, the brightly stained cell body of a Lucifer yellow-injected neuron was still observed with the filters for 568- and 647-nm excitation (Fig. 27). Most likely this reflects the slight excitation at these wavelengths possible with Lucifer yellow because of its much broader excitation spectrum. The use of alternate intracellular markers, such as biotin derivatives and fluorophore-conjugated avidins (Horikawa and Armstrong, 1988; Kita and Armstrong, 1991), or fluorophore-conjugated dextrans (Mesce *et al.*, 1993), that can be visualized with more specific fluorophores is preferable for multicolor studies.

Although each of the red fluorophores could be imaged with the filters for 568-nm excitation, the shorter wavelength red fluorophores could not be

---

**Fig. 28** Specificity of visualization of red fluorophores, using the microscope filters for three-color imaging with a krypton–argon ion laser. Rat spinal cord sections were stained with a mouse monoclonal antibody against synaptophysin and either cyanine 3.18 (CY3.18)-, tetramethylrhodamine (TRITC)-, Lissamine rhodamine (LRSC)-, or Texas Red (TRSC)-conjugated donkey anti-mouse IgGs. Single optical sections are shown for each of the fluorophores. The intensity of laser illumination used to acquire the images is given in milliwatts (mW). The relative increase in photomultiplier gain and contrast for the images of each fluorophore is indicated in the upper right of each image. Scale bar = 25 μm. Nikon ×60 NA 1.4.

## 488 nm Excitation (522 DF 35)   568 nm Excitation (605 DF 32)   647nm Excitation (680 DF 32)

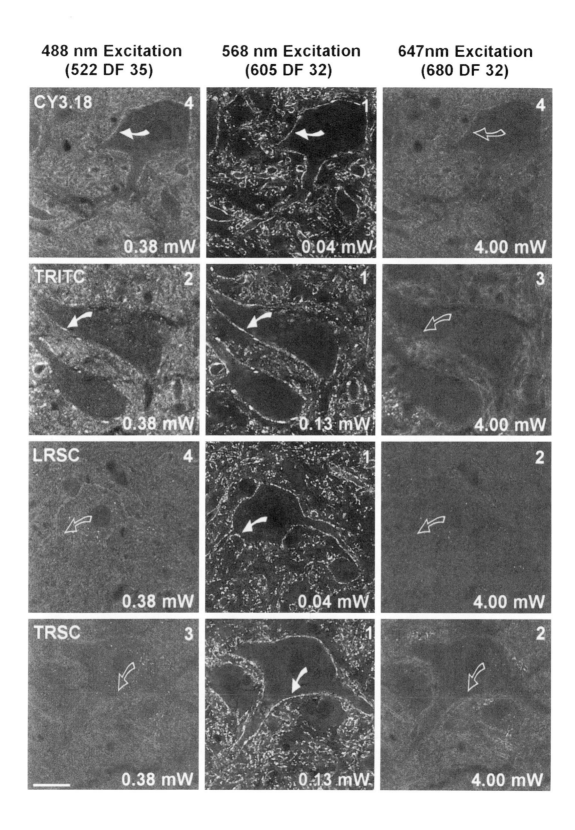

specifically visualized by using the filter configuration for three-color imaging with a krypton–argon ion laser (Fig. 28). Similar to the argon ion laser (Figs. 19 and 20), both cyanine 3.18 and tetramethylrhodamine were visible in the green fluorescence images because of the slight overlap between their emission spectra and the green fluorescence emission filter (Fig. 18). However, it should be noted that the detection of cyanine 3.18 in the green fluorescence images has been possible only for intensely stained specimens. The longer wavelength Lissamine rhodamine and Texas Red were not observed with the filters for 488-nm excitation. In addition, red fluorescence images of cyanine 3.18 and Lissamine rhodamine could be obtained by using a lower illumination intensity (0.04 vs 0.13 mW). This probably reflects the superior brightness of cyanine 3.18 compared to the rhodamine conjugates (Wessendorf and Brelje, 1992; Mujumdar *et al.*, 1993) and the nearly maximal excitation of Lissamine rhodamine by 568-nm light. No staining beyond the normal tissue autofluorescence was observed for these red fluorophores with the filters for 647-nm excitation (Fig. 28). With the reduction in autofluorescence at longer excitation wavelengths, a 10-fold increase in laser illumination intensity was necessary to obtain comparable green and far red autofluorescence images for Lissamine rhodamine and Texas Red.

Each of the far red fluorophores examined was easily imaged with the filters for 647-nm excitation and the detection of far red fluorescence (Fig. 29). Although allophycocyanin was extremely bright when imaged with the far red filters, its broad excitation and emission spectra make it visible in both the red and far red fluorescence images, using the same illumination intensity. In contrast, a 10-fold increase in illumination intensity for 568- compared to 647-nm excitation was required to observe cyanine 5.18 in the red fluorescence image. Except for a few specimens with particularly bright staining, this has not been a problem when staining for other substances, using cyanine 5.18-conjugated antibodies. In contrast, the aluminum tetrabenztriazaporphyrin derivative could be visualized only with the far red filters, probably because of its narrow emission peak.

In summary, it appears possible to specifically visualize fluorophores with the krypton–argon ion laser if the combinations of fluorophores are carefully chosen. For two-color imaging, it is expected that FITC used in combination with Lissamine rhodamine or Texas Red should permit specific visualization of the fluorophores. Although cyanine 3.18 can be detected in the green fluorescence filters with intensely stained specimens, it should be preferable to the rhodamines when a red fluorophore must be used to visualize an antigen that gives relatively weak staining. In this case, the superior brightness of cyanine 3.18 should improve the detection of specific staining. Similarly, it should be possible to use cyanine 5.18 or phthalocyanine derivatives as far red fluorophores for three-color imaging. However, because LSCM has sufficient sensitivity to image some of these fluorophores under suboptimal conditions, corresponding control specimens stained with a single fluorescent dye should be

**488 nm Excitation** | **568 nm Excitation** | **647nm Excitation**
**(522 DF 35)** | **(605 DF 32)** | **(680 DF 32)**

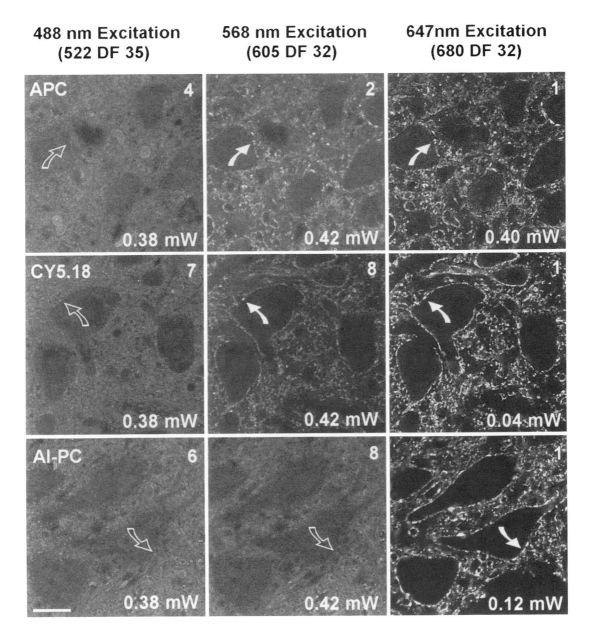

**Fig. 29** Specificity of visualization of far red fluorophores, using the microscope filters for three-color imaging with a krypton–argon ion laser. Rat spinal cord sections were stained wtih a mouse monoclonal antibody against synaptophysin and either allophycocyanin (APC)-conjugated goat anti-mouse IgG (Biomeda), cyanine 5.18 (CY5.18)-conjugated donkey anti-mouse IgG (Jackson ImmunoResearch Laboratories), or aluminum tetrabenztriazaporphyrin (Al-PC)-conjugated goat anti-mouse IgG (Ultralight T680). Single optical sections are shown for each of the fluorophores. The intensity of laser illumination used to acquire the images is given in milliwatts (mW). The relative increase in photomultiplier gain and contrast for the images of each fluorophore is indicated in the upper right of each image. Scale bar = 25 $\mu$m. Nikon ×60 NA 1.4.

examined to verify the specific visualization of the fluorophores for multiple-labeled specimens. This is especially important for specimens in which the coexistence of staining will be examined.

## 2. Observations on Two-Color Laser Scanning Confocal Microscopy with Krypton–Argon Ion Laser

To demonstrate the superiority of specific visualization of fluorophores with the krypton–argon ion laser, rat spinal cord sections stained for serotonin and substance P were imaged with the two-color filter configuration for the krypton–argon ion laser (Fig. 17). Unlike the differences in distribution of these neurotransmitters observed after switching the fluorophores with the argon ion laser (see Section V,A,2), both specimens appear similar except for the switching of the colors (Color Plate 7). The ability to specifically visualize each of the fluorophores removes the requirement to carefully select and carefully balance the relative staining intensity of the fluorophores used with double-labeled specimens.

It should be noted, however, that it is difficult to observe the smaller number of red fibers in the presence of the larger number of green fibers. This is not the result of actual differences in the specimens or the imaging, but results from the colors assigned to each image when printing the merged, color image (see Section VI,B).

## 3. Simultaneous vs Sequential Imaging of Double-Labeled Specimens

The consequences of using simultaneous vs sequential imaging of fluorophores in a double-labeled specimen can be demonstrated by using the filter configuration for two-color imaging with a krypton–argon ion laser (Fig. 17). Human islets of Langerhans were double labeled for somatostatin and glucagon, using fluorescein- and Lissamine rhodamine-conjugated secondary antibodies, respectively. By sequential excitation with 488- and 568-nm light, the distinct populations of somatostatin-containing $\delta$ cells and glucagon-containing $\alpha$ cells can be clearly observed (Fig. 30). The green fluorescence image observed with 488-nm excitation shows the $\delta$ cells at the periphery of the islets stained with fluoroscein (Fig. 30A). Similarly, the red fluorescence image observed with 568-nm excitation shows the $\alpha$ cells (Fig. 30C). No double-labeled cells are observed when the green and red fluorescence images are compared.

In contrast, these fluorophores cannot be specifically visualized when both 488- and 568-nm light is used to simultaneously excite fluorescein and Lissamine rhodamine (Fig. 30). Because 568-nm light is at a wavelength longer than those used to obtain the green fluorescence image (505 to 539 nm), the red fluorescence simultaneously emitted by the Lissamine rhodamine is not observed in the green fluorescence image (not shown). However, the red fluorescence image contains the emissions from both Lissamine rhodamine and fluoroscein (Fig. 30B). Although less than 10% of the fluoroscein emission spectra overlaps with the red

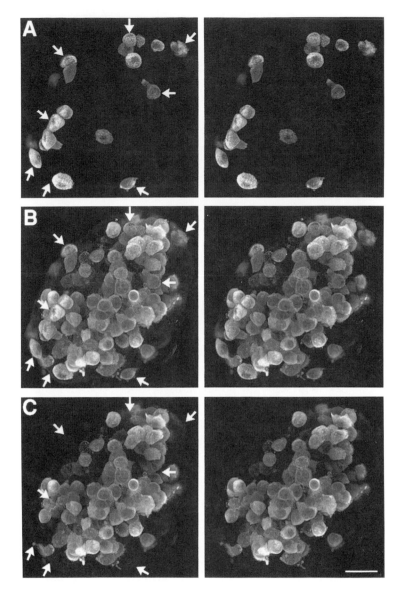

**Fig. 30**  Stereo images of a double-labeled human islet of Langerhans, using sequential vs simultaneous excitation with the 488- and 568-nm lines of a krypton–argon ion laser with the filter configuration shown in Fig. 17. Human islets were stained with rabbit anti-somatostatin antiserum and fluorescein-conjugated donkey anti-rabbit IgG, and a mouse anti-glucagon monoclonal antibody and Lissamine rhodamine-conjugated donkey anti-mouse IgG. (A) The somatostatin-containing δ cells are clearly visible in the green fluorescence image observed with 488-nm excitation. (B) The same cells (arrows) are also observed in the red fluorescence image observed with simultaneous excitation with the 488- and 568-nm lines. (C) The glucagon-containing α cells can, however, be specifically visualized in the red fluorescence image when observed with only 568-nm excitation. In this case, the δ cells (arrows) are not visible because of the inefficient excitation of fluorescein with 568-nm light. The stereo images were constructed from 21 optical sections acquired at 1.0-μm intervals. Scale bar = 25 μm. Olympus ×40  NA 0.85. [Human islets provided by Drs. D. Scharp and P. Lacy (Washington University, St. Louis, MO).]

fluorescence emission filter (Fig. 17), similar fluorescence intensities for both fluorophores may result from more intense fluorescein staining or the superior brightness of fluorescein conjugates. This situation is similar to that observed with the simultaneous excitation of multiple fluorophores with an argon ion laser but with more efficient excitation of the rhodamine.

Therefore sequential excitation and imaging of each fluorophore in a multiple-labeled specimen will usually be necessary to spectrally isolate their fluorescence emissions. Unfortunately, this approach is rather time consuming because the specimen must be scanned several times with different excitation and emission wavelengths. Temporal resolution could be improved by the automatic switching of excitation filters and detectors between successive frames or even individual scan lines. Besides providing more immediate results, this approach would help minimize the problem of specimen movement changing the volume sampled for each pixel with each filter set.

## 4. Examples of Multicolor Laser Scanning Confocal Microscopy with Krypton–Argon Ion Laser

The usefulness of a krypton–argon ion laser for multicolor LSCM was tested by further examining lumbar spinal cord sections stained for serotonin and substance P. In the superficial dorsal horn, these neurotransmitters appear to exist in separate populations of fibers (Color Plate 9A). A few instances of apparent coexistence can be seen in the stereo images to be separate fibers superimposed on top of each other. In contrast, in the ventral horn, both neurotransmitters appear to stain the same nerve fibers and varicosities (Color Plate 9B). These processes are oriented around large cells resembling motor neurons and appear to occupy the same space when viewed in the stereo images. This suggests that the observed double labeling does not result from the apposition of different fibers of similar morphology. The difference in colors among different varicose fibers suggests that different neurons contain different molar ratios of serotonin and substance P.

The identity of the large cells surrounded by these nerve fibers in the ventral horn of the spinal cord was further investigated. Motor neurons of the lumbar spinal cord were stained by injection of the sciatic nerve with the retrograde tract-tracer hydroxystilbamidine (Fluoro-gold; Fluorochrome, Englewood, CO; Schmeud and Fallon, 1986; Wessendorf, 1991). In 300-$\mu$m vibratome sections of the spinal cord, individual hydroxystilbamidine-labeled motor neurons were identified by conventional fluorescence microscopy and intracellularly injected with Lucifer yellow. After staining for substance P, numerous nerve fibers containing substance P immunoreactivity were observed around the individual motor neurons (Color Plate 9C). These fibers appeared as a series of varicosities in close apposition to the surface of the motor neuron. From these projections, the distribution and number of varicosities containing various neurotransmitters on individual neurons can be more easily examined than by conventional fluorescence microscopy.

Control studies were undertaken to determine whether the observed double labeling was due to the neurotransmitter immunoreactivity or whether it was artifactual. The most likely source of artifactual double labeling would be the failure to specifically visualize each fluorophore or the secondary antibodies to specifically recognize only one of the primary antibodies. As previously discussed (see Section II,B), both of these artifacts can be tested by staining individual specimens with a single primary antibody and all of the fluorophore-conjugated secondary antibodies used. Spinal cord sections were singly stained with either goat anti-serotonin or rabbit anti-substance P antisera alone, followed by incubation with both the fluorescein-conjugated donkey anti-goat IgG and Lissamine rhodamine-conjugated donkey anti-rabbit IgGs. If the secondary antibodies recognized the inappropriate primary antisera or each other, it would be expected that double labeling would be observed. Similarly, double labeling would also be observed if the fluorophores could not be visualized specifically with the microscope filters. Although the latter appeared unlikely, using sequential excitation with the filter configuration for two-color imaging with a krypton–argon ion laser (see Section V,B,3), a lack of specificity will be more likely observed with brighter staining. Thus it is good practice to always test for this artifact by using the same tissue and antibodies as will be used in experimental situations.

When the sections stained for serotonin were examined, the typical pattern of serotonin immunoreactivity in the superficial dorsal horn was observed by 488-nm excitation and the green fluorescence detector (Fig. 31). Even when the illumination intensity of the 568-nm light was increased 100-fold and photon counting was used, no staining whatsoever was observed beyond normal tissue autofluorescence in the red fluorescence detector. Similarly, staining for substance P could be observed only by 568-nm excitation and the red fluorescence detector (Fig. 31). This suggests that the fluorophores can be specifically visualized and that the secondary antibodies are specific with respect to recognition of the primary antisera and have little affinity for each other. Although not shown here, these primary antibodies have already been shown to have specific immunoreactivity for the appropriate antigens (Wessendorf and Elde, 1985; Wessendorf et al., 1990a).

Similarly, the krypton–argon ion laser allows the distribution of three different neurotransmitters to be examined in triple-labeled specimens. For example, spinal cord sections were stained for serotonin, substance P, and Met-enkephalin by using fluorescein-, cyanine 3.18-, and cyanine 5.18-conjugated secondary antibodies, respectively. The overall staining pattern of these neurotransmitters can be observed in a low-magnification image of a section of the lumbar spinal cord (Color Plate 10A). Although it has been infrequently mentioned, the intense and even illumination achieved with LSCM allows the acquisition of low-magnification images that would be difficult to photograph by conventional fluorescence microscopy. Because the entire section could not be viewed with a ×4 objective, overlapping images of each half of the spinal cord were collected and subsequently combined into one large image for each

# Green Fluorescence

# Red Fluorescence

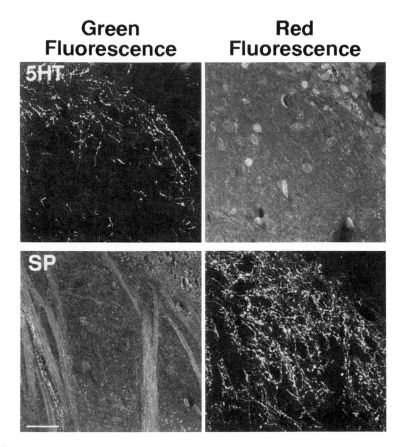

**Fig. 31** Tests of the specificity of the secondary antibody and fluorophore used for double labeling the spinal cord. Rat spinal cord sections were stained with either goat anti-serotonin (5-HT) or rabbit anti-substance P (SP) antisera. All sections were then stained with both fluorescein-conjugated donkey anti-goat and Lissamine rhodamine-conjugated donkey anti-rabbit IgGs (multiple species adsorbed). The sections were examined with the filter configuration for two-color imaging with the krypton–argon ion laser (Fig. 17). If either the secondary antibodies or the fluorophores lacked specificity, double labeling would be expected. For 5-HT, only 0.05 mW of 488-nm light was required to obtain an image of the fluorescein staining in the green fluorescence detector. In contrast, even with 4.5 mW of 568-nm light and using the photon-counting mode of the Bio-Rad MRC-600, only the autofluorescence from the tissue was observed in the red fluorescence detector. Similarly, for SP only 0.05 mW of 568-nm light was required to obtain an image of the Lissamine rhodamine staining in the red fluorescence detector. In contrast, it was necessary to use 0.45 mW of 488-nm light and photon counting to obtain an image of the autofluorescence in the green fluorescence detector. This suggests that the secondary antibodies are specific in the recognition of the primary antibodies and that the fluorophores can be specifically visualized. Each image was formed from the projection of 10 optical sections acquired at 1.0-$\mu$m intervals. Scale bar = 25 $\mu$m. Nikon ×60 NA 1.4.

fluorophore. Minimal photobleaching of the fluorophores was observed even with the intense illumination (~4mW) necessary to collect these images because of the low magnification and scanning times. Although individual nerve fibers cannot be observed in low-magnification images, they can be resolved when smaller regions are examined at higher magnifications (Color Plate 10B). In this case, these neurotransmitters appear to exist primarily in separate populations of nerve fibers and varicosities in the region around the central canal of the spinal cord.

In our initial study, using LSCM to investigate the three-dimensional structure of islets of Langerhans, we observed in double-labeled specimens that the somatostatin-containing $\delta$ cells appeared adjacent to the glucagon-containing $\alpha$ cells (Brelje *et al.*, 1989). Although the relationship between these two cell types could be examined with the argon ion laser, it was not possible to examine simultaneously the orientation of $\delta$ cells with respect to the insulin-containing $\beta$ cells. With the krypton–argon ion laser, the distribution of these islet cell types in the same islet could be easily examined by imaging islets triple labeled for insulin, somatostatin, and glucagon, using fluorescein-, cyanine 3.18-, and cyanine 5.18-conjugated secondary antibodies, respectively (Fig. 32). These images should be compared to those obtained with an argon ion laser (Fig. 26). Besides the absence of cross-talk between the fluorescence images, the more efficient imaging of the fluorophores with a krypton–argon ion laser dramatically improves the contrast and detail observed. In particular, the presence of long cytoplasmic processes on the irregularly shaped $\delta$ cells is quite noticeable (Fig. 32B). In addition, the relationship between these different islet cell types can be easily appreciated by merging the individual fluorescence images to form a color stereo image (Color Plate 11A). The somatostatin-containing $\delta$ cells are observed only in direct apposition between the glucagon-containing $\alpha$ cells on the exterior surface of the islet and the insulin-containing $\beta$ cells that compose the majority of cells in the islet. Note that the amount of detail for each fluorophore apparent in the color merged image is less than that in the separate images (see Section VI,B,3). The advantage of three-dimensional reconstructions is particularly evident in human islets, in which the relationship between the different islet cell types is less distinguishable (Color Plate 11B).

Besides the examination of the relationship between different populations of cells and/or nerve fibers, the krypton–argon ion laser can also be used to examine the distribution of intracellular staining at higher magnifications. The utility of multicolor LSCM in approaching this type of problem can be easily appreciated from the stereo images of the cytoskeleton of individual cells from dorsal root ganglion cell cultures (Color Plate 11C). For this cell, the actin filaments were observed at the periphery of the cell near the plasma membrane and as stress fibers parallel to the surface of the culture substrate. In contrast, the microtubules were observed as a radiating network surrounding the nucleus of the cell and extending out toward the attached surfaces of the cell. In both cases, the efficient imaging of the staining allowed images with high signal-to-noise ratios to be collected.

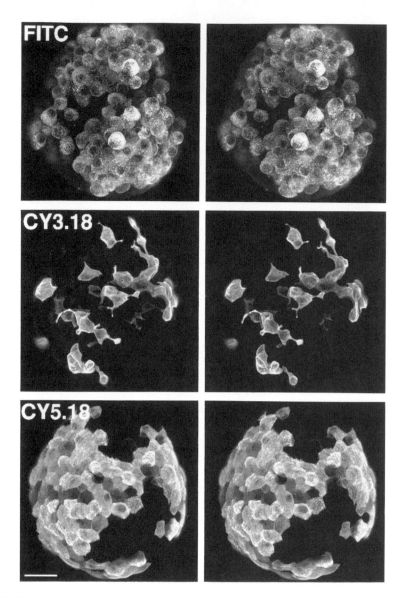

**Fig. 32**  Stereo images of a triple-labeled rat islet of Langerhans, using the three-color filter configuration of the krypton–argon ion laser shown in Fig. 18. Neonatal rat islets were stained with guinea pig anti-insulin serum, rabbit anti-somatostatin serum, and a mouse anti-glucagon monoclonal antibody. The staining was visualized with the following secondary antibodies: fluorescein (FITC)-conjugated donkey anti-guinea pig, cyanine 3.18 (CY3.18)-conjugated donkey anti-rabbit, and cyanine 5.18 (CY5.18)-conjugated donkey anti-mouse IgGs (multiple species adsorbed). In the individual stereo projections, note the presence of considerable detail and the absence of cells stained with the other fluorophores. The stereo projections were constructed from 25 optical sections acquired at 1.0-$\mu$m intervals across the top of the islet. Scale bar = 25 $\mu$m. Olympus ×40 NA 0.85.

===================    # VI. Multicolor Laser Scanning Confocal Microscopy Considerations

The general problems of imaging biological specimens by LSCM are discussed by Majlof and Forsgren ([3] in this volume). Therefore, the various artifacts incurred by the optical sectioning of thick specimens by LSCM will not be discussed in this article. Instead, the specific problems that occur when using a broad range of excitation and detection wavelengths with LSCM will be addressed.

## A. Effect of Excitation/Emission Wavelength Differences

The use of different excitation/emission wavelengths with multicolor fluorescence microscopy complicates the comparison of images acquired in different spectral regions. Because many biological studies require optical resolutions approaching or beyond the diffraction limit, the wavelength dependence of resolution must be considered. The effect of chromatic and spherical aberration in the optics of the microscope are important regardless of the magnification. Although these wavelength-dependent imaging properties must be considered with conventional fluorescence microscopy, it is often much easier to observe their effects with the improved performance of confocal microscopy. Even if filter configurations are used that attempt to maintain registration, these effects will still complicate the comparison of the observed intensities of apparently corresponding pixels in images acquired with different excitation and emission wavelengths.

## 1. Resolution

To demonstrate the effect of different excitation/emission wavelengths on the appearance of structures near the minimal resolution possible with LSCM, intact *Giardia* cysts were double labeled with two antibodies specific for cyst wall antigens, using fluorescein- and cyanine 5.18-conjugated secondary antibodies. Previously, transmission and field emission scanning electron microscopy has shown that the cyst wall is formed by numerous 20-nm filaments in a layer with an overall thickness of 200 to 250 nm (Erlandsen *et al.*, 1990). When examined by multicolor LSCM, the green and red fluorescence images collected through the center of the same cyst appeared similar (Fig. 33). However, measuring the thickness of the cyst wall in these images showed an increase from $295 \pm 50$ nm ($n = 8$) in the green fluorescence image (i.e., fluorescein staining) to $388 \pm 35$ ($n = 8$) in the red fluorescence image (i.e., cyanine 5.18 staining; $p < 0.05$). Although this may reflect actual differences in staining, this difference is similar to the 30% decrease in lateral resolution expected when using the longer wavelengths used to visualize the cyanine 5.18 staining (Table II). Additional evidence for this conclusion is that a similar difference in cyst wall thickness was observed when the fluorophores used to visualize the staining were switched (data not shown).

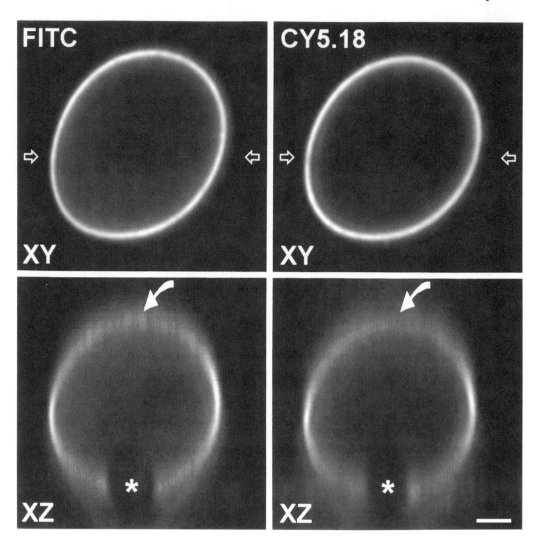

**Fig. 33** The effect of using different imaging wavelengths on the observation of structures near the optical resolution of the microscope. *Giardia* cysts were stained with rabbit and mouse antibodies against cyst wall antigens followed by fluorescein (FITC)-conjugated donkey anti-mouse and cyanine 5.18 (CY5.18)-conjugated donkey anti-rabbit IgGs (multiple species adsorbed). *Top:* Single *xy* images acquired through the center of a double-labeled cyst. Open arrows indicate location of the *xz* images. *Bottom: xz* images acquired through the same cyst by collecting a single scan line at different depths along the optical (*z*) axis. The region across the top of the cyst with differences in intensity is indicated by solid arrows. The unstained region at the bottom of the cyst line in the *xz* images (asterisks) is from their attachment to the slide. Scale bar = 2 $\mu$m. Nikon ×60 NA 1.4. (Specimen courtesy of S. Erlandsen, University of Minnesota.)

Similar to the *xy* images, an apparent increase in the thickness of the cyst wall also occurs in the *xz* images through the same cyst (Fig. 33). However, the cyst wall appears to be at least 700 nm thick across the top of the cyst in these *xz* images. This occurs because the thickness of the cyst wall is below the minimal axial resolution expected at these wavelengths (Table II). As a result, the cyst wall appears brighter when oriented parallel rather than when oriented perpendicular to the optical axis because the thickness of the cyst wall is below the axial resolution of this objective (~700 nm). This is an example of how the apparent staining intensity of structures observed with LSCM can vary depending on its orientation with respect to the optical axis (Van Der Voort and Brakenhoff, 1990).

These differences in resolution observed between images acquired at multiple wavelengths could be compensated for by adjusting the size of the detector apertures. By increasing the size of the detector apertures for the shorter wavelengths, the resolution for each imaging condition can be reduced to that observed with the longest wavelength. Although this facilitates a more direct comparison of the images acquired at different wavelengths, it is typically more desirable to adjust the detector apertures to obtain the best resolution possible with the intensity of staining for each fluorophore.

## 2. Spherical Aberration

Although confocal microscopy allows the collection of optical sections within thick specimens, the high-numerical aperture objectives typically used for fluorescence microscopy are corrected for the observation of specimens positioned immediately underneath a coverslip of the appropriate thickness. Spherical aberration is often introduced by focusing through a specimen mounted in a material whose refractive index varies only slightly from that of the immersion medium for an objective lens. In this case, light rays will be refracted at these boundaries and will not be properly focused on the detector aperture. This will reduce the observed intensities in the deeper optical sections and introduces discrepancies between stage and focal plane movements (see [3], this volume; see also Carlsson, 1991). Besides reducing the observed intensity of staining, the presence of extremely small amounts of spherical aberration is sufficient to produce a more substantial degradation of axial rather than lateral resolution in a confocal microscope as the focal plane is moved deeper into the specimen (Sheppard and Gu, 1991).

A dramatic example of this effect is apparent in *xz* images through islets of Langerhans with their peripheral $\alpha$ cells stained for glucagon (Fig. 34). Because the amount of spherical aberration introduced by the mismatch of refractive indexes is wavelength dependent, the attenuation of signal intensity and loss of axial resolution with deeper imaging into the islets is much more noticeable for the islet stained with fluorescein rather than cyanine 5.18. In double-labeled specimens, this effect can alter the relative intensities and position of stained structures in images collected at different excitation/emission wavelengths.

## 3. Chromatic Aberration

It should also be noted that even the best achromatic and apochromatic lenses have residual chromatic aberration that is more apparent when used with confocal microscopy (Wells *et al.*, 1990; Akinyemi *et al.*, 1992). Traditionally, chromatic aberration has been corrected by careful selection of objective lens elements to bring two or three selected wavelengths to the same focus. Intermediate wavelengths have slightly different focal planes depending on the lens design. Although the differences in focal plane are well within the depth of field for conventional fluorescence imaging, the lack of correction at these intermediate wavelengths will result in misalignment of the illumination and fluorescence paths with confocal fluorescence microscopy. Axial chromatic aberration can result in a 50% loss in the observed signal intensity and in a doubling of the practical optical section thickness at various wavelengths (Fricker and White, 1992). Although less attractive for multiline lasers, the individual lines can be separated and additional prefocusing elements used for each beam to counteract the axial chromatic aberration introduced by other optical components (Kuba *et al.*, 1991). Similarly, lateral chromatic aberration will reduce the intensity of fluorescence observed at positions located further from the optical axis (Wells *et al.*, 1990). Depending on the objective, the extent of this aberration can vary dramatically for the various wavelengths used for LSCM. Because these chromatic aberrations are still observable for the corrected objective lenses typically used with LSCM, the performance of individual objectives should be verified when images will be acquired at different excitation/ emission wavelengths for quantitative comparisons (Wells *et al.*, 1990).

## 4. Depth of Optical Sectioning

Because differences in excitation and emission wavelengths alter numerous aspects of imaging with LSCM, the apparent depth to which specimens may be optically sectioned is also affected. A common misconception is that LSCM allows the acquisition of optical sections as deep into the specimen as the working distance of the objective allows (Cheng and Summers, 1990; Visser *et al.*, 1991).

However, the actual depth to which a specimen can be optically sectioned is dependent on absorption and scattering within the specimen being examined. Besides spherical aberration induced by mismatches between the immersion and mounting medium, structures within the specimen can produce effects similar to spherical aberration when their refractive index is different than that of the mounting medium. This will have the effect of reducing observed intensity and resolution of optical sections acquired at greater depths in the specimen.

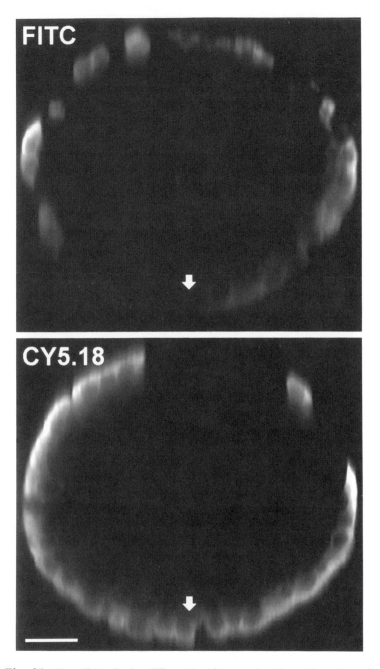

**Fig. 34** The effect of using different imaging wavelengths on the extent of spherical aberration observed. Neonatal rat islets of Langerhans were stained with a mouse monoclonal antibody against glucagon and either fluorescein (FITC)- or cyanine 5.18 (CY5.18)-conjugated donkey anti-mouse IgGs. The islets were mounted in glycerol and the correction collar on the objective set for the highest contrast and detail observed midway through the fluorescein-stained islet. Each image was then corrected for refractive index differences by stretching by a factor of 1.47 in the depth dimension. The arrows indicate positively stained cells at the bottom of the islets that are barely discernible when stained with fluorescein. Scale bar = 25 $\mu$m. Olympus ×40, NA 0.85.

Because the extent of this induced spherical aberration is wavelength dependent, the use of longer excitation wavelengths with far red fluorophores is particularly useful for the imaging of especially thick specimens (see Section VI,A,2).

The observed intensity of stained structures in deeper optical sections can also be decreased by a reduction in the excitation (i.e., inner filter effect) or the reabsorption of fluorescence emission from fluorophores in deeper layers by overlying regions of the specimen (Van Oostveldt and Baumens, 1990; Visser *et al.*, 1991). The simplest approach to reduce this "shadowing" of deeper structures by overlying regions is to reduce the overall intensity of staining (i.e., reduce the local absorbance value). Because autofluorescence and scattering will decrease for longer excitation wavelengths, the far red fluorophores allow the collection of images with acceptable contrast with the lower staining intensities required for the optical sectioning of especially thick specimens (Mesce *et al.*, 1993). Although computationally intensive, a restoration filter for absorption and scattering correction in optical sections acquired with fluorescence confocal microscopy has been described (Visser *et al.*, 1991).

## B. Image Processing and Presentation

Multicolor LSCM is used to acquire monochromatic images of several fluorophores in different spectral regions. If the independent detection of signals from each fluorophore was achieved, then each image contains information on the localization of staining of different substances for the same field of view. Typically, it is advantageous to merge these monochromatic images into a single color image to facilitate the detection of double labeling or relationships between stained structures. In addition, color images are generally much more pleasant to look at than black-and-white images. Although the normal corrections required after the acquisition of digitized images are not usually required with confocal images (i.e., background subtraction, flat field correction), there are several corrections that facilitate the comparison of images acquired in different spectral regions.

## 1. Image Registration

Because even slight variations in the position of the dichroic mirror cause translational shifts in the resulting images, the misregistration of images acquired with multiple filter sets is a common problem. Although individual images can be translated by simple address operations when they are overlaid in different colors, the occurrence of a shift along the optical axis between the data sets must be considered for three-dimensional reconstructions. Finding the exact translation vector giving optimal registration may be further complicated by small shifts in the scanning axis with respect to the optical axis between the collection of data sets. To reduce this type of registration error, it is preferable to use filter configurations in which images of each fluorophore are acquired with the same dichroic mirror.

## 2. Image Contrast

The comparison of images of multiple fluorophores is frequently complicated by differences in contrast of the individual monochromatic images. Ideally, each image should properly fill the available dynamic range and be of comparable contrast before merging into a color image. The use of linear image processing transformations to more fully utilize the available dynamic range can dramatically improve the quality of each image (i.e., remapping the minimum pixel value to black and the maximum pixel value to peak white). A limitation of these transformations is that all pixels of the same intensity are similarly remapped. This is less successful if the intensity of desired details varies in different regions of an image. In this case, the use of adaptive contrast enhancement techniques that are dependent on the local characteristics of an image (e.g., subregions of $n \times n$ pixels) can improve the retention of contrast and subtle details in individual images and projections (Schormann and Jovin, 1991; Mesce *et al.,* 1993). Because these filters do not maintain relative pixel intensities, they are not suitable for quantitative studies based on the observed pixel intensities.

## 3. Image Display

After acquiring and processing the images, the question remains as to how to display the multiple images acquired of each fluorophore. A good solution is to merge the individual monochromatic images into a color image, so that they can be displayed simultaneously. Typically, the primary colors of the additive color system (i.e., red, green, and blue) are assigned to individual images because they produce the widest range of colors. However, it should be noted that this process quickly surpasses the capacity of the viewing medium and the observer. Often, the colors assigned to each image can have considerable effect on the appearance of the individual structures within the merged image. For example, the bright green microtubules are easily followed against the darker red background of actin filaments in the previously shown color projection of the cytoskeleton (Color Plate 11C). In contrast, when the colors are assigned to more closely match the fluorophores (i.e., fluorescein-stained actin filaments in green and the cyanine 3.18-stained microtubules in red), it is difficult to observe the dark red microtubules against a background of bright green actin filaments. Because of these differences in discerning the relative intensities of one color against different backgrounds, it is useful to switch the colors assigned to individual images in a merged color image to prevent visualization artifacts.

Even after considering the colors assigned to each image, adjusting the brightness and contrast of each image can dramatically affect the appearance of a merged color image. Often it is difficult to obtain acceptable merged images when one of the images is colored blue because of the difficulty in detecting pure blue against a black background. This is especially true for color printers, which are usually designed to give dark primary colors. Because a lighter blue contrasts better with the black background, we typically add a fraction (0.3–0.5) of the blue image to the green image before merging the individual monochrome images into a single color image.

Even with these adjustments, a loss of detail within the individual images is usually observed in the merged color images. For example, the number of optical sections in the projections of the glucagon-containing $\alpha$ cells can be easily counted in the black-and-white stereo pair (Fig. 32, CY5.18). However, when colored blue in the merged three-color stereo image, it is no longer possible to count the individual optical sections even though no color reduction was done during the printing process (Color Plate 11A). Although it is obvious that lightly stained structures may not be visible in merged images, this example demonstrates that information can also be lost from brightly stained structures in merged color images. Therefore it may be preferable to show the individual monochrome images to demonstrate the actual contrast and detail present, and the merged color image to emphasize the relationships between stained structures.

The techniques for the display and analysis of the multiple data sets collected by multicolor LSCM are still being developed. Although many options currently exist for two-dimensional reconstructions, further work is required to permit the display and analysis of the multiple data sets as three-dimensional reconstructions. Hopefully, advances in the hardware and software for the manipulation of graphics will make this type of software available to more biologists in the near future. Fortunately, the development of multicolor LSCM has coincided with the availability of more capable graphics workstations and 24-bit color printers (such as the Kodak XL7700 used for the images in this article) for hard copy output.

## VII. Conclusions

The use of LSCM for multicolor immunofluorescence studies is a complex task involving a thorough knowledge of immunohistochemistry, confocal microscope operation and instrumentation, and image presentation. We have presented background information that forms the basis for using these technologies for multicolor LSCM. We have also described what, in our experience, are the practical issues and limitations of doing multicolor immunofluorescence studies with the currently available confocal microscopes. From the examples shown, the advantages of using lasers with a broad selection of emission lines for the multiwavelength excitation compared to single-wavelength excitation of several fluorophores has been demonstrated. With the development of an air-cooled krypton–argon ion laser, the ability to use confocal imaging with triple-labeled specimens is now available to researchers for a cost comparable to the previous argon ion laser-equipped microscopes. Although this article is limited to the use of LSCM for multicolor immunofluorescence studies, the issues discussed in this article should enable researchers to more fully exploit the capabilities of the available instruments for other types of studies (i.e., live-cell imaging and *in situ* hybridization) that require the detection of multiple signals from a single specimen.

## Acknowledgments

We would like to thank our colleague Robert Elde for continued guidance and support in the use of LSCM for multicolor immunofluorescence studies. We also wish to thank Bio-Rad Microscience (Cambridge, MA) and Ion Laser Technology (Salt Lake City, UT) for collaborating in the development of the krypton–argon ion laser suitable for LSCM; Alan Waggoner (Carnegie-Mellon University, Pittsburgh, PA) for providing the cyanine dyes and unpublished data on various fluorophores; William Stegeman (Jackson ImmunoResearch Laboratories, West Grove, PA) for performing the various conjugations with cyanine 3.18, cyanine 5.18, and the R-phycoerythrin/cyanine 5.18 tandem conjugate; Debra Schindele and George Renzoni (formerly of Ultra Diagnositics Corp., Seattle, WA) for providing samples of various Ultralight dyes; Diether Recktenwald (Becton Dickinson, San Jose, CA) for providing samples of PerCP and its conjugates; Rosaria Haugland and Sam Wells (Molecular Probes, Eugene, OR) for providing samples of various BODIPY and Cascade Blue conjugates. The many helpful discussions and critical reading of this article by William Stegeman, Cynara Ko, Alan Waggoner, and Brian Matsumoto are gratefully acknowledged. We would like to thank Paul Letourneau, Stanley Erlandsen, David Scharp, and Paul Lacy for donating various specimens. We also wish to thank Jianlin Wang, Celest Roth, Steve Schnell, and Jane Wobken for excellent technical assistance, and Jerry Sedgewick for photographic assistance.

This work was supported by PHS Grants DK-33655 from NIH (R.L.S.), DA-05466 from ADAMHA (M.W.W.), and the Department of Cell Biology and Neuroanatomy (University of Minnesota). The donation of the large number of fluorophore-conjugated secondary antibodies used in these studies by Jackson ImmunoResearch Laboratories, and the payment of the publication costs by Bio-Rad Microscience for the color plates in this article are gratefully acknowledged.

## References

Afar, B., Merrill, J., and Clark, E. A. (1991). *J. Clin. Immunol.* **11**, 254–261.

Akinyemi, O., Boyde, A., Browne, M. A., Hadravsky, M., and Petran, M. (1992). *Scanning* **14**, 136–143.

Akner, G., Mossberg, K., Wikström, A. C., Sundquist, K. G., and Gustafsson, J. Å. (1991). *J. Steroid Biochem. Mol. Biol.* **39**, 419–432.

Amos, W. B. (1988). *Cell Motil. Cytoskeleton* **10**, 54–61.

Arndt-Jovin, D. J., Robert-Nicoud, M., and Jovin, T. M. (1990). *J. Microsc. (Oxford)* **157**, 61–72.

Art, J. (1990). *In* "Handbook of Biological Confocal Microscopy" (J. B. Pawley, ed.), Rev. Ed., pp. 127–139. Plenum, New York.

Aubin, J. E. (1979). *J. Histochem. Cytochem.* **27**, 36–43.

Benson, R. C., Meyer, R. A., Zaruba, M. E., and McKhann, G. M. (1979). *J. Histochem. Cytochem.* **27**, 44–48.

Blakeslee, D., and Baines, M. G. (1976). *J. Immunol. Methods* **13**, 305–320.

Bliton, C., Lechleiter, J., and Clapham, D. E. (1993). *J. Microsc.* **169**, 15–26.

Brakenhoff, G. H., Blom, P., and Barends, P. (1979). *J. Microsc.* (*Oxford*) **117**, 219–232.

Brakenhoff, G. H., Van Der Voort, H. T. M., Van Spronsen, E. A., and Nanninga, N. (1989a). *J. Microsc.* (*Oxford*) **153**, 151–159.

Brakenhoff, G. H., Van Spronsen, E. A., Van Der Voort, H. T. M., and Nanninga, N. (1989b). *Methods Cell Biol.* **30B**, 379–398.

Brakenhoff, G. H., Visscher, K., and Van Der Voort, H. T. M. (1990). *In* "Handbook of Biological Confocal Microscopy" (J. B. Pawley, ed.), 2nd Ed., pp. 87–91. Plenum, New York.

Brelje, T. C., and Sorenson, R. L. (1991). *Endocrinology* **128**, 45–57.

Brelje, T. C., and Sorenson, R. L. (1992). U.S. Pat. 5,127,730.

Brelje, T. C., Sharp, D. W., and Sorenson, R. L. (1989). *Diabetes* **38**, 808–814.

Brodin, L., Ericsson, M., Mossberg, K., Hökfelt, T., Ohta, Y., and Grillner, S. (1988). *Exp. Brain Res.* **73**, 441–446.

Buurman, E. P., Sanders, R., Draaijer, A., Gerritsen, H. C., Van Veen, J. J. F., Houpt, P. M., and Levine, Y. K. (1992). *Scanning* **14**, 155–159.

Carlsson, K. (1990). *J. Microsc.* (*Oxford*) **157**, 21–27.

Carlsson, K. (1991). *J. Microsc.* (*Oxford*) **163**, 167–178.

Carlsson, K., and Mossberg, K. (1992). *J. Microsc.* (*Oxford*) **167**, 23–37.

Chapple, M. R., Johnson, G. D., and Davidson, R. S. (1988). *J. Immunol. Methods* **111**, 209–217.

Chen, R. F. (1969). *Arch. Biochem. Biophys.* **133**, 263–276.

Cheng, P. C., and Summers, R. G. (1990). *In* "The Handbook of Confocal Imaging" (J. Pawley, ed.), Rev. Ed., pp. 179–195. Plenum, New York.

Cogswell, C. J., Hamilton D. K., and Sheppard, C. J. R. (1992). *J. Microsc.* **165**, 49–60.

Coons, A. H., and Kaplan, M. H. (1950). *J. Exp. Med.* **91**, 1–13.

DeBiasio, R., Bright, G. R., Ernst, L. A., Waggoner, A. S., and Taylor, D. L. (1987). *J. Cell Biol.* **105**, 1613–1622.

Delia, D., Martinez, E., Fontanella, E., and Aiello, A. (1991). *Cytometry* **12**, 537–544.

Denk, W., Strickler, J. H., and Webb, W. W. (1990). *Science* **248**, 73–76.

Elde, R., Cao, Y., Cintra, A., Brelje, T. C., Pelto-Huikko, M., Junttila, T., Fuxe, K., Pettersson, R. F., and Hökfelt, T. (1991). *Neuron* **7**, 349–364.

Erlandsen, S. L., Bemrick, W. J., Schupp, D. E., Shields, J. M., Jarroll, E. L., Sauch, J. F., and Pawley, J. B. (1990). *J. Histochem. Cytochem.* **38**, 625–632.

Fehon, R. G., Kooh, P. J., Rebay, I., Regan, C. L., Xu, T., Mushkavitch, M. A. T., and Artavanis-Tsakonas, S. (1990). *Cell* **61**, 523–534.

Feston, R., Björkland, A., and Tötterman, T. H. (1990). *J. Immunol. Methods* **126**, 69–78.

Fox, M. H., Arndt-Jovin, D. J., Jovin, T. M., Bamann, P. H., and Robert-Nicoud, M. (1991). *J. Cell Sci.* **99**, 247–253.

Fricker, M. D., and White, N. S. (1992). *J. Microsc.* **166**, 29–42.

Fritschy, J. M., Benke, D., Mertens, S., Oertel, W. H., Bachi, T., and Möhler, H. (1992). *Proc. Natl. Acad. Sci. U.S.A.* **89**, 6726–6730.

Gailbraith, G. M., Gailbraith, R. M., and Faulk, W. P. (1978). *J. Clin. Lab. Immunol.* **1**, 163–167.

Galbraith, W., Ernst, L. A., Taylor, D. L., and Waggoner, A. S. (1989). *Soc. Photo-Opt. Instrum. Eng.* **1063**, 19–20.

Galbraith, W., Wagner, M. C. E., Chao, J., Abaza, M., Ernst, L. A., Nederlof, M. A., Hartsock, R. J., Taylor, D. L., and Waggoner, A. S. (1991). *Cytometry* **12**, 579–596.

Giloh, H., and Sedat, J. W. (1982). *Science* **217**, 1252–1255.

Glazer, A. N. (1989). *J. Biol. Chem.* **264**, 1–4.

Glazer, A. N., and Stryer, L. (1983). *Biophys. J.* **43**, 383–386.

Goller, B., and Kubbies, M. (1992). *J. Histochem. Cytochem.* **40**, 451–456.

Gratton, E., and van de Ven, M. J. (1990). *In* "Handbook of Biological Confocal Microscopy" (J. B. Pawley, ed.), 2nd Ed. pp. 53–67. Plenum, New York.

Hansen, P. A. (1967). *Acta Histochem., Suppl* **8**, 167–180.

Haugland, R. P. (1983). *In* "Excited States of Biopolymers" (R. F. Steiner, ed.), pp. 29–58. Plenum, New York.

Haugland, R. P. (1990). *In* "Optical Microscopy for Biology" (B. Herman and K. Jacobson, eds.), pp. 143–157. Wiley, New York.

Haugland, R. P. (1992). "Handbook of Fluorescent Probes and Research Chemicals." Molecular Probes, Inc., Eugene, Oregon.

Hiramoto, R., Bernecky, J., Jurand, J., and Hamlin, M. (1964). *J. Histochem. Cytochem.* **12,** 271–274.

Hoffman, R. A. (1988). *Cytometry, Suppl.* **3,** 18–22.

Horikawa, K., and Armstrong, W. E. (1988). *J. Neurosci. Methods* **25,** 1–11.

Houser, C. R., Barber, R. P., Crawford, G. D., Matthews, D. A., Phelps, P. E., Salvaterra, P. M., and Vaughn, J. E. (1984). *J. Histochem. Cytochem.* **32,** 395–402.

Jahn, R., Schiebler, W., Ouiment, C., and Greengard, P. (1985). *Proc. Natl. Acad. Sci. U.S.A.* **82,** 4137–4141.

Johnson, G. D., and deC. Nogueira Araujo, G. M. (1981). *J. Immunol. Methods* **43,** 349–360.

Johnson, G. D., Davidson, R. S., McNamee, K. C., Russel, G., Goodwin, D., and Holborow, E. J. (1982). *J. Immunol. Methods* **55,** 231–242.

Khalfan, H., Abuknesha, R., Rand-Weaver, M., Price, R. G., and Robinson, D. (1986). *Histochem. J.* **18,** 497–499.

Kita, H., and Armstrong, W. (1991). *J. Neurosci. Methods* **37,** 141–150.

Kronick, M. N. (1986). *J. Immunol. Methods* **92,** 1–13.

Kuba, K., Hua, S. Y., and Nohmi, M. (1991). *Neurosci. Res.* **10,** 245–256.

Lang, M., Stober, F., and Lichtenthaler, H. K. (1991). *Radiat. Environ. Biophys.* **30,** 333–347.

Lanier, L. L., and Recktenwald, D. J. (1991). *Methods: Companion to Methods in Enzymol.* **2,** 192–199.

Lansdorp, P. M., Smith, C., Safford, M., Terstappen, L., and Thomas, T. E. (1991). *Cytometry* **12,** 723–730.

Larsson, L.-I. (1983). *In* "Handbook of Chemical Neuroanatomy" (A. Björklund and T. Hökfelt, eds.), Vol. 1, pp. 147–209. Elsevier, Amsterdam.

Lechleiter, J., and Clapham, D. E. (1992). *Cell* **69,** 283–294.

Loken, M. R., Parks, D. R., and Herzenberg, L. A. (1977). *J. Histochem. Cytochem.* **25,** 899–907.

Lynch, R. M., Fogarty, K. E., and Fay, F. S. (1991). *J. Cell Biol.* **112,** 385–395.

McKay, I. C., Forman, D., and White, R. G. (1981). *Immunology* **43,** 591–602.

Mathies, R. A., and Stryer, L. (1986). *In* "Applications of Fluorescence in the Biomedical Systems" (D. L. Taylor, A. S. Waggoner, F. Lanni, R. F. Murphy, and R. R. Birge, eds.), pp. 129–140. Alan R. Liss, New York.

Mesce, K. A., Klukas, K. A., and Brelje, T. C. (1993). *Cell Tissue Res.* **271,** 381–397.

Montag, M., Kukulies, J., Jorgens, R., Gundlach, H., Trendelenburg, M. F., and Spring, H. (1991). *J. Microsc. (Oxford)* **163,** 201–210.

Morgan, C. G., Mitchell, A. C., and Murray, J. G. (1992). *J. Microsc. (Oxford)* **165,** 49–60.

Mossberg, K., and Ericsson, M. (1990). *J. Microsc. (Oxford)* **158,** 215–224.

Mossberg, K., Arvidsson, U., and Ulfhake, B. (1990). *J. Histochem. Cytochem.* **38,** 179–190.

Mujumdar, R. B., Ernst, L. A., Mujumdar, S. R., Lewis, C. J., and Waggoner, A. S. (1993). *Bioconjugate* (in press).

Oi, V. T., Glazer, A. N., and Stryer, L. (1982). *J. Cell Biol.* **93,** 981–986.

Paddock, S. W. (1991). *Proc. Soc. Exp. Biol. Med.* **198,** 772–780.

Pagano, R. E., Martin, O. C., Kang, H. C., and Haugland, R. P. (1991). *J. Cell Biol.* **113,** 11267–1279.

Pawley, J. B. (1990). *In* "Handbook of Biological Confocal Microscopy" (J. B. Pawley, ed.), 2nd Ed., pp. 15–26. Plenum, New York.

Pearse, A. G. E. (1980). *In* "Histochemistry: Theoretical and Applied," 4th Ed. Vol. 1, pp. 159–252. Churchill Livingstone, London.

Recktenwald, D. J. (1989). U.S. Pat. 4,876,190.

Renzoni, G. E., Schindele, D. C., Theodore, L. J., Leznoff, C. C., Fearon, K. L., and Pepich, B. V. (1992). U.S. Pat. 5,135,717.

Robitaille, R., Adler, E. M., and Charlton, M. P. (1990). Strategic location of calcium channels at transmitter release sites of frog neuromuscular synapses. *Neuron,* **5,** 773–779.

Schindele, D. C., and Renzoni, G. E. (1990). *J. Clin. Immunoassay* **13,** 182–186.

Schmeud, L. C., and Fallon, J. H. (1986). *Brain Res.* **377,** 147–154.

Schormann, T., and Jovin, T. M. (1991). *J. Microsc. (Oxford)* **166,** 155–168.

Schotten, D. M. (1989). *J. Cell Sci.* **94,** 175–206.

Schubert, W. (1991). *Eur. J. Cell Biol.* **55,** 272–285.

Schweitzer, E. S., and Paddock, S. (1990). *J. Cell Sci.* **96,** 375–381.

Shapiro, H. M. (1988). "Practical Flow Cytometry," 2nd Ed. Alan R. Liss, New York.

Sheppard, C. J. R., and Gu, M. (1991). *Appl. Opt.* **30,** 3563–3568.

Sorenson, R. L., Garry, D., and Brelje, T. C. (1991). *Diabetes* **40,** 1365–1374.

Southwick, P. L., Ernst, L. A., Tauriello, E. W., Parker, S. R., Mujumdar, R. B., Mujumdar, S. R., Clever, H. A., and Waggoner, A. S. (1990). *Cytometry* **11,** 418–430.

Spack, E. G., Packard, B., Wier, M. C., and Edidin, M. (1986). *Anal. Biochem.* **158,** 233–237.

Staines, W. A., Meister, B., Melander, T., Nagy, J. I., and Hökfelt, T. (1988). *J. Histochem. Cytochem.* **36,** 145–151.

Stamatoglou, S. C., Sullivan, K. H., Johansson, S., Bayley, P. M., Burdett, I. J., and Hughes, R. C. (1990). *J. Cell Sci.* **97,** 595–606.

Stelzer, E. H. K. (1990). *In* "Handbook of Biological Confocal Microscopy" (J. B. Pawley, ed.), 2nd Ed., pp. 93–103. Plenun, New York.

Sternberger, L. A. (1986). "Immunocytochemistry," 3rd Ed. Wiley, New York.

Stewart, W. (1978). *Cell* **14,** 741–759.

Szarowski, D. H., Smith, K. L., Herchenroder, A., Matuszek, G., Swann, J. W., and Turner, J. N. (1992). *Scanning,* **14,** 104–111.

Titus, J. A., Haugland, R., Sharrow, S. O., and Segal, D. M. (1982). *J. Immunol. Methods* **50,** 193–204.

Tsien, R. Y., and Waggoner, A. (1990). *In* "Handbook of Biological Confocal Microscopy" ( J. Pawley, ed.), 2nd Ed. pp. 169–178. Plenum, New York.

Ulfhake, B., Carlsson, K., Mossberg, K., Arvidsson, U., and Helm, P. J. (1991). *J. Neurosci.* **40,** 39–48.

Van Dekken, H., Van Rotterdam, A., Jonker, R., Van Der Voort, H. T. M., Brakenhoff, G. J., and Bauman, J. G. J. (1990). *J. Microsc. (Oxford)* **158,** 207–214.

Van Der Voort, H. T. M., and Brakenhoff, G. J. (1990). *J. Microsc. (Oxford)* **158,** 43–54.

Van Oostveldt, P., and Baumens, S. (1990). *J. Microsc. (Oxford)* **158,** 121–132.

Vassy, J., Rigaut, J. P., Hill, A. M., and Foucrier, J. (1990). *J. Microsc. (Oxford)* **157,** 91–104.

Vincent, S. L., Sorensen, I., and Benes, F. M. (1991). *BioTechniques* **11,** 628–634.

Visser, T. D., Groen, F. C. A., and Brakenhoff, G. J. (1991). *J. Microsc. (Oxford)* **163,** 189–200.

Waggoner, A., DeBiasio, R., Conrad, P., Bright, G. R., Ernst, L., Ryan, K., Nederlof, M., and Taylor, D. (1989). *Methods Cell Biol.* **30B,** 449–478.

Wang, X., and Kurtz, I. (1990). *Am. J. Physiol.* **259,** C365–C373.

Weidenmann, B., and Franke, W. W. (1985). *Cell* **41,** 1017–1028.

Wells, K. S., Sandison, D. R., Strickler, J., and Webb, W. W. (1990). *In* "Handbook of Biological Confocal Microscopy" (J. B. Pawley, ed.), 2nd Ed. pp. 27–39. Plenum, New York.

Wells, S., and Johnson, I. (1993). *In* "Three-Dimensional Confocal Microscopy" (J. K. Stevens, L. R. Mills, and J. E. Trogadis, eds.), Academic Press, San Diego. In press.

Wessendorf, M. W. (1990). *In* "Handbook of Chemical Neuroanatomy" (A. Björklund, T. Hökfelt, F. G. Wouterlood, and A. N. van den Pol, eds.), Vol. 8, pp. 1–45. Elsevier, Amsterdam.

Wessendorf, M. W. (1991). *Brain Res.* **553,** 135–148.

Wessendorf, M. W., and Brelje, T. C. (1992). *Histochemistry* **98,** 81–85.

Wessendorf, M. W., and Elde, R. P. (1985). *J. Neurosci.* **7,** 2352–2363.

Wessendorf, M. W., Appel, N. M., Molitor, T. W., and Elde, R. P. (1990a). *J. Histochem. Cytochem.* **38,** 1859–1877.

Wessendorf, M. W., Tallaksen-Greene, S. J., and Wohlhueter, R. M. (1990b). *J. Histochem. Cytochem.* **38,** 87–94.

Wessendorf, M. W., Tallaksen-Greene, S. J., and Wohlhueter, R. M. (1990c). *J. Histochem. Cytochem.* **38,** 741.

Wetmore, C., and Elde, R. (1991). *J. Comp. Neurol.* **305,** 148–163.

Whitaker, J. E., Haugland, R. P., Moore, P. L., Hewitt, P. C., Reese, M., and Haugland, R. P. (1991a). *Anal. Biochem.* **198,** 119–130.

Whitaker, J. E., Haugland, R. P., and Prendergast, F. G. (1991b). *Anal. Biochem.* **194,** 330–344.

White, J. C., and Stryer, L. (1987). *Anal. Biochem.* **161,** 442–452.

White, J. G., Amos, W. B., and Fordham, M. (1987). *J. Cell Biol.* **105,** 41–48.

Wilson, T. (1989). *J. Microsc.* (*Oxford*) **154,** 143–156.

Wilson, T., and Sheppard, C. (1984). ''Theory and Practice of Scanning Optical Microscopy.'' Academic Press, San Diego.

Wories, H. J., Koek, J. H., Lodder, G., Lugtenburg, J., Fokkens, R., Driessen, O., and Mohn, G. R. (1985). *Recl. Trav. Chim. Pays-Bas* **104,** 288–291.

Yu, H., Ernst, L., Wagner, M., and Waggoner, A. (1992). *Nucleic Acids Res.* **20,** 83–88.

## CHAPTER 5

# Measurement of Intracellular pH with a Laser Scanning Confocal Microscope

## Ira Kurtz* and Cheryl Emmons*,†

*Division of Nephrology
Department of Medicine
UCLA School of Medicine
University of California, Los Angeles
Los Angeles, California 90024

†Wadsworth VA Medical Center
Los Angeles, California 90024

## I. Introduction

### A. pH Probes

Optical fluorescent methods for measuring intracellular pH ($pH_i$) in single cells are advantageous because these techniques yield spatial information and have a high sensitivity and rapid response time (Tanasugarn *et al.*, 1984). Since the introduction of carboxyfluorescein by Thomas *et al.* (1979), several new fluorescent pH probes have been developed that differ in their spectral properties and $pK_a$ (*Bioprobes*, 1991). The most widely used pH probe is

2′,7′-bis(carboxyethyl)-5,6-carboxyfluorescein (BCECF) (Rink *et al.*, 1982). Following its introduction in 1982, BCECF has been used to measure intracellular pH in a diverse variety of cell types. With a p$K_a$ of approximately 6.9 and a slow leakage rate, BCECF comes close to being the ideal pH$_i$ probe. To measure the pH$_i$, cells are exposed to the lipid-soluble acetoxymethyl ester form (BCECF-AM). Intracellular esterases hydrolyze the dye to the less permeant free acid, BCECF, within the cell. The BCECF is excited at approximately 490 nm (pH-sensitive wavelength) and at 440 nm (isosbestic wavelength) and the emission is measured at 530 nm. The 490/440 fluorescence excitation ratio is a function of pH$_i$. Intracellular calibration of BCECF is accomplished with high $K^+$ nigericin-containing solutions to clamp pH$_i$ at specific values (Thomas *et al.*, 1979).

Microscopic approaches allow the measurement of pH$_i$ in single cells configured as an epithelium or as a monolayer in culture (Tanasugarn *et al.*, 1984; Wang and Kurtz, 1990). Several methods have been described for switching the excitation wavelength with a white light source coupled to a microscope, including (1) a filter wheel stepping motor system (Tanasugarn *et al.*, 1984), (2) mechanical monochromator (Tsien *et al.*, 1985), (3) intensity modulator (Kurtz, 1987), and (4) acousto-optical tunable filters (Kurtz *et al.*, 1987). By coupling a two-dimensional detector such as an intensified silicon-intensified tube (ISIT) or charge-coupled device (CCD) camera instead of a photomultiplier tube to the emission port of the microscope, the pH$_i$ can be measured in various spatial locations in the *xy* plane (Tanasugarn *et al.*, 1984). Problematic, however, is that regular fluorescent microscopes have poor resolution in the depth (*z*) dimension. In epithelia composed of several cell types in the *z* dimension, such as the cylindrical kidney tubule or gastric gland, accurate pH measurements from a small volume of the cell becomes difficult because of the potential acquisition of out-of-focus fluorescence information. This is also true for the study of spatial pH differences in various compartments within a single cell, that is, cytoplasm vs nucleus, and endocytic vesicles. In these situations, it is preferable to use an optical approach, which offers the best resolution in the *z* dimension.

## B. Advantages and Disadvantages of Measuring pH$_i$ with a Confocal Microscope

The confocal microscope has markedly improved resolution in the *z* dimension (approximately 0.5 $\mu$m under optimal conditions) (Wells *et al.*, 1989; Wang and Kurtz, 1990). The resolution varies with the pinhole size, excitation wavelength vs emission wavelength (Stokes shift), and objective used (Wells *et al.*, 1989). Two types of excitation light are utilized: (1) scanning laser source and (2) white light source. The laser-based systems have a greater throughput with less overall light loss, and also have less image pixel-to-pixel variation because a single photomultiplier tube is used as the detector. However, slow image acquisition rates (one to four per second) and limited choice of excitation wavelengths are disadvantages of the laser-based systems. Typically a 25-mW argon laser that emits two wavelengths, 488 and 514 nm, is used. The 488-nm excitation wavelength is used to excite BCECF at its pH-sensitive wavelength; however, the isosbestic wavelength, 440 nm, is not excitable with an argon laser. As discussed below, a helium–cadmium laser (He–Cd) is needed as well. 7'-chloro-3'-ethylamino-2'-methylspiro [(isobenzofuran-1(3H),9'-(9H)-xanthen]-3-one-6-carboxylic acid (Cl-NERF) and 2',7'-dimethyl-6-hydroxyspiro-[isobenzofuran-1(3H),9'-(9H)-xanthen]-3-one (DM-NERF) transferrin and dextran conjugates are excited at 488 and 514 nm, respectively, and are ideally suited for measurement of pH in endocytic compartments with a confocal microscope coupled to an argon laser (Dunn *et al.*, 1991). A confocal microscope, with a two-dimensional detector, that is, ISIT or CCD camera, and with a Petran disk (Technical Instruments Co., San Jose, CA) coupled to a white light source, has several advantages: (1) wide wavelength selection and (2) a rapid image acquisition rate (30/sec). However, the white light-based systems suffer from decreased sensitivity and approaches to increasing the throughput thus far have led to decreased resolution in the $z$ dimension.

Because of the time it takes to acquire an image with some laser-scanning confocal microscopes, movement of the preparation is a serious problem and must be corrected before useful two- and three-dimensional measurements can be acquired. The microscope should be placed on a vibration-free table. In addition, the hose connecting the cooling fan to the laser source must be secured so as not to touch the table. An additional source of vibration is from solutions flowing through chambers containing biological preparations on the microscope stage. Laminar flow perfusion chambers will help decrease movement of the preparation due to turbulent solution flow.

## II. Materials and Methods

### A. Description of a Dual-Excitation Laser Scanning Confocal Microscope for Measuring $pH_i$

A dual-excitation laser scanning confocal microscope was designed in our laboratory for measuring intracellular pH with BCECF (Wang and Kurtz, 1990). In the original design, an MRC-500 lasing scanning unit (Bio-Rad, Richmond, CA) and more recently an MRC-600 scanning unit was coupled to the emission side port of a Nikon Diaphot microscope (Nikon Inc., Garden City, NY; Fig. 1). A ×1 projection lens was inserted in the optical path. This port was used to both excite and collect the flourescence information from the biological preparation on the microscope stage. A 25-mW polarized argon laser (model 5425A; Ion Laser Technology, Salt Lake City, UT) emitting at 488 and 514 nm and a 15-mW polarized helium–cadmium laser (He–Cd) (model 4214B; Liconix, Santa Clara, CA) emitting at 442 nm were coupled to the input port of the laser scanning system. The beams from the two lasers were combined by reflecting the 442 nm He–Cd laser with a 100% mirror (Oriel Corp., Stratford, CT) onto a dichroic

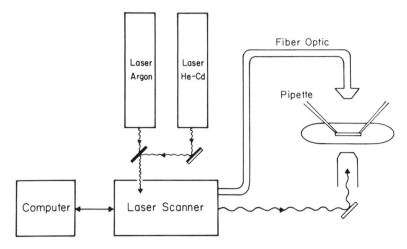

**Fig. 1**  Block diagram of a dual-excitation laser scanning confocal microscope. (After Wang and Kurtz, 1990.)

mirror (Omega Optics, Brattleboro, VT) placed at a 45° angle in front of the argon laser. The dichroic mirror transmitted the argon beam and reflected the 442-nm He–Cd laser to the input port of the laser scanner (Fig. 2). An electronic shutter (Vincent Assoc., Rochester, NY) under computer control was placed at an angle in front of each laser to prevent laser light from reflecting backward into the laser cavity. The shutters were alternately opened and closed by the computer. The timing parameters (duration of shutter opening, time between shutter 1 closing and shutter 2 opening) were software selectable. A ×40 fluorite objective [numerical aperture (NA) 0.8; Nikon] was used in all experiments. This objective was selected for its high throughput and minimal longitudinal chromatic aberration (Keller, 1989). An excitation filter cube that contained a dichroic mirror that reflected 442- and 488-nm light to the preparation was inserted in the MRC-600 scanner. A barrier filter (transmission, 500–650 nm) minimized scattered excitation light from impinging on the photomultiplier tubes in the MRC-600 scanner.

The preparation could be observed in the fluorescent mode (photomultiplier tube 1) and in the bright-field mode (photomultiplier tube 2) simultaneously. To acquire a bright-field image, the light above the preparation was collected with a fiber bundle and was detected with photomultiplier tube 2 in the MRC-600 scanner. The fluorescence information (excited with the argon and He–Cd lasers alone or sequentially) was measured confocally with photomultiplier tube 1 in the MRC-600 scanner. In an earlier version of the system, spatial information was sacrificed by focusing the lasers on a 0.6-$\mu$m spot in a single cell. The data from this voxel was digitized (20,000 samples/sec) with a Labmaster DMA board (Scientific Solutions, Cleveland, OH). The cell was exposed to laser light for a brief duration of time (2 msec/excitation ratio) to minimize bleaching. More

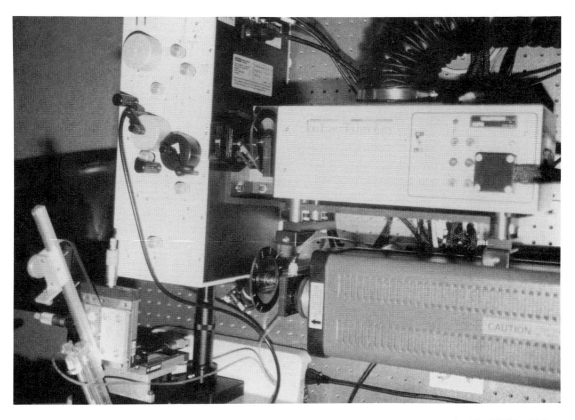

**Fig. 2**  Close-up view of the coupling of a 25-mW argon laser (*right*) and a 15-mW He–Cd laser (*left*) to the MRC-600 laser scanning unit.

recently, software has been written that uses the analog-to-digital (A/D) board in the MRC-600 system computer to control the timing parameters of the shutters and to digitize fluorescence images alternately at 488- and 442-nm excitation. A zoom factor of 1.5 to 8 times can be used. Initially, the computer captures a fluorescence image at 488-nm excitation. Up to eight regions of interest in the $xy$ plane (e.g., eight cells, or eight regions within a cell) are circled, using a mouse. The computer digitizes the data from these eight regions and stores the fluorescence intensity at 488- and 442-nm excitation from each of the eight selected regions as a function of time in an ASCII file, which can later be imported into a spreadsheet program. Background intensity due to scattered excitation light is measured outside the preparation and is digitized and subtracted from the fluorescence data at each wavelength. The excitation ratio from any of the eight regions is displayed as function of time (in real time) with or without background subtraction. Images (511 × 767 pixels) can be stored at software-selectable specified times throughout an experiment for later reference.

## B. Optical Properties of the Instrument

The following analysis applies to the MRC-500 scanner-based system. Radial and longitudinal chromatic aberrations and curvature of field reduce the resolution of confocal images (Keller, 1989; Wells *et al.,* 1989). To minimize radial chromatic aberration and curvature of field, data are acquired as close to the optical axis of the objective as possible (Wells *et al.,* 1989). Longitudinal chromatic aberration is minimized by using a fluorite objective (Keller, 1989).

The *z*-axis resolution (50% intensity value) of the system was measured in the fluorescence and reflected light mode. Figure 3A depicts the *z*-axis resolution in the reflected light mode at 488 nm, using the ×40 fluorite objective as a function of detector pinhole size. The resolution with the pinhole at 0.96 mm was approximately 1 $\mu$m. In the fluorescence mode, unlike reflected light imaging, the excitation and emission wavelengths are not identical and chromatic aberration prevents the excitation and emitted light from following the same optical path

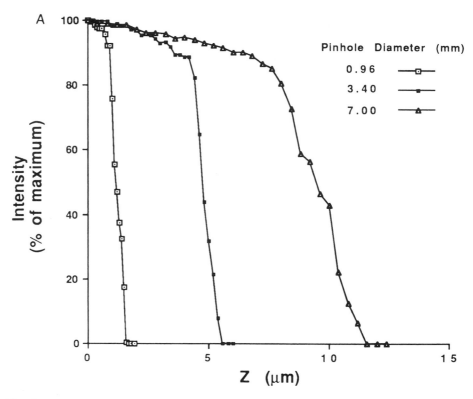

**Fig. 3** (A) *z*-Axis resolution of the system vs detector pinhole size (488-nm excitation). Measurement of the reflected intensity of a flat mirror was made at 0.1-$\mu$m steps on the optical axis. (After Wang and Kurtz, 1990). (B) *z*-Axis resolution, using a thin sample of fluorescing BCECF. Measurements in the fluorescence mode at 488-nm excitation (*top*) and 442-nm excitation (*bottom*) were made at 0.1-$\mu$m steps on the optical axis. (After Wang and Kurtz, 1990.)

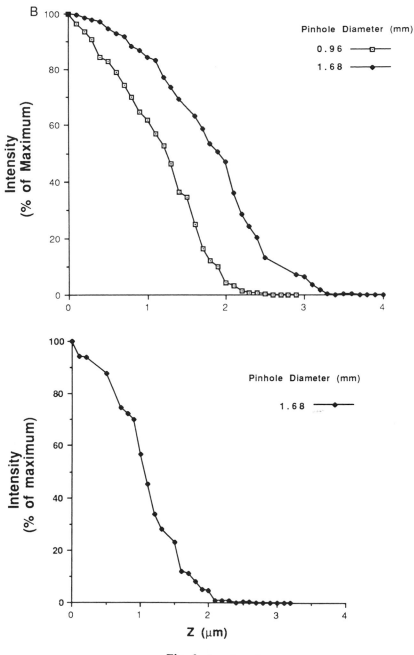

**Fig. 3** (*continued*)

(Wells *et al.*, 1989). The emitted light will not be imaged at the detector pinhole, causing the $z$-axis resolution to be less than in reflected light imaging. The decrease in the $z$-axis resolution will be a function of the Stokes shift of the dye (the separation in nanometers between the excitation and emission wavelengths). With a thin layer of BCECF excited at 488 nm and with the detector pinhole at 0.96 mm, the $z$-axis resolution was approximately 1.2 $\mu$m (Fig. 3B). With the pinhole at 0.96 mm, the signal-to-noise ratio was too low to acquire useful data. Therefore during any cell measurements, the detector pinhole was opened to 1.68 mm. The $z$-axis resolution at 488- and 442-nm excitation at this pinhole size is depicted in Fig. 3B. At 442-nm excitation, $z$-axis resolution is 1.1 $\mu$m, whereas at 488-nm excitation the $z$-axis resolution is 1.8 $\mu$m.

## C. Biological Applications

### Cortical Collecting Tubule

The cortical collecting tubule (CCT) is a heterogeneous cylindrical epithelium consisting of two main cell types: intercalated and principal cells (Fig. 4). Approximately 70% of the cells are principal cells. Thus fluorescent measurements with a laser scanning confocal microscope are ideal for the study of individual cells in this heterogeneous cylindrical epithelium. Traditionally, the principal cell has been thought to function in $Na^+$ and $K^+$ transport, whereas acid–base and $Cl^-$ transport has been attributed to intercalated cells. To study $pH_i$ regulation in individual principal cells, perfused CCTs were loaded with BCECF-AM. Basolateral BCECF-AM application results in homogeneous uptake of all cells (principal and intercalated) in the perfusing CCT. Principal cells were then identified by their smooth appearance with Nomarski optics. With the device described in this article, we have identified three types of basolateral $H^+$/base transport processes in the principal cells: $Na^+$-independent $Cl^-$/base exchange, $Na^+/H^+$ antiporter, and a $Na^+$/base cotransporter (Wang and Kurtz, 1990). Because the nucleus stains with BCECF in cells in the collecting duct, nuclear pH could also be measured. No difference was found between nuclear and cytoplasmic pH under resting conditions. Although we have not yet been able to identify an apical $H^+$/base transporter in principal cells, it may be that, under certain conditions, principal cells also participate in transepithelial CCT $H^+$/base transport.

Principal cells fluoresce less intensely than intercalated cells when exposed to luminal BCECF. However, principal cells and intercalated cells initially fluoresce similarly when exposed to basolateral dye, but subsequently principal cells lose fluorescence at a greater rate than intercalated cells (Weiner *et al.*, 1989). To explore the mechanism of the different patterns of fluorescence, CCTs were exposed to 30 $\mu$M basolateral BCECF-AM for 5 min and then the flowing bath was changed to a dye-free solution. The more rapid loss of BCECF from principal cells was found to be due to a basolateral $Na^+$-dependent, probenecid-

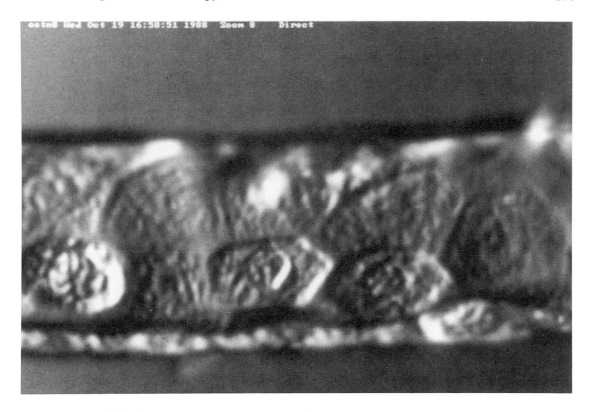

**Fig. 4** Pseudo-Nomarski image of an isolated perfused rabbit cortical collecting tubule. The larger polygonal cells are principal cells whereas the smaller cells are intercalated cells.

and stilbene-inhibitable organic anion transporter that transports BCECF (Emmons and Kurtz, 1990).

In separate experiments, the $Cl^-$-dependent base transport properties of intercalated cells were studied. The majority of CCT intercalated cells were thought to have an apical $Cl^-$/base exchanger, with a minority having a basolateral $Cl^-$/base exchanger. Using a laser scanning confocal microscope, it has been demonstrated that most intercalated cells in the rabbit outer cortical collecting tubule have both apical and basolateral $Cl^-$/base exchangers (Emmons and Kurtz, 1991).

## III. Future Directions

*Advances in pH dyes:* The most widely used intracellular pH dye is BCECF. As described earlier, this dye requires excitation with two different lasers. New pH dyes, called carboxy SNARF (seminaphthorhodafluor) and carboxy

SNAFL (seminaphthofluorescein), have been designed that are excited at a single wavelength (514 nm) and these dyes emit at two peak wavelengths with the intensity varying reciprocally with pH (*Bioprobes*, 1991). The two photomultiplier tubes in most confocal microscopes can be used to measure the intensity of the two emission peaks. The difficulty with these dyes is their high $pK_a$ values (7.5–7.9), which will likely preclude widespread use. Future development of intracellular cytoplasmic pH dyes based on rhodol derivatives with lower $pK_a$ values could lead to dual-excitation dyes that are excited at the 488- and 514-nm lines of a single argon laser.

*Measurement of pH in endocytic compartments:* Dunn *et al.* have designed a series of flourescent conjugates of dextran and transferrin based on two new rhodol dyes, Cl-NERF and DM-NERF (Dunn *et al.*, 1991). These dyes demonstrate a pH dependence at 514 nm and an isosbestic wavelength at 485 nm. The new compounds are trapped within endocytic vesicles and can be used to measure the pH of different acidic compartments in the endocytic pathway. The $pK_a$ of the Cl-NERF derivative is 3.0–3.5, whereas the DM-NERF conjugate have a $pK_a$ of 5.0–5.5. With these dyes it should be possible to generate three-dimensional maps of endocytic vesicle pH. This will require taking a set of images at both 488- and 514-nm excitation at various levels in the $z$ dimension and reconstructing, in three dimensions, the ratio images at each $z$ level.

*Future developments in optics hardware:* In most laser-based confocal microscopes, a single laser is mechanically coupled to the laser scanning unit. In the future fiber optic coupling will provide greater flexibility in the number of lasers that can be coupled to the scanner. Having the lasers in a separate area will free space on the floating table near the microscope. The ability to couple two or more lasers to the scanner will increase the number of excitation wavelengths that can be utilized.

To monitor biological phenomena that occur on a millisecond time scale in three dimensions (three-dimensional maps of cytoplasmic pH changes as a function of time) it will be necessary to increase the speed of data acquisition. One approach would be to acquire the images on an analog optical disk for digitization at a later time. This approach is still limited by the approximately one to four images/sec scanning speed of most laser-based systems. The latter will likely be increased in the near future so that these systems will be able to acquire 30 or more images per second. It is also expected that the sensitivity of white light-based confocal microscopes will improve, allowing a wider range of excitation wavelengths to be chosen and the data to be acquired with one or two two-dimensional CCT detectors (two detectors for dual-emission imaging).

## Acknowledgments

This work is supported by VA Career Development Research Associate Award (C.E.) and NIH Grant #851 IG-4 (I.K.). Dr. Kurtz is an Established Investigator of the American Heart Association.

# References

*Bioprobes*. (1991). Molecular Probes, Inc., Eugene, Oregon.

Dunn, K. W., Maxfield, F. R., Whitaker, J. E., and Haughland, R. P. (1991). *Biophys. J.* **59,** 345a. (Abstr.)

Emmons, C., and Kurtz, I. (1990). *J. Am. Soc. Nephrol.* **2,** 697. (Abstr.)

Emmons, C., and Kurtz, I. (1991). *J. Am. Soc. Nephrol.* **2,** 699. (Abstr.)

Keller, H. E. (1989). *In* "The Handbook of Biological Confocal Microscopy" (J. Pawley, ed.), pp. 69–77. IMR Press, Madison, Wisconsin.

Kurtz, I. (1987). *J. Clin. Invest.* **80,** 928–935.

Kurtz, I., Dwelle, R., and Katzka, P. (1987). *Rev. Sci. Instrum.* **58,** 1996–2003.

Rink, T. J., Tsien, R. Y., and Pozzan, T. (1982). *J. Cell Biol.* **95,** 189–196.

Tanasugarn, L., McNeil, P., Reynolds, G. T., and Taylor, D. L. (1984). *J. Cell Biol.* **98,** 717–724.

Thomas, J. A., Buchsbaum, R. N., Zimniak, A., and Racker, E. (1979). *Biochemistry* **18,** 2210–2218.

Tsien, R. Y., Rink, T. J., and Poenie, M. (1985). *Cell Calcium* **6,** 145–157.

Wang, X., and Kurtz, I. (1990). *Am. J. Physiol.* **259,** C365–C373.

Weiner, I. D., and Hamm, L. L. (1989). *Am. J. Physiol.* **256,** F957–F964.

Wells, K. S., Sandison, D. R., Strickler, J., and Webb, W. W. (1989). *In* "The Handbook of Biological Confocal Microscopy" (J. Pawley, ed.), pp. 23–35. IMR Press, Madison, Wisconsin.

# CHAPTER 6

# Confocal Microscopy of Potentiometric Fluorescent Dyes

**Leslie M. Loew**

Department of Physiology
University of Connecticut Health Center
Farmington, Connecticut 06030

## I. Introduction

### A. Overview of Fluorescent Methods for Measuring Membrane Potential

The use of fluorescent dyes to measure membrane potential was pioneered by Cohen and co-workers (Cohen *et al.*, 1974; Ross *et al.*, 1977; Gupta *et al.*, 1981; London *et al.*, 1986; Wu *et al.*, 1989) in an effort to develop methods for mapping activity in complex neuronal systems. Naturally, the indicators were required to respond rapidly in order to monitor the rapid voltage changes associated with action potentials. The fast potentiometric indicators are generally membrane stains that respond to changes in the electric field within the membrane via subtle conformational or electronic rearrangements. The fluorescence changes associated with an action potential correspond to 10–20% of the resting fluorescence for the best (i.e., most sensitive) of these indicators. This low sensitivity, together with the need for high-enough fluorescence intensities to give good signals in the milisecond time range, have dictated that electrical activity in excitable systems could be measured only with low spatial resolution.

A second class of dyes emerged from these studies and were developed by Waggoner (Sims *et al.*, 1974; Waggoner, 1979, 1985). These are positively charged cyanine dyes whose spectral properties have high sensitivities to membrane potential, albeit over slow time scales. The delocalization of the positive charge on these molecules renders them membrane permeant. Therefore the equilibrium distribution across the membrane may be governed by the Nernst equation:

$$\Delta V = -60 \log([dye]_{in}/[dye]_{out}) \text{ mV} \tag{1}$$

Thus the potential difference across the membrane, $\Delta V$, drives an uneven distribution of dye between the cell interior and the extracellular medium. For the cyanines, the dye distribution generally deviates significantly from that predicted by the Nernst equation because of significant binding to the plasma and organelle membranes and the tendency of these compounds to form aggregates when their concentrations exceed a threshold. Indeed, it is these features of the chemistry of the cyanines that make their spectral properties so sensitive to potential: membrane-bound dye displays enhanced fluorescence whereas dye aggregates have low fluorescence quantum yields. The cyanine dyes can therefore have complex spectral responses to potential that depend strongly on the cell to dye ratio, the hydrophobicity of the dye, and the particular cell type. Binding to mitochondria and possible responses to mitochrondrial potential changes add further complications. Still, with careful calibration protocols, these indicators have been extremely successful for studies of bulk cell populations and remain the best choice for such applications. They have only rarely been used for microphotometric measurements of membrane potential in single cells.

Using another delocalized cationic dye, rhodamine-123, Chen has developed methods for specifically staining mitochondria (Johnson *et al.*, 1980, 1981; Chen, 1988). The brightness provides a qualitative or relative correlation with the membrane potential of the mitochondria and mitochondrial uncouplers inhibit dye uptake. In a typical protocol, the cells are stained with 10 $\mu M$ rhodamine-123 in the presence of high extracellular $K^+$ to depolarize the plasma membrane. Excess dye is then washed away, so that the influence of mitochondrial potential on dye uptake is kinetic rather than steady state; the dye is not in true equilibrium (i.e., the Nernst equation cannot be rigorously applied) but remains essentially irreversibly bound to the mitochondria. The resultant fluorescent micrographs display the mitochondria in beautiful contrast, especially for the flat portions of cells spread on a substrate. Chen has introduced (Reers *et*

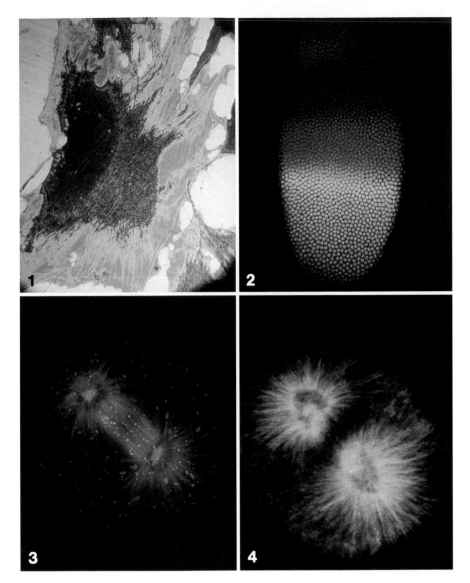

**Color Plate 1** (Chapter 1) Tandem scanning reflected light micrograph of a single optical section of Swiss 3T3 cells stained with Coomassie blue. The image was focused with a ×60 Plan-Apo, 1.4 NA objective at the cell–substratum interface and shows the striking color effect caused by reflection at the glass interface. The "real" image colors were photographed with a 35-mm camera equipped with a 55-mm lens mounted over the eyepiece as described by Paddock (1989). Stress fibers appear golden in color. [Printed with permission from Paddock, S. W. (1989). *J. Cell Sci.* **93**, 143–146.] **Color Plate 2** (Chapter 1) Confocal fluorescence image of a single optical section of a *Drosophila* embryo. The embryo was imaged with the Bio-Rad MRC-600 confocal microscope equipped with a krypton–argon ion laser. The distribution of *hunchback* and *Krüppel* segmentation proteins is shown in the cellular blastoderm-stage *Drosophila* embryo labeled with antisera raised against the *hunchback* (green label) and *Krüppel* (red label) proteins. The overlap region of expression is yellow. **Color Plate 3** (Chapter 1) Confocal fluorescence image of a single optical section of a double-labeled sea urchin (*Lytechinus pictus*) embryo in first mitosis. The embryo was imaged with a Bio-Rad MRC-600 confocal microscope equipped with a krypton–argon ion laser. Microtubules are labeled in green and centrosomes in red. **Color Plate 4** (Chapter 1) Confocal fluorescence image of microtubules (green), centrosomes (yellow), and chromosomes (blue), in a mitotic sea urchin (*Strongylocentrotus purpuratus*) embryo imaged with the tandem scanning confocal microscope. [Printed with permission from Wright, S. J., *et al.* (1989). *J. Cell Sci.* **94**, 617–624.]

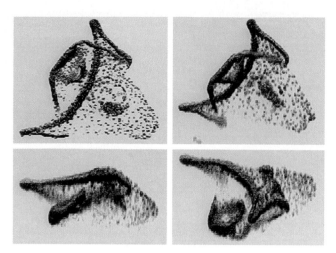

**Color Plate 5**   (Chapter 1) Portion of an animated sequence of a three-dimensional reconstruction, in which a *z* series of ~130 optical sections (taken 1.2 mm apart) of a sea urchin (*Strongylocentrotus purpuratus*) pluteus was volume rendered, generating 40 volumes at 9° increments. The sea urchin pluteus, stained with thiazole orange to label the nuclei, is rotated approximately every 45° in each panel. Individual optical sections of this volume can be observed in Fig. 16. [Printed with permission from Wright, S. J., and Schatten, G. (1991). *J. Electron Microsc. Tech.* **18,** 2–10.]

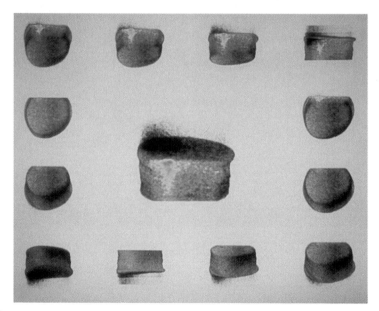

**Color Plate 6**   (Chapter 1) Reconstructions of optical sections taken (at the same focal plane) of a sea urchin (*Lytechinus pictus*) egg microinjected with the calcium-indicating dye, calcium green. Every 2 sec for a 10-min duration, optical sections were generated with a video-rate CLSM at a focal plane of the egg equator. During this time, the egg was fertilized. The individual optical sections (some of which are shown in Fig. 18) were then stacked together and rendered to yield a cylindrical reconstruction that shows alterations in the calcium green fluorescence of the selected focal plane over time. The center image is a longitudinal section of the cylinder and shows the specific pattern of fluorescence of calcium green induced by fertilization. The smaller peripheral images represent different views of the same three-dimensional reconstruction displayed in the center image, and show fluctuations in calcium green fluorescence as viewed from the outside of the egg over time.

**5-HT / FITC
SP / LRSC**

**SP / FITC
5-HT / LRSC**

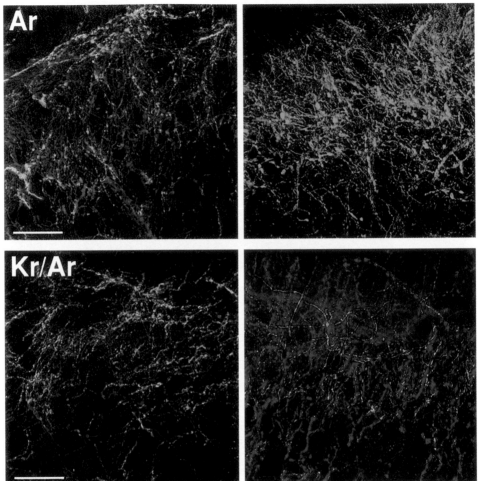

**Color Plate 7** (Chapter 4) Comparison of two-color imaging, using simultaneous excitation of fluorescein and Lissamine rhodamine with the 514-nm line of an argon ion laser (Fig. 10) and sequential excitation with the 488- and 568-nm lines of a krypton–argon ion laser (Fig. 17). Rat spinal cord sections were stained with goat antiserotonin (5-HT) and rabbit antisubstance P (SP) antisera, and visualized with the combination of fluorescein (FITC)-conjugated donkey anti-goat IgG and Lissamine rhodamine (LRSC)-conjugated donkey anti-rabbit IgG (left), or Lissamine rhodamine-conjugated anti-goat IgG and fluorescein-conjugated donkey anti-rabbit IgG (right). All secondary antibodies were used as 1:100 dilutions. With the argon ion laser (Ar), a separate population of fibers appears to be stained with the first combination of secondary antibodies (top, left), but they appear to coexist in the same fibers when the fluorophores were switched (top, right). In the latter case, the bright SP staining with fluorescein contributes more to the red fluorescence signal than the weaker 5-HT staining with Lissamine rhodamine. The considerable differences observed between these two images demonstrate how the choice of fluorophores can dramatically affect conclusions, using the argon ion laser. In contrast, when the same specimens were examined with the krypton–argon ion laser, separate populations of fibers are observed for both combinations of fluorophores (bottom, left and right). Each image is a projection of either 16 (top) or 20 (bottom) optical sections acquired at 1.0 μm. Nikon ×60, NA 1.4.

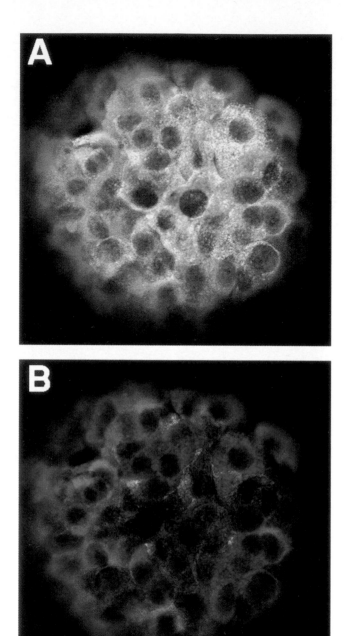

**Color Plate 8** (Chapter 4) Merged display of the observed and "corrected" images shown in Fig. 26 of a triple-labeled rat islet of Langerhans, using an argon ion laser. The green (green), red (red), and far red (blue) fluorescence images are shown as collected (A) and after correction for cross-talk between the images (B). Although the cross-talk compensation dramatically improves the separation of the fluorescence signals, several cells still appear to be possibly double-labeled. These images were manually shifted to correct for the misalignment of the individual images resulting from the use of separate filter sets. Scale bar = 25μm.

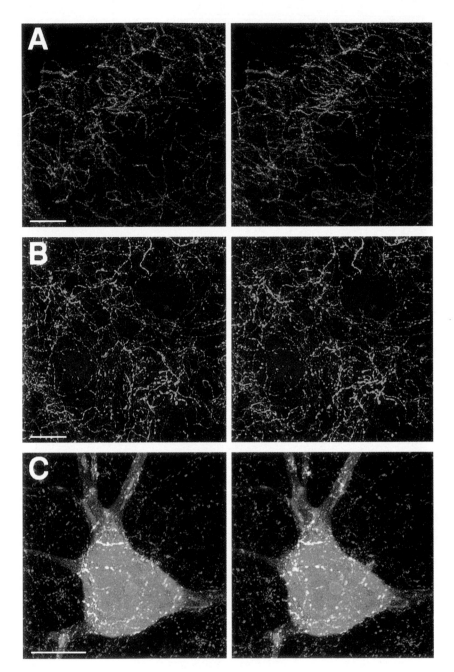

**Color Plate 9** (Chapter 4) Stereo images of double-labeled rat spinal cord specimens, using a krypton–argon ion laser. Rat spinal cord sections were stained with goat antiserotonin and rabbit antisubstance P antisera, followed by fluorescein-conjugated donkey anti-goat (green) and Lissamine rhodamine-conjugated donkey anti-rabbit (red) IgGs (multiple species adsorbed). In the dorsal horn (A), the neurotransmitters are observed in separate populations of fibers. In contrast, in the ventral horn (B) the co-existence of serotonin and substance P is observed. Note that the nerve fibers appear to be positioned around large cells resembling motor neurons. To examine whether these cells might be motor neurons, the motor neurons were stained by retrograde labeling from the sciatic nerve with hydroxystilbamidine (Fluoro-Gold). In spinal cord sections, individual fluorogold-labeled motor neurons were intracellularly injected with Lucifer yellow, and subsequently stained with a rat antisubstance P monoclonal antibody and cyanine 5.18-conjugated donkey anti-rat IgG. This allowed the visualization of both the motor neuron (yellow) and the substance P fibers (blue) wrapping around its surface with the confocal microscope (C). The stereo projections were constructed from 25, 29, and 51 optical sections, respectively, acquired at 0.8-μm intervals. Scale bars = 25 μm. Nikon ×60, NA 1.4.

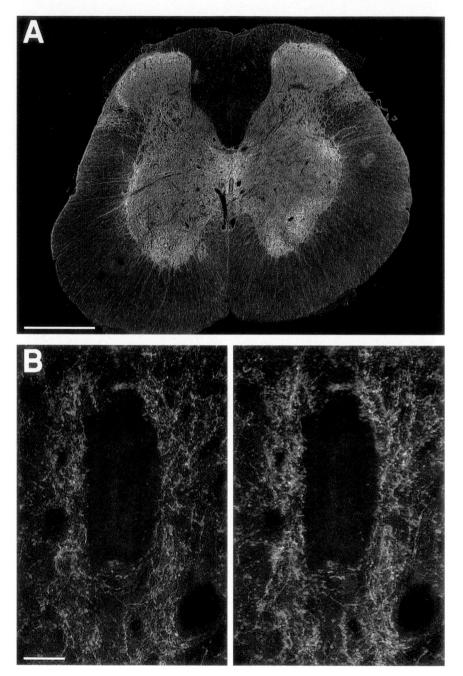

**Color Plate 10** (Chapter 4) Merged images of a triple-labeled rat spinal cord, using a krypton–argon ion laser. Spinal cord sections were stained with goat antiserotonin antiserum and fluorescein-conjugated donkey anti-goat IgG (green), a rat antisubstance P monoclonal antibody and cyanine 3.18-conjugated donkey anti-rat IgG (red), and rabbit anti-Met-enkephalin antiserum and cyanine 5.18-conjugated donkey anti-rabbit IgG (blue). The fluorophore-conjugated secondary antibodies were adsorbed against serum proteins from multiple species to reduce cross-reactivity. (A) A low-magnification image obtained by combining images collected from two fields of view. Laser illumination intensity was 4 mW for the imaging of all three fluorophores. Scale bar = 100 μm. Olympus ×4, NA 0.13. (B) A stereo pair of the region around the central canal of the spinal cord at higher magnification. The stereo projections were constructed from 17 images acquired at 0.6-μm intervals. Laser illumination intensity was 0.4 mW for the imaging of all three fluorophores. Scale bar = 25 μm. Nikon ×60, NA 1.4. (Specimen courtesy of J. Wang and R. Elde.)

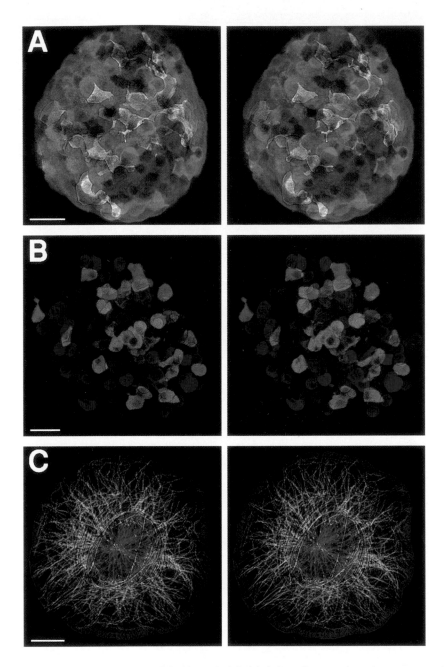

**Color Plate 11** (Chapter 4) Stereo images of double- and triple-labeled specimens, using a krypton–argon ion laser. (A) Triple-labeled rat islet of Langerhans. This stereo pair was formed from the merging of the images of the insulin (green), somatostatin (red), and glucagon (blue) shown in Fig. 32. In this merged image, the somatostatin-containing δ cells can be seen to be positioned between the glucagon-containing α cells on the surface of the islet and the insulin-containing β cells that comprise the majority of cells in the islet. Scale bar = 25 μm. (B) Double-labeled human islet of Langerhans. Islets were stained with rabbit anti-somatostatin antiserum and cyanine 3.18-conjugated donkey anti-rabbit IgG (red), and a mouse anti-glucagon monoclonal antibody and cyanine 5.18-conjugated donkey anti-mouse IgG (blue). The stereo projections were constructed from 62 optical sections acquired at 1.0-μm intervals. Scale bar = 25 μm. Olympus ×40, NA 0.85. (C) A non-neuronal cell from a chicken dorsal root ganglion culture. Actin filaments were stained with fluorescein-conjugated phalloidin (red) and microtubules with a mouse antitubulin monoclonal antibody and cyanine 3.18-conjugated donkey anti-mouse IgG (green). The stereo projections were constructed from 12 optical sections acquired at 0.6-μm intervals. Scale bar = 10 μm. Nikon ×60, NA 1.4. (Specimen courtesy of P. Letourneau.)

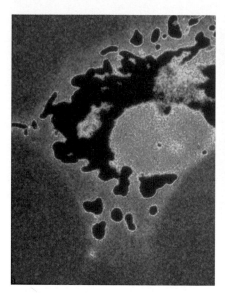 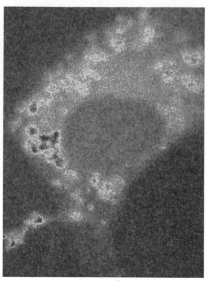

**Color Plate 12** (Chapter 6) (Left) The data of Fig. 3b after 20-fold expansion of the intensity scale and application of a spectral pseudocolor map. The mitochondrial regions of the cell are all saturated at the red end of the scale but the fluorescence from the nucleus and extracellular medium is now apparent. The relative fluorescence between the cytosol (i.e., nucleus) and the extracellular medium is 8.5:1. (Right) The same cell after treatment with a medium containing 1 μm valinomycin and in which $Na^+$ is replaced with $K^+$. This treatment effectively depolarizes both the plasma and mitochondrial membranes. Again the scale is expanded and a pseudocolor map is applied in order to visualize the contrast between the cytosol and the extracellular medium. The relative fluorescence is 2.5:1, indicating a small level of nonpotentiometric binding of dye. Dye association with depolarized mitochondria amounts to another factor of 3.

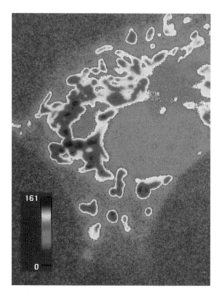 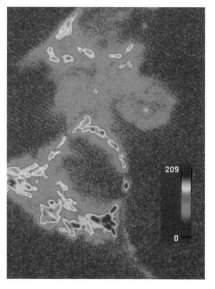

**Color Plate 13** (Chapter 6) Potential distributions via a logarithmic transformation of the intensity data. A pair of images are shown in which the intensities are corrected for nonpotentiometric binding and then transformed via Eq. (2). The scales indicate the level of polarization (negative potentials in millivolts) represented by the spectral color map. The image on the left is derived from the same cell as in Figs. 3 and Color Plate 12. Because a given mitochondrion is not necessarily well centered in the plane of focus or may be smaller than the effective depth of focus, mitochondrial potential may be underestimated while the width of the distribution of potentials among them may be exaggerated by these images.

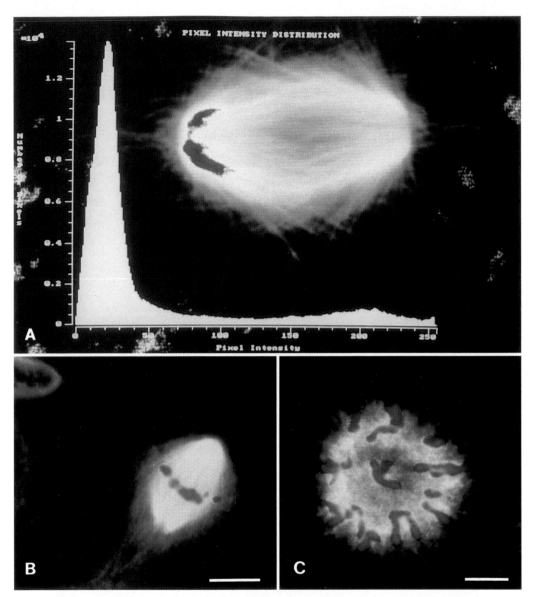

**Color Plate 14**   (Chapter 9) (A) Optimizing gain and black level: using a false-color LUT during image collection. The spindle shown in Fig. 1F is displayed, using a false-color LUT in which peak pixel values (255) are displayed as red, minimum pixel values (0) are green, and intermediate pixel values are displayed in shades of cyan (the setcol . cmd supplied with the Bio-Rad MRC-600: R 245 = 0; G 1 = 255, 5 = 5, 245 = 245, 250 = 0, 255 = 0; B 245 = 245, 250 = 0, 255 = 0). Used during image collection, this LUT aids setting of the photomultiplier gain and black level to optimize use of the gray scale (note that all pixel values are represented in the overlying intensity distribution). (B and C) Dual fluorescence of microtubules and chromosomes, using propidium iodide. Metaphase II meiotic spindles [note the polar body in (A), upper left] stained with antitubulin and propidium iodide are shown in both lateral (B) and polar views (C) (from Gard, 1992). Although the methanol fixation used for these samples is not optimal for microtubules, the overall preservation of spindle morphology is acceptable. Images were collected with a dual-wavelength filter set for fluorescein and Texas Red (supplied with the MRC-600) and were merged with a 7-bit interlaced pixel algorithm (the nmerge command in SOM 4.6 software supplied with the Bio-Rad MRC-600). Scale bars = 10 μm in (B) and 5 μm in (C).

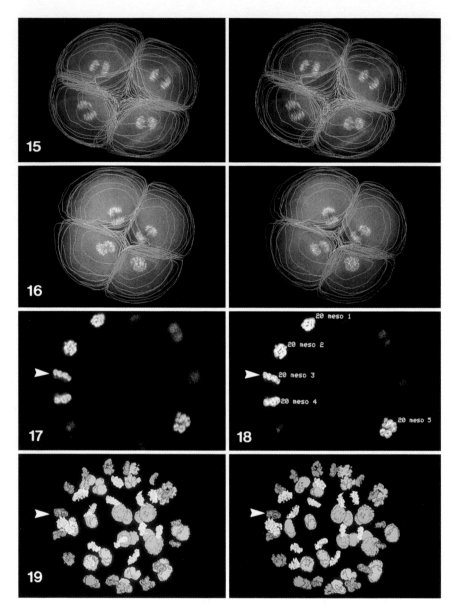

**Color Plate 15** (Chapter 10) Stereo pair of animal hemisphere of an embryo in anaphase of fourth cleavage and viewed from the blastocoel, in which original confocal projections and STERECON contours are displayed simultaneously. Outlines of animal blastomeres (green), cleavage cavity (blue), and nuclear division axes (red) are shown. Projection prepared from 43 serial optical sections at 1-μm intervals. (Reproduced from Summers *et al.,* 1993, with permission of *Jpn. Soc. Dev. Biol.*) **Color Plate 16** (Chapter 10) Vegetal hemisphere of same embryo and with colors as in Color Plate 15. Projection prepared from 43 serial optical sections. (Reproduced from Summers *et al.,* 1993, with permission *Jpn. Soc. Dev. Biol.*) **Color Plates 17 and 18** (Chapter 10) An optical section (number 20 of 81) through the vegetal hemisphere of an *S. purpuratus* embryo that is undergoing sixth cleavage division. Color Plate 17 has been contoured by contrast thresholding producing Color Plate 18. Each of the contours is encoded and stored in an overlay plane. Arrowheads indicate chromosomes labeled by arrows in Color Plate 19. **Color Plate 19** (Chapter 10) From the contours, as shown in Color Plate 18, three-dimensional renditions can be prepared. In this sixth, cleavage embryo, the macromere derivatives (blue) and mesomere derivatives (yellow and green) are dividing, while the micromeres (pink) remain in interphase. Arrowheads correspond to chromosomes in optical sections shown in Color Plates 17 and 18.

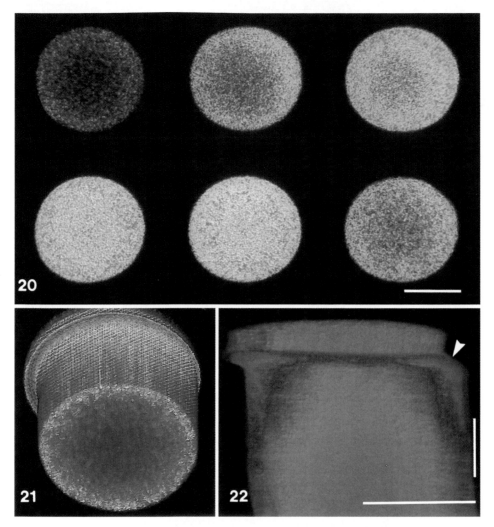

**Color Plate 20** (Chapter 10) A time-lapse laser scanning confocal microscope sequence of a single optical section through a fluo-3-loaded *L. pictus* egg that was undergoing fertilization. The upper left-hand frame shows the egg prior to the addition of sperm. Blue images in this pseudocolored figure represent relatively low fluo-3 fluorescence intensities. Note the increase in free calcium following fertilization as indicated by the increased fluo-3 fluorescence (red and white regions of the egg). The lower right-hand image shows the fertilized egg, after it had returned to prefertilization resting levels of free calcium. Scale bar = 50 μm.    **Color Plate 21** (Chapter 10) A volumetric reconstruction of the time-lapse data set such as shown in Color Plate 20. The individual optical sections of a fluo-3-loaded sea urchin egg have been stacked on top of each other to form a cylinder that represents the optical section over time. The red region toward the top of the cylinder corresponds to the fertilization-induced calcium wave. **Color Plate 22** (Chapter 10) A reconstructed cylinder of time-lapse confocal optical sections through a fluo-3-loaded *L. pictus* egg undergoing fertilization. The cylinder has been cleaved longitudinally to show the fertilization-induced calcium wave (arrowhead). Horizontal scale bar = 50 μm; vertical scale bar = 1 min.

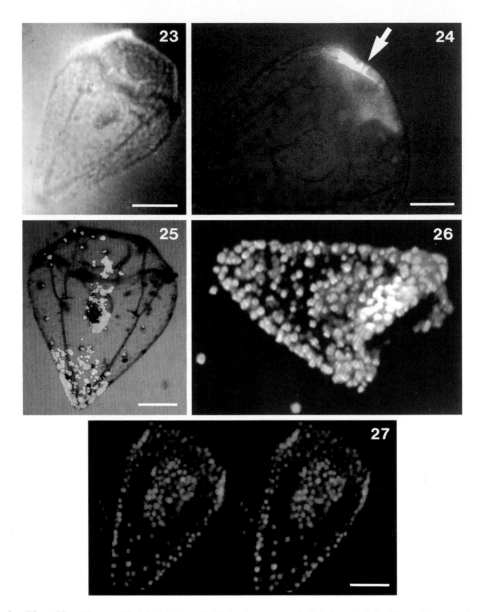

**Color Plate 23**   (Chapter 10) A facial view of a 72-hr pluteus turned slightly to the left of the embryo. The image was photographed on 35-mm film from the video monitor. This particular example is labeled in the ciliated band on the viewer's upper left. The labeled cells are derived from the right NL2 eight-cell blastomere. Bar = 30 μm.
**Color Plate 24**   (Chapter 10) A facial view of a double-labeled embryo rendered as a three-color 24-bit image. The blue portion is the bright-field image, the green portion is the fluorescein-conjugated lineage tracer, and the red portion is the rhodamine-conjugated lineage tracer. Bar = 20 μm.      **Color Plate 25**   (Chapter 10) A confocal microscope projection series of fluorescent images superimposed on a bright-field image. The embryo is viewed from the anal side and the anterior is toward the upper right. Labeled cells are represented in yellow and the bright-field image is in green. Bar = 30 μm.      **Color Plate 26**   (Chapter 10) A three-dimensional reconstruction of the abanal half of a sea urchin pluteus. The embryo was prepared with a nuclear stain, propidium iodide, and a through-focus series prepared on a confocal microscope. The series of image planes were then processed with a three-dimensional rendering package (VoxelView). The completed image was printed on a Tektronics printer and the paper copy photographed.      **Color Plate 27**   (Chapter 10) A stereo pair of a propidium iodide-stained pluteus photographed from the monitor of a confocal microscope. The image planes spanned the central third of the embryo and eliminated the aboral ectoderm on both the anal and abanal sides. The cells of the left coelomic pouch can clearly be seen. Bar = 30 μm.

*al.,* 1991; Smiley *et al.,* 1991) a new dye, JC-1, which actually changes its fluorescence emission wavelength above a threshold mitochondrial potential; again, these studies have been limited to qualitative correlations.

Work in this laboratory has aimed at extending the use of permeant cationic dyes to permit quantitative imaging of membrane potential in individual cells (Ehrenberg *et al.,* 1987; 1988; Farkas *et al.,* 1989; Gross and Loew, 1989; Loew *et al.,* 1990). The idea was simply to substitute fluorescence intensities for dye concentrations in the Nernst equation to calculate the membrane potential. It became necessary, therefore, to find a dye whose fluorescence intensity both inside and outside the cell is proportional to its concentration. Thus the cyanines, which have the tendency to form nonfluorescent aggregates, are generally unsuitable. Similarly, dyes that bind strongly to membranes would distribute in a more complex manner than predicted by the Nernst equation. Also, the Nernst equation describes a steady state equilibrium rather than irreversible dye uptake, so rhodamine-123 cannot be employed in this way. Several commercially available delocalized cationic dyes were screened, including additional members of the rhodamine and cyanine class, in an effort to identify suitable "Nernstian" dyes for imaging of membrane potential (Ehrenberg *et al.,* 1987, 1988). Although none of these dyes were ideal, the data from these experiments permitted us to design and synthesize a pair of new dyes, tetramethylrhodamine methyl and ethyl esters (TMRM and TMRE respectively), which closely meet the requirements for Nernstian distributions.

Both of these new dyes are members of the rhodamine class and are in fact closely related to rhodamine-123. They are more hydrophobic than the latter and do not contain any hydrogen bond-donating groups; we believe these differences are what permit a reversible Nernstian equilibrium to be readily established with TMRE and TMRM. The time for equilibration varies somewhat with cell type over a range of about 20 sec to 3 min. Because of their high brightness, the dyes can be used at low enough concentrations so that dye aggregation is insignificant—even in the mitochondria, where dye can be concentrated up to 10,000 fold. The dyes are quite resistant to photobleaching and photodynamic effects (Farkas *et al.,* 1989) but should still be used with the minimum possible light exposure. The degree of background (i.e., nonpotentiometric) binding to intracellular components is relatively low compared to other delocalized cations. Corrections for background binding must be made, however, in order to obtain accurate membrane potentials; procedures will be described below.

Structures of some of the most important potentiometric fluorescent dyes are given in Fig. 1, together with brief descriptive data. Figure 1 serves to summarize how each class of dye can be utilized for different types of measurements. A series of comprehensive reviews on the chemistry and applications of potentiometric dyes can be found in Loew, (1988), in which additional details on this general subject may be found. However, with the above perspective in mind, the remainder of this article will concentrate on the use of the Nernstian dyes to quantitate membrane potential with the aid of confocal microscopy.

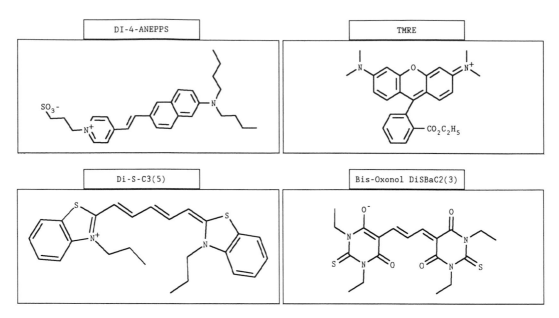

**Fig. 1** Structures and properties of some popular potentiometric dyes (TMRE is the focus of most of this chapter). DI-4-ANEPPS is a fast membrane-staining dye with excitation maximum at 470 nm and emission at 640 nm, (see Fluhler *et al.*, 1985). Dual-wavelength excitation may be used to ratiometrically map potential (Montana *et al.*, 1989). TMRE is a redistribution dye for single-cell measurements. Rhodamine filters are perfect for fluorescence microscopy (Ehrenberg *et al.*, 1988; Farkas *et al.*, 1989; Loew *et al.*, 1990). Di-S-C3(5) is a slow redistribution dye used for cells in suspension with a spectrofluorometer with high sensitivity. Many cyanine dyes with a choice of spectral properties are available for such applications (Waggoner, 1985). Bis-oxonol DiSBaC2(3) is a negatively charged redistribution dye that has been used mainly for cell suspensions but also in flow cytometry applications. Excitation and emission maxima are 535 and 560 nm, respectively, in ethanol (Brauner *et al.*, 1984).

## B. Application of Confocal Microscopy to Quantitative Imaging of Membrane Potential

The physical, chemical, and spectral properties of TMRE and TMRM make them appropriate dyes for microphotometric determination of membrane potential via a simple variant of the Nernst equation:

$$\Delta V = -60 \log(F_{in}/F_{out}) \text{ mV} \qquad (2)$$

The ratio of the fluorescence intensities, $F_{in}/F_{out}$, is taken to be equal to the ratio of the free cytosolic to extracellular dye concentrations used in the Nernst equation. As described above, this condition is met by TMRE or TMRM after a correction for a small amount of background binding. However, in practice, limitations of the optics, rather than the dye chemistry, have placed constraints on how readily the approach can be used. Specifically, it is difficult to determine fluorescence from a compartment as small as a cell and at the same time measure fluorescence from an equal volume in the extracellular medium. This is because a wide-field microscope will tend to dilute the in-focus intracellular fluorescence with the lower fluorescence from above or below the cell; the fluorescence from a point to the side of the cell is not so diluted because the concentration of dye is uniform in the extracellular medium at all points within the depth of the specimen. To fully appreciate this critical point it may be useful to consider an analogy with small and large cuvettes in a conventional fluorometer. If one wishes to compare the concentrations of a fluorophore in two different solutions with a fluorometer, it is necessary to measure fluorescence from solutions in cuvettes with identical dimensions. A large cuvette, with a longer path for the exciting light, will produce more fluorescence than a small cuvette for a given fluorophore concentration. In the fluorescence microscope, attempting to compare fluorescence from inside a cell to fluorescence outside is equivalent to using small and large cuvettes. Therefore, $F_{in}/F_{out}$ may be severely underestimated. On the other hand, in trying to quantitate fluorescence from the cytosol, the presence of mitochondria above or below the plane of focus can lead to artifactually high $F_{in}$; this is because the high mitochondrial potential can lead to intramitochondrial dye concentrations 1000 times higher than in the cytosol. These problems have been addressed with a microphotometer incorporating pinhole field and measuring apertures, to optically restrict the depth of focus, coupled with complex calibration procedures to correct for residual out-of-focus contributions (Ehrenberg et al., 1988).

A microphotometer is capable only of single spot measurements, however. To obtain spatial information with a wide-field microscope, one must be content to monitor qualitative changes in potential whether from mitochondrial or plasma membrane (Farkas et al., 1989). The confocal microscope offers a nearly ideal solution to this problem. The most distinctive feature of the confocal microscope—its ability to reject light originating from outside the plane of focus—is precisely what is required to measure fluorescence quantitatively from a compartment as small as the cell. This property is well demonstrated in Fig. 2A, which shows the exclusion of fluoresceinated dextran from a fibroblast. The dextran is used to mark the extracellular bathing medium surrounding the cell. With the focus centered 2 $\mu$m below the coverslip to which the cell adheres, almost no fluorescence can be measured intracellularly, whereas extracellular fluorescence at the same focus nearly saturates the digitizer circuit. The chamber to which the coverslip is attached provides a 200-$\mu$m blanket of medium bathing the cells. A comparable image from a wide-field microscope shows almost no contrast between the intracellular and extracellular space. The narrow depth of focus of the confocal microscope effectively defines a "cuvette" smaller than the intracellular compartment so that equivalent volumes of dye-containing solution are sampled outside and inside the cell. Figure 2B shows the distribution of fluorescence after TMRE is allowed to equilibrate with the same cell. It is clear from the result of Fig. 2A that it is possible to measure $F_{in}/F_{out}$ in

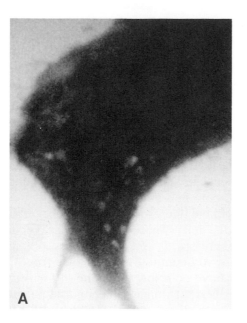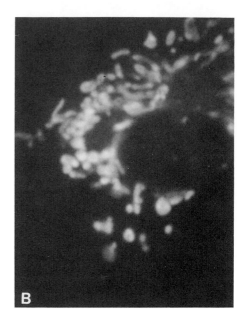

**Fig. 2** Confocal images of NIH-3T3 cells. A Bio-Rad MRC-600 laser confocal microscope was used with a Zeiss Axioskop microscope and a Nikon ×60 NA 1.4 Plan-Apochromat objective; the slow scan mode was employed with the confocal pinhole set at position 2. (A) Confocal image of a cell bathed in 4 mg FITC–dextran ($M_r$ 45,000) per ml, which marks the extracellular medium but does not penetrate the cell. A fluorescein filter set was employed to demonstrate the ability of the confocal microscope to exclude extracellular fluorescence from an optical section centered on the middle of the cell. The intensity measured from the center of the cell is at least a factor of 10 lower than the extracellular fluorescence. This image was obtained after a series of measurements with TMRE. (B) The same cell as in (A), showing the distribution of fluorescence from TMRE. The optical set-up was the same as in (A) except that a rhodamine filter set was employed. The cells were equilibrated with 0.1 $\mu M$ TMRE at 37°C for 5 min and a series of 30 laser scans was accumulated into a 16-bit image. A no-light background image was subtracted and the resultant image is displayed with a linear gray scale. Punctate fluorescence, corresponding to mitochondria, is prominent but, with this linear scale, the intensities from the cytosol, nucleus, and extracellular medium are barely perceptible.

Fig. 2B with confidence. In fact, it is even possible to approach the measurement of voltage across membranes of objects as small as mitochondria with Nernstian dyes (Farkas *et al.,* 1989; Loew *et al.,* 1990).

The use of confocal images to obtain precise information on the physiological state of a cell has been relatively rare; indeed, most of the articles in this volume deal with the ability of confocal microscopy to increase the definition of cellular and subcellular morphology. Therefore issues relating to the treatment of living cells in a confocal microscope and the extraction of precise fluorescence intensities from confocal images are not often considered. But consideration of such concerns is critical to the validity of membrane potential measurement. The remainder of this article describes how this laboratory approaches these issues;

the discussion should be helpful to any application of confocal microscopy requiring accurate fluorescence intensity measurements in living cells.

## II. Protocols

### A. Overview

The primary quantity to be measured is $F_{in}/F_{out}$ [Eq. (2)]. After equilibration with TMRE or TMRM, the intensities of light associated with the cytosol and an adjacent extracellular region can be obtained directly from a digital confocal image. These intensities need to be corrected for dark current and stray light. Any potential-independent binding of dye to the cell must be determined and the measured intensities appropriately adjusted. If potentials in mitochondria or thin cellular processes are to be determined, it should be established that these compartments are thicker than the limiting depth of focus of the microscope.

For the measurement to be meaningful, it is important to assure that the cells are maintained in physiological conditions during the experiment. Temperature, pH, $CO_2$, and oxygen tensions should all be controlled. Practical considerations may limit how well this ideal can be met. Also, even though TMRE and TMRM are relatively benign fluorophores, the high concentrations that are attained in mitochondria can lead to phototoxic effects. These are generally thought to arise from photosensitization of singlet oxygen production and can be especially severe with the high intensity of the exciting laser light in confocal microscopes (Tsien and Waggoner, 1990).

The studies in this laboratory were performed with a Bio-Rad (Richmond, CA) MRC-500 or MRC-600 laser scanning confocal microscope attached to a Zeiss (Thornwood, NY) Axioskop microscope. TMRE and TMRM are both rhodamine dyes that are readily excited with the 514-nm line of the argon ion laser; the standard rhodamine dichroic mirror and emission filter work well. Data analysis can be performed with the basic Bio-Rad software running on a 386 personal computer. It is advantageous to be able to analyze 16-bit images to deal with a wide dynamic range of fluorescence intensities (mitochondria can be 10,000 times brighter than the extracellular medium). We have employed a Silicon Graphics (Mountain View, CA) workstation for this reason, although PC and Macintosh software exists that can accommodate 16-bit images.

### B. Specimen Preparation

Studies in this laboratory have employed adherent cell lines, which can be grown on glass coverslips. Coverslips are used when cells reach approximately 20% confluency, so that ample cell-free regions can be found. After washing with a protein-free, well-buffered balanced salt solution containing 10 m$M$ glucose, the cells are mounted on a microscope chamber that permits temperature control and the exchange of extracellular medium. An example of a chamber used in our laboratory is shown in Fig. 3. The design can easily be modified for an inverted microscope or for rectangular coverslips. To avoid vibrations during image acquisition low flow rates from a high-quality thermostatted circulator should be employed. We prefer the use of this chamber for temperature control as opposed to a heated stage or a chamber in which heat exchange takes place around the perimeter of the coverslip. The latter cannot guarantee effective heat exchange in the region of the cells under observation; this is of special concern with high-numerical aperture immersion objectives, which act as efficient heat sinks. Ideally, continuous slow perfusion of medium will maintain concentrations of dissolved gases and nutrients; in practice, flow of medium is stopped before image acquisition to avoid agitation that would disturb the focus.

After acquisition of images in the absence of dye (usually identical to dark images because of the negligible autofluorescence of most cells at the rhodmaine

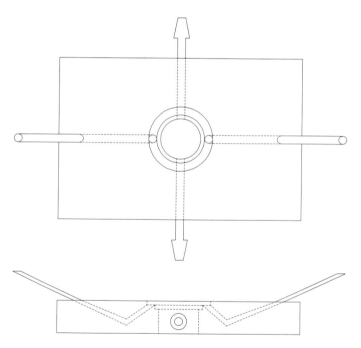

**Fig. 3** Diagram of a Plexiglas chamber, top view above and front view below, for maintenance of living cells during microscopic observation. Thermostatted water is circulated from the front to the back of the chamber via the hose nipples. The water is contained via a round coverslip glued into the inner ledge at the top and a glass plate glued onto the bottom (neither of these is shown). Cells are grown on a large glass coverslip that is then sealed onto the top of the chamber. This forms a narrow closed channel under the cells through which media can be perfused and exchanged via the metal tubes protruding from the sides of the chamber. The outer dimensions of the Plexiglas are $4 \times 3 \times 0.25$ in.

wavelengths), a solution of either TMRE or TMRM in the same balanced salt solution is perfused through the chamber. We have found little difference in the properties of these two dyes (Ehrenberg *et al.*, 1988; Farkas *et al.*, 1989); most of our work has been with TMRE. Above approximately 0.3 $\mu M$, we have observed some self-quenching of dye associated with mitochondria as well as indications of enhanced photodynamic damage. Therefore all of our work is carried out with dye concentrations of 50–100 n$M$. The time required for the dye to equilibrate across the plasma and mitochondrial membranes, thereby attaining a steady state fluorescence, varies with cell type and should be determined, especially if studies of the kinetics of potential changes are planned. About a dozen cell lines have been examined with TMRE in this laboratory and equilibration has always been complete in under 5 min at 37°C.

## C. Data Acquisition

The choice of parameters for image acquisition necessitates a decision pitting the four issues of spatial resolution, precision, minimal light exposure, and speed against each other. Each of these may be of critical importance depending on specific experimental requirements. In all cases, an objective with the highest possible numerical aperture should be used to minimize the depth of focus and achieve the greatest brightness. We have found that any of the various ×60 or ×63 Plan-Apochromat lenses with a numerical aperture of 1.4 provide excellent results in almost any situation. With such a lens, offered by many of the manufacturers of research microscopes, the size of the field of view can be adjusted over a range encompassing most animal cells by controlling the extent of the laser scan.

The measurement of plasma membrane potential can be achieved with rapid laser scanning over a low-magnification field of view. Because the potential is rarely over −80 mV, both the cytosolic fluorescence and the extracellular fluorescence can be determined within the normal 256 gray levels of an 8-bit confocal image. Care should be taken that the optical slice is centered around the middle of the cell. $F_{in}$ and $F_{out}$ may be determined as an average over many pixels within the respective compartments to increase the precision of the measurement. Color Plate 12 shows an image that may form the basis for this measurement. In many cells it is impossible to find a region of cytosol that is free of contaminating fluorescence from the bright and abundant mitochondria, even at a minimum setting of the confocal pinhole. In such cases we resort to measurement of fluorescence from the nucleus on the assumption that the large nuclear membrane pores preclude a potential difference between cytosol and nucleoplasm [this assumption may not be always valid (Mazzanti *et al.*, 1990)].

The dynamic range and resolution requirements are significantly more stringent if mitochondrial membrane potential is the subject of study. With a potential as high as −180 mV (Rottenberg, 1986; Brand and Murphy, 1987), the concentration of dye, and therefore the fluorescence intensity, may be three orders of magnitude higher in a mitochondrion than in the cytosol. Both intensities must be obtained to calculate membrane potential from Eq. (2). This may be achieved by measuring the mitochondrial potential with a strongly absorbing calibrated neutral density filter in the laser light path; this filter would then be removed to permit measurement of cytosolic (or intranuclear) fluorescence. Alternatively, data may be acquired into a 16-bit image to provide sufficient dynamic range for both compartments within a single frame. Also, the small size of mitochondria, typically 0.25–2 $\mu$m in diameter, requires a high pixel density and a minimum confocal pinhole for maximum three-dimensional resolution. It is important to be sure that the intensities are measured from mitochondia that are well centered in the plane of focus; a mitochondrion that is slightly off focus will display artifically low intensities. The acquisition of a limited three-dimensional data set consisting of a series of about five focal planes obviates this problem by delineating the disposition of mitochondria along the $z$ (i.e., optical) axis. These requirements force multiple exposure of the cell to the laser scan and necessitate long acquisition times. Therefore phototoxicity, photobleaching, or motion artifacts may become limiting factors in the success of mitochondrial membrane potential measurements. Color Plate 13 exemplifies the mitochondrial membrane potential distribution imaged with a confocal microscope.

To determine the level of nonpotentiometric binding, the potential across plasma and mitochondrial membranes can be set to 0 by treatment of the preparation with 1 $\mu$M valinomycin in a high-potassium medium. Valinomycin is a $K^+$-selective ionophore that clamps the membrane potential to the potassium equilibrium potential. It will depolarize the mitochondria, which have membranes with normally low potassium permeability. It will also depolarize the plasma membrane if the extracellular medium has a $K^+$ concentration comparable to the cytosolic $K^+$. This is illustrated in Color Plate 12 (*right*), in which the cell of Fig. 2 and Color Plate 12 (*left*) has been so depolarized. A small amount of dye remains bound to mitochondria and other intracellular membraneous organelles. This residual fluorescence can be used to correct Eq. (2) for nonpotentiometric binding according to the procedure outlined in the next section.

## D. Data Analysis

A prerequisite for quantitation of fluorescence intensities from a microscope image is a digital format to which an image analysis software package may be applied. Digital images are the direct output of laser scanning confocal microscopes and may also be obtained from the Nipkow disk systems by digitization of video output from a low light level camera. Any image analysis software capable of 16-bit arithmetic will then serve to extract quantitative information from these images. Background images obtained before the addition of the dye to the chamber, and acquired under the same instrument settings, should be subtracted from all fluorescence images prior to analysis. To determine $F_{in}/F_{out}$, small regions of uniform fluorescence inside and outside the cell are chosen, respectively, and the average intensities within them is calculated. After correction of this ratio for any nonpotentiometric accumulation of dye in the cell, the plasma membrane potential can be calculated from Eq. (2). This latter correction factor is obtained by depolarizing the cells with a medium containing high [K$^+$] and the potassium-selective ionophore valinomycin.

Color Plate 12 illustrates how this scheme is put into practice. The image in Color Plate 12 (*left*) was generated from the same data as Fig. 2B, by scaling up the data by a factor of 20 and applying a pseudocolor map to accentuate the contrast between the cytosolic fluorescence and the extracellular fluorescence. Naturally, the mitochondria-rich regions of the cell are pegged at the maximum brightness of the video display (i.e., fully red in the spectral pseudocolor scale). To avoid contamination from mitochondrial fluorescence, the cytosolic fluorescence intensity is taken as an average within a small nuclear region. The ratio of fluorescence intensities between the intracellular and extracellular spaces is 8.5:1. Color Plate 12 (*right*) shows the same cell after depolarization with high [K$^+$] and valinomycin. The intra- to extracellular fluorescence intensity ratio is now 2.5:1, indicating a small level of nonspecific binding. This binding is still reversible (i.e., linearly related to the amount of extracellular dye) and can therefore be used to directly normalize $F_{in}/F_{out}$ to 8.5/2.5 = 3.4. A full discussion of this analysis has been published (Ehrenberg *et al.*, 1988). The membrane potential calculated from Eq. (2) is − 32 mV.

Fluorescence associated with mitochondria is several orders of magnitude higher than nuclear or extracellular fluorescence. To correct for nonpotentiometric binding to mitochondria, the binding to depolarized mitochondria is determined [Color Plate 12 (*right*)]; typically, the residual fluorescence after depolarization is a factor of three higher in the mitochondria than in the surrounding cytosol. A logarithmic transformation of the corrected intensity distribution produces a new image with an intensity scale proportional to potential (Color Plate 13).

A pair of important caveats must be considered in interpreting such images, however. First, the image represents data from a single focal plane. Not all the mitochondria captured within this optical section will be well centered in this plane. An off-center mitochondrion may produce an artifically low intensity, resulting in an underestimate of its potential. Ideally, therefore, three-dimensional images containing several planes of data should be acquired and only those mitochondria that are wholly encompassed within the three-dimensional field of view should be analyzed.

The second caveat has to do with the inherent limitations of even a confocal microscope in attempting to quantify fluorescence from objects as small as mitochondria. For all practical purposes, the narrowest depth of focus that may be attained is about 0.6 $\mu$m. Therefore, to quantitate fluorescence without any correction, an object must have a width along the optical ($z$) axis greater than 0.6 $\mu$m. It is important to obtain electron micrographs to determine the size distribution of mitochondria in a cell line under investigation; this will establish whether the depth of focus is sufficiently narrow to lie within most of the mitochondria. If it is not, correction schemes can be devised with calibrated subresolution fluorescent microspheres, which are available from several manufacturers.

## III. Perspectives

### A. Limitations and Potential Improvements

An important problem for confocal microscopy of living cells results from the high excitation light levels required for adequate signal. In addition to the problem of dye bleaching, which cannot be countered with the toxic antifade reagents employed for fixed specimens, the high light levels produce photodynamic damage that can rapidly kill living cells (Tsien and Waggoner, 1990). This is believed to arise from photosensitization of singlet oxygen by the dye. In mitochondria, with their high TMRE concentrations, this is manifested as a dramatic swelling and release of dye to the cytosol. This problem severely limits the ability of the technique to follow changes over time by collecting a series of time-lapse images; the light dose absorbed by the cell under study limits such an experiment to only a few time points. In some cases, even a single three-dimensional data set is compromised.

The time required to acquire a single plane of 16-bit data, such as in Fig. 2B, can be as long as 30 sec, and this also may place limitations on the scope of questions the technique may be able to address. An obvious constraint is placed on the time resolution of any kinetic phenomenon that may be of interest, but this is also an inherent limitation of the dye, which can require minutes for a significant reequilibration. In addition, mitochondria are often highly motile within the cell and can move significantly during the time required for acquisition of an image. The resultant intensity will be blurred over a distance larger than the mitochondrion, resulting in an artifactually low estimate of its membrane potential.

Improvements in the sensitivity of confocal microscopes and the photostability of potentiometric probes may help alleviate both of these problems. In discussing sensitivity, it should be appreciated that the signal size per se is not at issue; a stronger laser can give a higher signal—at least to the point at which the excited states become saturated. Using stronger excitation will also increase the rate of photobleaching and phototoxicity, however. What is needed is additional optimization at the emission side to collect the fluorescence with maximum efficiency without sacrifice of spatial resolution. On the other hand, if more photostable dyes were available, higher light levels could be employed for excitation to produce amplified signals. In either case, more extensive data sets could be acquired more rapidly.

In measuring intensities from objects as small as mitochondria, the resolution limit of the confocal microscope does remain an important inherent limitation that cannot be overcome with any conceivable improvements. As noted above, it may be possible to estimate and correct for such limitations via careful calibration with a series of uniformly fluorescent microspheres with narrow size distributions. However, if electron micrographic examination of a cell line reveals the mitochondria to have a wide size distribution with dimensions significantly smaller than the confocal depth of field, it will be necessary to settle for an average estimate of the potential for the population of mitochondria within a cell; with larger, more uniformly sized mitochondria, assignment of potentials to individuals should be an attainable goal.

## B. Alternative Methods

Quantitative three-dimensional imaging can be achieved with a wide-field microscope by using computational methods to remove the out-of-focus blur (Agard, 1984; Carrington and Fogarty, 1987; Fay *et al.*, 1989). In this method, the optical characteristics of the microscope are defined by its point spread function, the three-dimensional distribution of light collected from a point source, such as a subresolution fluorescent bead. The point spread function is used to deconvolve a three-dimensional image data set by an iterative process often called image restoration. In effect, the out-of-focus haze collected by the microscope is restored to its point of origin within the imaged three-dimensional volume of the specimen. This can create images with resolutions as good as or better than confocal microscopy. In addition, this approach has the significant advantage of being much more efficient in collection of fluorescence emission. Confocal microscopy is based on the use of a pinhole to block out all the emission that does not originate from the focal plane; if sensitivity is defined (see above) as the efficiency of light collection relative to the level of the exciting light, it can be appreciated that confocal microscopy is inherently insensitive. Image restoration of wide-field images is based on the collection of all the emission from a three-dimensional specimen—the computation then places the light into its appropriate place. Therefore a much higher sensitivity and dynamic range are attained with a lower dose of exciting light.

Commercially available software has been introduced that uses a limited "nearest neighbor" deconvolution to remove out-of-focus blur and improve the quality of images from wide-field microscopes. To obtain quantitative intensity data on small fluorescent objects, however, a more extensive restoration must be performed on a data set containing sufficient optical sections to fully sample and bracket all the bright objects along the optical axis of the specimen. The approach, therefore, requires long computation times on powerful workstations or array processors. It also requires input images that are of high accuracy and low noise; this is usually possible only with slow-readout cooled charge-coupled device (CCD) cameras (Hiraoka *et al.*, 1987). The expense of this equipment and the complexity of the software have limited the spread of the image restoration approach. Rapid improvements in the software and hardware are progressing and will soon make the image restoration approach a viable and attractive alternative to confocal microscopy.

For some experimental applications, the use of membrane-staining potentiometric probes may provide an alternative to redistribution probes such as TMRE. Dual-wavelength ratio imaging has been demonstrated with these probes (Montana *et al.*, 1989), permitting the development of maps indicating variations in membrane potential along a cell surface. Coupling this approach with confocal microscopy will significantly improve the accuracy of these images and may permit the detection of membrane potential distributions and changes within subcellular organelles such as the endoplasmic reticulum (see [7] of this volume). Improvements in the sensitivity of fast membrane-staining probes will be required to realize such applications.

## Acknowledgments

The assistance of Dr. Mei-de Wei and Mr. Frank Morgan in obtaining the images in Fig. 2 and Color Plates 12 and 13 is gratefully acknowledged. This work was supported by the U.S. Public Health Service under Grant GM35063 and, for the purchase of the confocal microscope, under Grant RR03976.

## References

Agard, D. A. (1984). *Annu. Rev. Biophys. Bioeng.* **13,** 191–219.
Brand, M. D., and Murphy, M. P. (1987). *Biol. Rev. Cambridge Philos. Soc.* **62,** 141–193.
Brauner, T., Hulser, D. F., and Strasser, R. J. (1984). *Biochim. Biophys. Acta* **771,** 208.
Carrington, W., and Fogarty, K. E. (1987). *Northeast Bioeng. Conf., 13th, IEEE* pp. 108–111.
Chen, L. B. (1988). *Annu. Rev. Cell Biol.* **4,** 155–181.
Cohen, L. B., Salzberg, B. M., Davila, H. V., Ross, W. N., Landowne, D., Waggoner, A. S., and Wang, C. H. (1974). *J. Membr. Biol.* **19,** 1–36.
Ehrenberg, B., Wei, M.-d., and Loew, L. M. (1987). *In* "Membrane Proteins" (S. C. Goheen, ed.), pp. 279–294. Bio-Rad Lab., Richmond, California.
Ehrenberg, B., Montana, V., Wei, M.-d., Wuskell, J. P., and Loew, L. M. (1988). *Biophys. J.* **53,** 785–794.
Farkas, D. L., Wei, M.-d., Febbroriello, P., Carson, J. H., and Loew, L. M. (1989). *Biophys. J.* **56,** 1053–1069.
Fay, F. S., Carrington, W., and Fogarty, K. E. (1989). *J. Microsc. (Oxford)* **153,** 133–149.
Gross, D., and Loew, L. M. (1989). *Methods Cell Biol.* **30,** 193–218.
Gupta, R. K., Salzberg, B. M., Grinvald, A., Cohen, L. B., Kamino, K., Lesher, S., Boyle, M. B., Waggoner, A. S., and Wang, C. (1981). *J. Membr. Biol.* **58,** 123–137.
Hiraoka, Y., Sedat, J. W., and Agard, D. A. (1987). *Science* **238,** 36–41.
Johnson, L. V., Walsh, M. L., and Chen, L. B. (1980). *Proc. Natl. Acad. Sci. U.S.A.* **77,** 990–994.
Johnson, L. V., Walsh, M. L., Bockus, B. J., and Chen, L. B. (1981). *J. Cell Biol.* **88,** 526–535.
Loew, L. M. (1988). "Spectroscope Membrane Probes." CRC Press, Boca Raton, Florida.
Loew, L. M., Farkas, D. L., and Wei, M.-d. (1990). *In* "Optical Microscopy for Biology" (B. Herman and K. Jacobson, eds.), pp. 131–142. Wiley-Liss, New York.
London, J. A., Zecevic, D., Loew, L. M., Ohrbach, H. S., and Cohen, L. B. (1986). *In* "Fluorescence in the Biological Sciences" (D. L. Taylor, A. S. Waggoner, F. Lanni, R. F. Murphy, and R. Birge, eds.), pp. 423–448. Alan R. Liss, New York.

Mazzanti, M., DeFelice, L. J., Cohen, J., and Malter, H. (1990). *Nature (London)* **343,** 764–767.

Montana, V., Farkas, D. L., and Loew, L. M. (1989). *Biochemistry* **28,** 4536–4539.

Reers, M., Smith, T. W., and Chen, L. B. (1991). *Biochemistry* **30,** 4480–4486.

Ross, W. N., Salzberg, B. M., Cohen, L. B., Grinvald, A., Davila, H. V., Waggoner, A. S., and Wang, C. H. (1977). *J. Membr. Biol.* **33,** 141–183.

Rottenberg, H. (1986). *In* ''Biomembranes, Part M: Transport in Bacteria, Mitochondria, and Chloroplasts: General Approaches and Transport Systems'' (S. Fleischer and B. Fleischer, eds.), Methods in Enzymology, Vol. 125, pp. 1–15. Academic Press, Orlando, Florida.

Sims, P. J., Waggoner, A. S., Wang, C.-H., and Hoffman, J. F. (1974). *Biochemistry* **13,** 3315–3330.

Smiley, S. T., Reers, M., Mottola-Hartshorn, C., Lin, M., Chen, A., Smith, T. W., Steele, G. D., and Chen, L. B. (1991). *Proc. Natl. Acad. Sci. U.S.A.* **88,** 3671–3675.

Tsien, R. Y., and Waggoner, A. S. (1990). *In* ''Handbook of Biological Confocal Microscopy'' (J. B. Pawley, ed.), pp. 169–178. Plenum, New York.

Waggoner, A. S. (1979). *Annu. Rev. Biophys. Bioeng.* **8,** 847–868.

Waggoner, A. S. (1985). *In* ''The Enzymes of Biological Membranes'' (A. N. Martonosi, ed.), pp. 313–331. Plenum, New York.

Wu, J. Y., London, J. A., Zecevic, D., Loew, L. M., Ohrbach, H. S., Catarelli, M., and Cohen, L. B. (1989). *In* ''Cell Structure and Function by Microspectrofluorometry'' (E. Cohen, ed.), pp. 329–346. Academic Press, San Diego.

**CHAPTER 7**

# Imaging Endoplasmic Reticulum in Living Sea Urchin Eggs

## Mark Terasaki* and Laurinda A. Jaffe†

\* Laboratory of Neurobiology
National Institute for Neurological Diseases and Stroke
National Institutes of Health
Bethesda, Maryland 20892

† Department of Physiology
University of Connecticut Health Center
Farmington, Connecticut 06032

## I. Introduction

This article describes a way to label the endoplasmic reticulum (ER) of living sea urchin eggs so that it can be imaged by confocal microscopy. This involves intracellular injection of the dicarbocyanine DiI dissolved in oil. DiI spreads in the ER of the egg and then is observed by confocal microscopy. This article is essentially an expanded version of the Materials and Methods section of the publication describing this technique (Terasaki and Jaffe, 1991).

## A. Properties of DiI

The name *DiI* refers to either $DiIC_{16}(3)$ or $DiIC_{18}(3)$ (Molecular Probes, Eugene, OR). These are dicarbocyanine dyes that consist of a fluorescent portion and two long alkyl chains (Fig. 1). Both dyes seem to behave similarly in labeling the ER. DiI is a bright dye that photobleaches relatively slowly. DiI becomes incorporated into the membrane bilayer through intercalation of the long hydrocarbon chains (Axelrod, 1979) (Fig. 1). The dye is able then to diffuse freely within the bilayer, but does not transfer out of the membrane. DiI was first used to trace the plasma membrane of neurons by Honig and Hume (1986), and since then has been used successfully for this purpose (see Haugland, 1992, for references). DiI has also been used to label the t-tubular system of muscle (Flucher *et al.*, 1991).

## B. Use of DiI in Sea Urchin Eggs

Aqueous suspensions of DiI label the ER of isolated cortices prepared from sea urchin eggs (Henson *et al.*, 1989). DiI labels the ER by a "random hit" mechanism in which DiI aggregates collide with and then spread in the continuous membranes of the cortical ER (Terasaki *et al.*, 1991). It was thought that the ER in a living sea urchin egg could be labeled by microinjecting DiI into an egg. Microinjection of aqueous suspensions of DiI failed, partly because of clogging of the pipette tip by DiI aggregates. We then found that DiI dissolves well in Wesson oil, an oil commonly used in microinjection experiments with

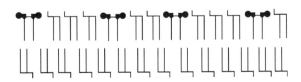

**Fig. 1** *Top:* Molecular structure of DiI [$DiIC_{18}(3)$]. *Bottom:* How DiI associates with membrane bilayers. DiI intercalates in the leaflet of the membrane that is nearest to the source of DiI. DiI diffuses freely in that leaflet but does not transfer significantly to the other leaflet or to membranes that are not continuous with the membrane with which DiI was first associated.

marine eggs. When DiI-saturated oil was microinjected into eggs, DiI spread throughout the egg in the ER.

What probably happens is that the oil droplet contacts and stains many different membranes in the cell (Fig. 2). Many organelles, such as ER, mito-chondria, lysosomes, or yolk platelets, should be stained in the vicinity of the oil drop. However, of the organelles in the cell, the only organelle that has extensive continuity is the ER. The dye should spread in the continuous membranes of the ER, so that in regions sufficiently far from the oil drop only the ER should be stained.

## C. Does This Method Label the Endoplasmic Reticulum?

Whether this method labels the ER is dealt with more fully in Terasaki and Jaffe (1991). Briefly, the method labels membranes that are part of the ER, including the nuclear envelope and the cortical ER network, and the method produces similar staining as seen with immunocytochemical localization of a calsequestrin-like protein that was isolated from sea urchin egg microsomes (Oberdorf *et al.*, 1988; Henson *et al.*, 1989). Also, DiI does not label yolk

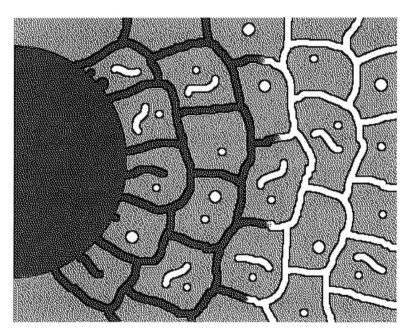

**Fig. 2** Probable mechanism of staining by DiI-saturated oil drop in sea urchin eggs. The oil drop (large half-circle) contacts various organelles, transferring DiI to them. DiI diffuses in the organelle membranes. The ER is an organelle with extensive continuity. At a distance sufficiently far from the oil drop, only the ER should be stained.

platelets or cortical granules, which are abundant in sea urchin eggs. There are two significant precautions about the use of this method. First, bright punctate labeling accumulates with time and may represent dye leaving the ER network via membrane traffic with the Golgi apparatus. Second, although we have shown that DiI labels many parts of the ER, it is not possible at this time to show that DiI labels all of the ER. If the ER is a single interconnected membrane, then this method probably labels all of the ER.

## II. Protocols

### A. Sea Urchins

The original experiments were done with the California sea urchin *Lytechinus pictus*. The animals were obtained from Marinus, Inc. (Venice, CA). Although cleavage proceeded normally in this series of experiments done at room temperature (22–24°C), the ocean temperature at which these eggs develop in nature is probably about 15°C. To avoid possible problems related to temperature (Schroeder and Battaglia, 1985), later experiments were done with *Lytechinus variegatus,* a sea urchin from the southern Atlantic coast. Eggs of this species are more tolerant of higher temperatures. Animals from North Carolina were obtained from E. Bachman (Duke University; season from April to October). Animals from Florida can be obtained from S. Decker (Hollywood, FL; season from November to April). The results we obtained with eggs of this species are essentially identical to results obtained with *L. pictus* eggs.

### B. Preparation of DiI

To prepare a saturated solution of DiI in oil, crystals of DiI (several milligrams) were sprinkled into the bottom of a 1.5-ml Eppendorf tube. Approximately 300 $\mu$l of Wesson oil was then added. After about 5 min with some shaking, the oil was a bright red solution, with some crystals remaining. Because the crystals can clog up the microinjection pipette, the tube was centrifuged at 10,000 $g$ for 3 min. The DiI in oil was then stored at room temperature protected from light. It is better to make a new solution after 1 or 2 weeks. Because Wesson oil eventually becomes rancid, it is probably better to buy a new stock within 6 months to 1 year.

Wesson oil is advertised as 100% soybean oil. Because Wesson oil is unavailable in Europe, DiI was dissolved in corn oil to do one experiment and compared later with Wesson oil. DiI dissolved better in corn oil, but it did not spread as well (A. Speksnyder *et al.*, unpublished observations). Wesson oil was toxic for work with plant cells (P. Hepler, personal communication); therefore for some preparations it may be necessary to test different oils.

## C. Preparation of Microinjection/Observation Slide

Some details of the procedures we use to prepare a slide of eggs for microinjection and observation are described below. These procedures have been developed for many uses by many people; previous descriptions by Hiramoto (1974), Kiehart (1982), Kishimoto (1986), and Lutz and Inoué (1986) are particularly useful.

Sea urchin eggs (*L. pictus* or *L. variegatus*) are placed between two coverslips separated by a piece of double-stick scotch tape, in an arrangement that leaves one side open for introduction of the microinjection pipette (Fig. 3). This assembly is mounted on a 3 × 1 in. plastic support with a U-shaped cut-out, as described by Kiehart (1982); these slides can be purchased from B. Knudson (Instrument Development Laboratory, Marine Biological Laboratories, Woods Hole, MA). For sea urchin eggs approximately 100 μm in diameter, a single piece of double-stick tape forms a space between the coverslips that compresses the egg just enough to hold it in place.

To assemble such a slide, we use No. 0 coverslips (about 100 μm thick) to allow maximum focusing depth into the egg. The coverslips should be cleaned as described by Lutz and Inoué (1986); uncleaned coverslips are toxic. We soak coverslips for 30 min in a dilute detergent solution (Alconox) in warm water, into which coverslips are individually dropped. The coverslips are then individually transferred to a coverslip rinser consisting of a 50-ml plastic test tube with holes cut in the lid and a piece of Tygon tubing attached at the other end. Deionized water is allowed to flow through the rinser for about 1 hr, with occasional shaking. After a final rinse in distilled water, the coverslips are individually transferred to 85% ethanol for storage. Coverslips are dried with a Kimwipe just before use. We use 22 × 22 mm coverslips for the top and bottom of the assembly, and cut the coverslip shelf (about 5 × 10 mm) from these, using a diamond pencil.

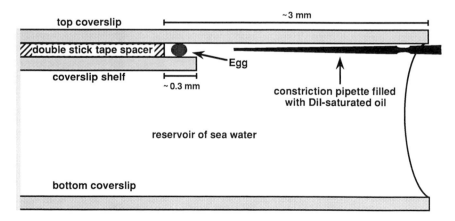

**Fig. 3**  Diagram of chamber used for microinjecting sea urchin eggs.

In assembling the top coverslip, the coverslip shelf, and the double-stick tape, it is important to pay careful attention to the dimensions. The tape should be about 3 mm from the front of the top coverslip, because an oil immersion objective will be used for later observation. However, if the tape is >3 mm back from the front, it is difficult to bring in the microinjection pipette. The coverslip shelf should be relatively narrow (about 0.3 mm), to facilitate microinjection and also to allow sperm to reach the egg. Of course, these dimensions will vary depending on the design of the experiment. It is convenient to put this assembly together on a piece of black Plexiglas. The coverslip pieces and tape should be pressed together firmly with forceps. The eggs are then introduced into the space between the coverslips, using a mouth pipette to deposit them near the edge; capillary action moves the eggs into the space.

The two coverslips (top and bottom) are adhered to the plastic support slide with silicone vacuum grease. Use enough grease to create a tight seal, but too much grease can result in drift during observation. It is convenient to pre-assemble the greased plastic slide and bottom coverslip, such that after the top coverslip is loaded with eggs it can be inverted and attached to the support slide without delay. After assembly, the space between the top and bottom coverslips is filled with a reservoir of sea water.

Except during microinjection and observation, this assembly should be kept in a moist chamber to avoid drying out. The eggs should be maintained at an appropriate temperature (a condition that is not always easy to obtain with a common-use confocal microscope). Evaporation of solution during observation is not usually a problem, but for continuous observations of 1–2 hr, a drop of sea water can be added to the front of the slide to replace lost solution (but not more than once or twice, to avoid hypertonicity).

The solution in the reservoir of the observation slide can be changed during observation (e.g., to introduce sperm or fixative) by carefully introducing a Pasteur pipette to withdraw the solution and then to replace it. A 9-in. pipette works best, because it is narrower than a 6-in. pipette. It should be brought into the reservoir space near the edge of the plastic to avoid contact with the coverslip shelf. If rapid access of the exchanged solution to the egg is needed, the shelf supporting the egg should be narrow (about 150 $\mu$m for a sea urchin egg).

## D. Microinjection

Microinjection can be performed in several ways. We use the constriction pipette technique described by Hiramoto (1974) and Kishimoto (1986). A constriction of about 5-$\mu$m width is made a few millimeters back from the tip of the micropipette. This serves to slow the flow of oil as pressure is applied to the back of the pipette. We apply pressure by means of a 2-ml micrometer syringe (Gilson Instruments, Inc., Great Neck, NY) coupled to the pipette by way of Teflon tubing filled with oil (Fluorinert, FC-70; Sigma, St. Louis, MO).

The pipette is coupled to the Teflon tubing by way of a microinstrument holder (E. Leitz, Rockleigh, NJ), held horizontally by a micromanipulator (Narishige SM-20; Narashige Scientific Instruments Laboratory, Tokyo, Japan). Before inserting the pipette in the microinstrument holder, we backfill it with an approximately 1-cm column of the DiI solution in Wesson oil. An air space is left between the Fluorinert and the DiI solution. The pipette tip is broken back to a diameter of about 3 $\mu$m by tapping it against the cut end of a piece of glass tubing while observing under a microscope.

Injections are made while observing the egg with a ×16 objective on an upright microscope. We rotate the microscope 90° from the front-facing eyepieces, in order to bring in the micropipette with the micromanipulator from the side. The amount of oil injected is determined by measurement with an eyepiece micrometer. The volume of oil injected was 4–20 pl.

## E. Confocal Microscopy

A Bio-Rad MRC-600 laser scanning confocal microscope was used with a krypton–argon laser. The 568-nm laser line was used with the yellow excitation filter (568 DF 10 laser line filter, 585 DRLP dichroic, and 585 EFLP emission filter) for imaging DiI, which has an excitation peak of 547 nm and emission peak at 565 nm. The confocal microscope software was run on a Dell system 325 computer. The confocal microscope scan head was attached to a Zeiss Axioplan microscope. A ×63 Plan-Apo NA 1.4 Zeiss lens was used

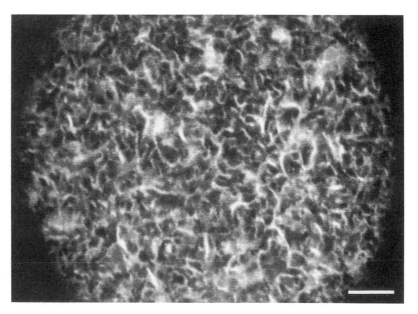

**Fig. 4**  Sea urchin egg ER stained by DiI and imaged by confocal microscopy. Bar = 10 $\mu$m.

for imaging because lower numerical aperture lenses were less able to resolve the structure of the ER. Some observations were also done with the same confocal system attached to a Nikon optiphot microscope with a Nikon ×60 Plan-Apo NA 1.4 lens. An example of a DiI-stained egg imaged by confocal microscopy is shown in Fig. 4.

## F. Optical Memory Disk Recorder Interface

The video output of the confocal microscope was wired to an optical memory disk recorder (OMDR) (model 3031F; Panasonic). The OMDR can record and play back images at video rates (i.e., 30 msec/frame) or it can record or play back one image at time. Image storage is rapid compared to the several seconds required to store an image on the computer hard disk. Also, time-lapse data are convenient to view with the OMDR and essentially impossible with the computer hard disk.

Images can be recorded on the OMDR manually but it is usually more advantageous to control the OMDR via a serial port connection. Both the computer and the OMDR are configured as DTE devices for serial port communication, therefore certain pins in the RS-232 cable linking them must be crossed in order to make one of them into a DCE device. Relevant information is in the OMDR manual. A computer program is required to send commands from the computer to the OMDR. Our BASIC program was four lines long:

```
Open "com2:2400, n, 8,1" for random as #1
com(2) on
Print #1, chr$(2) + command$ + chr$(3)
close
```

This program was named omdr, compiled as an exe file (using Microsoft Quick Basic), and stored in the cfocal directory on the hard disk. This program sends to the OMDR the ASCII values of the characters typed in the command line. For example, to send the command ON, which puts the omdr on line, type "omdr ON" at the DOS prompt, or use "$omdr ON" in the confocal macro command language. (*Note:* Use capital letters for the OMDR commands because capital vs lower-case letters have different values in ASCII code. Typing "omdr ON" at the DOS prompt will put the OMDR online, whereas "omdr on" at the DOS prompt will do nothing.)

For automated recordings, macros (.cmd files) were written with SOM software. The macros operated the OMDR by using the omdr.exe program described above. The macros used for time-lapse and *z*-series recordings are shown in Table 1. These macros were stopped by typing control U. The confocal software was then reset to normal operating mode with another macro, also shown in Table I. One disadvantage of the time-lapse macro is that the fastest image acquisition time with a 1-sec scan was only 2.6 sec. This was because of the time required to stop the scan and record the image. To record

**Table I**
**Macros for Data Collection Using an OMDR**

| Time series (no wait) | Time series (%1 = wait) | z and t series (%1 = steps; %2 = wait) | Reset |
|---|---|---|---|
| echo- | echo- | echo- | echo- |
| $omdr ON | $omdr ON | $omdr ON | live filter d |
| $omdr RM | $omdr RM | $omdr RM | $omdr RC |
| live filter a 1 | live filter a %1 | motor on | $omdr OF |
| for j = 1,10000 | for j = 1,10000 | live filter a 1 | motor off |
| clear | clear | for j = 1,10000 | |
| coll | coll | for i = 1, %1 | |
| $omdr GS | $omdr GS | clear | |
| next j | wait 0 | coll | |
| | wait %2 | $omdr GS | |
| | next j | motor step | |
| | | next i | |
| | | motor pos 0 | |
| | | wait 0 | |
| | | wait %2 | |
| | | next j | |

images faster, it is possible to use a continuous scan and to record images manually on the OMDR. Another possibility is to use faster scan rates with smaller box sizes and to record continuously onto a video tape recorder.

## G. Data Collection

On the one hand, it is crucial to minimize the amount of light to which the specimen is exposed. Light causes bleaching and, most important, causes damage to living eggs and may alter normal processes. On the other hand, lowering the light exposure usually reduces the quality or amount of data collected. Therefore optimization between light exposure and data collection is required. Because many factors are involved, there is no formula or rule to decide what is best. As an example, higher zoom can reveal more details but it also increases light damage to the sample.

The amount of light reaching the specimen is controlled by the neutral-density filter (0 = 100% transmission, 1 = 10%, 2 = 3%, and 3 = 1%). When the DiI-containing oil droplet was too small, the No. 1 neutral-density filter was required to obtain an image. With this filter, the dye usually bleaches quickly and there are toxic effects on the egg are visible. It is better to microinject a larger amount of dye so that the No. 2 or 3 neutral-density filter can be used.

Some processes seemed more susceptible to toxic damage than other processes. The change in ER organization at fertilization seemed the most able to withstand light damage. Mitosis was somewhat more sensitive and pronuclear migration and fusion seemed the most sensitive. One decided advantage of working with eggs is that there is a good standard for judging light damage: damage is considered minimal if the fertilized egg continues developing after observations are finished.

For some processes, it was important to be able to focus and then start recordings without missing too much of the phenomenon. It helps to be able to operate the confocal software rapidly, and it also helps to have uncomplicated macro programs for running the OMDR recordings.

In time-lapse experiments, the internal ER was found to be changing its distribution between every scan. Because of this, we usually collected images as a single scan without averaging.

*Additional note:* We have fixed eggs in glutaraldehyde and then injected DiI-saturated oil drops. The fixation precludes spread of the dye by membrane traffic. We observed that the dye spread throughout the fixed eggs, providing stronger evidence that the internal cisternae, cortical network, and nuclear envelope are all part of one membrane (Jaffe and Terasaki, 1993). We also observed that the dye spread throughout eggs fixed 10 min after fertilization, but that it did not spread significantly from the oil drop in eggs fixed 1 min after fertilization. This provides evidence that the ER is fragmented at the time of calcium release during fertilization, and that the ER subsequently regains its continuity.

## Acknowledgments

M.T. wishes to acknowledge Christian Sardet, Bob Silver, and Anneliese Speksnyder for help in early attempts to label the ER in sea urchin eggs.

## References

Axelrod, D. (1979). *Biophys. J.* **26,** 557–574.

Flucher, B. E., Terasaki, M., Chin, H., Beeler, T. J., and Daniels, M. P. (1991). *Dev. Biol.* **145,** 77–90.

Haugland, R. P. (1992). "Handbook of Fluorescent Probes and Research Chemicals." Molecular Probes, Inc., Eugene Oregon.

Henson, J. H., Begg, D. A., Beaulieu, S. M., Fishkind, D. J., Bonder, E. M., Terasaki, M., Lebeche, D., and Kaminer, B. (1989). *J. Cell Biol.* **109,** 149–161.

Hiramoto, Y. (1974). *Exp. Cell Res.* **87,** 403–406.

Honig, M. G., and Hume, R. I. (1986). *J. Cell Biol.* **103,** 171–187.

Jaffe, L. A., and Terasaki, M. (1993). *Dev. Biol.* **156,** 566–573.

Kiehart, D. P. (1982). *Methods Cell Biol.* **25,** 13–31.

Kishimoto, T. (1986). *Methods Cell Biol.* **27,** 379–394.

Lutz, D. A., and Inoué, S. (1986). *Methods Cell Biol.* **27,** 89–110.

Oberdorf, J. A., Lebeche, D., Head, J. F., and Kaminer, B. (1988). *J. Biol. Chem.* **263,** 6806–6809.

Schroeder, T. E., and Battaglia, D. E. (1985). *J. Cell Biol.* **100,** 1056–1062.

Terasaki, M., and Jaffe, L. A. (1991). *J. Cell Biol.* **114,** 929–940.

Terasaki, M., Henson, J., Begg, D., Kaminer, B., and Sardet, C. (1991). *Dev. Biol.* **148,** 398–401.

**CHAPTER 8**

# Membrane Glycolipid Trafficking in Living, Polarized Pancreatic Acinar Cells: Assessment by Confocal Microscopy

**A. H. Cornell-Bell, L. R. Otake, K. Sadler, P. G. Thomas, S. Lawrence, K. Olsen, F. Gumkowski, J. R. Peterson, and J. D. Jamieson**

Department of Cell Biology
Yale University School of Medicine
New Haven, Connecticut 06520

# I. Introduction

Our studies on membrane trafficking in epithelial cells have taken advantage of the development of two new technologies: the confocal laser scanning microscope (Pawley, 1990) and the synthesis of two fluorescent lipids that are vital stains for the Golgi apparatus (Pagano *et al.,* 1991; Lipsky and Pagano, 1985a,b; Pagano, 1989). Coupled with the use of well-defined *in vitro* preparations of secretagogue-responsive pancreatic acini, we have begun to image dynamics of Golgi-to-secretory granule transport of membrane glycolipids. This combination of new technology and a well-defined, functional secretory system (Jamieson and Palade, 1971; Bruzzone *et al.,* 1985; Amsterdam and Jamieson, 1974a,b; Palade, 1975) is valuable for examining the mechanisms and kinetics of intracellular transport in living, polarized regulated secretory cells and for visualizing factors controlling exocytosis.

## A. Confocal Laser Scanning Microscopy

The confocal scanning laser microscope (CLSM) is capable of capturing thin optical sections out of relatively thick ( up to 250 $\mu$m) intact tissues, allows exact microphotometry, gathers optically sectioned images for three-dimensional reconstructions and, most importantly, eliminates out-of-focus fluorescence in the plane of focus of the image. Unwanted light that expands the apparent depth of field in the conventional fluorescence microscope is exactly what confocal imaging eliminates. The resulting image is fully in focus within a shallow depth of field in the range of 0.5–1.0 $\mu$m. With the confocal laser scanning microscope there is also an increased effective optical resolution and an improved signal-to-noise ratio (Inoué, 1990). The light source for the laser confocal microscope is a laser beam focused to a spot of 0.26 $\mu$m in diameter (using a $\times 63$/NA 1.4 objective, spot size 1, zoom 1) that is scanned across the specimen during image acquisition. The beam has only a short dwell time on any one spot on the specimen, which results in a drastic decrease in phototoxicity.[1] Optical sectioning, the first step in production of

---

[1] With a Bio-Rad MRC-600 there are roughly 400,000 pixels/screen, that is, 768 pixels/line and 512 lines, and the image acquisition takes 1.0 sec. That means, roughly, 2.5 $\mu$sec is required to image each pixel; however, the computer is continuously scanning a line, so this time estimate is not precise. In the confocal microscope, the size of the illuminated spot is diffraction limited and is affected by the objective and wavelength of excitation. With the laser at a zoom of 1 (no electronic magnification), a $\times 63$ objective (NA 1.4), and excitation of 488 nm (FITC filter cube), the spot size calculated with the above settings would be 0.26 $\mu$m. If the laser were zoomed to 2, the spot size would decrease to 0.13 $\mu$m. The actual dwell time the laser would remain on a spot would be roughly 0.65 $\mu$sec.

three-dimensional images, is made possible by the small diameter of the illuminated spot on the specimen and the concomitant decrease in photobleaching.
As a consequence of the laser being focused on a single plane in the tissue,
thin optical sections can be made and stored of the entire specimen field without bleaching the out-of-focus regions. This then allows subsequent scans and
image acquisition through sequential optical planes that allow three-
dimensional reconstructions accomplished with computer programs designed
for three-dimensional image analysis, such as Voxel View (Vital Images, Inc.,
Fairfield, IA).

## Imaging Golgi in Living Cells

When the CSLM is equipped for video imaging through coupling to a digital
host computer with image processing capabilities and a shuttering system, it
becomes possible to image living cells with increased clarity and increased
resolution over that possible with conventional light microscopes. The drastic
reduction in laser dwell time noted above has made it possible to image with
exquisite detail the Golgi apparatus in living hippocampal astrocytes with
greater success than had previously been obtained with the conventional epifluorescence microscope and video intensification cameras (Cooper *et al.*,
1990). Once images obtained with the CSLM are stored in digitized form either
directly on the computer hard disk or more practically on a laser disk, they
can be subdivided into picture elements called *pixels*. All pixels in the image
are of equal area and spacing. An analogous division of the intensity range is
called the gray level. If an 8-bit storage system is used, the lowest intensity
value is 0 and the greatest is 255, resulting in a total gray scale of 256. Pixelation is the process of partitioning the image, both in space and intensity,
into discrete elements for storage, display, and quantitative analysis (Webb
and Dorey, 1990). Once pixels are assigned a value (gray level) and a position
in the array it is possible to carry out complex morphometric analyses of the
image. Measurements of pixel intensity become routine and numbers of pixels
involved in making an image can be described mathematically (area, volume,
etc.). We have made use of pixelation to quantify the ceramide fluorescence in
pancreatic acinar cells as it moves with time from the Golgi to membranes of
the post-Golgi compartments that compose the secretory pathway.

## B. Fluorescent Ceramide Analogs

In our current studies, we have taken advantage of fluorescent analogs of
ceramide and the vectorial secretory transport pathway in pancreatic acinar
cells in order to (1) define the kinetics of entry of the fluorescent lipid derivatives into elements of the Golgi complex and (2) examine the kinetics and
routes of post-Golgi transport of membrane glycolipids into the distal

compartments of the secretory pathway, terminating in secretory (zymogen) granules at the cell apex in rat pancreatic acinar cells.

## 1. NBD–Ceramide

A series of fluorescent glycolipid derivatives have been developed to study the synthesis, molecular sorting, and intracellular transport of membrane lipids (Pagano and Sleight, 1985). With these probes, glycolipid metabolism has been studied by conventional lipid biochemistry and then correlated with intracellular distribution by conventional fluorescence microscopy (Pagano and Sleight, 1985). The lipid *N*-[7-(4-nitrobenzo-2-oxa-1,3-diazole)]-6-aminocaproyl sphingosine (C6-NBD-ceramide) is one such vital fluorescent marker that localizes in the Golgi apparatus (Lipsky and Pagano, 1985a,b; Pagano, 1989). The site and mechanism of C6-NBD-ceramide accumulation in the Golgi apparatus is, however, unclear. Interactions with endogenous lipids and possibly with cholesterol in this organelle may result in the restriction of this fluorescent marker to what is believed to be the trans-Golgi cisternae (Pagano, 1990a,b). C6-NBD-ceramide is metabolized to sphingomyelin and glycosylceramide (Pagano *et al.*, 1991; Kobayashi and Pagano, 1989; Van Meer *et al.*, 1987; Van Meer, 1989; Van't Hof and Van Meer, 1990). Transport of these metabolites to the plasma membrane indicates that C6-NBD-ceramide and its metabolites are recognized by normal cellular sorting and transport machinery (Pagano *et al.*, 1991). Biophysical studies of the NBD-labeled lipids in model membrane systems suggest that although the NBD-fluorophore is attached to the acyl chain of the lipid, this dye is not totally intercalated in the membrane bilayer as a result of its polar nature (Chattopadahyay, 1990). This may limit the interpretation of results obtained with C6-NBD-ceramide for normal lipid-sorting events. The lack of intercalation in the membrane does not, however, appear to affect the metabolism of C6-NBD-ceramide or sorting of its metabolites. The major disadvantage to using the C6-NBD-ceramide probe lies in the fact that this fluorophore rapidly bleaches, using conventional fluorescence microscopy and higher apparent magnification (zoom) levels in the confocal laser scanning microscope. Leaving the laser at lower zooms (1–2) coupled with the use of neutral density filters in the laser path makes routine use of this fluoroprobe possible.

## 2. BODIPY–Ceramide

The combination of a new analog conjugate of D-erythrosphingosine and a fluorophore, boron dipyrromethene difluoride (BODIPY), attached to a fatty acid have overcome many of the problems associated with C6-NBD-ceramide (Pagano *et al.*, 1991). BODIPY-C5-DMB-ceramide, as it is termed, has a two- to threefold greater fluorescence yield and appears to be more photostable than NBD-labeled lipids. The BODIPY fluorophore is less polar than NBD and as a result it has been suggested that BODIPY-labeled lipid analogs may be more efficiently intercalated into the membrane bilayer than NBD-labeled analogs (Pagano *et al.*, 1991). The fluorescence of this new fluorophore is dramatically red shifted when concentrations of the dye are elevated. This dye is excited in the range of 450–490 nm and emits in either the green and red (520–560 nm) or in the red (>590 nm) range. Fluorescence ratio imaging measurements of red to green fluorescence after background subtraction are possible with this dye and these manipulations have resulted in plots whereby the ratio of red to green fluorescence is linear with respect to the concentration of C5-DMB-ceramide at a given subcellular site (Pagano *et al.*, 1991). This allows estimation of the concentration of the dye at a particular location. NBD and BODIPY differ structurally; accordingly, when these fluorophores are attached to ceramide and are loaded into structurally polar pancreatic acinar cells at 16 or 20°C over a 30-min period, there appear to be subtle differences in the initial site of accumulation in the Golgi region. Once cells are maintained at 37°C for more than 5 min these differences disappear and both dyes appear to label the perinuclear Golgi cisternae. In addition, there appear to be kinetic differences in dye loading and transport of the two lipid analogs during normal resting intracellular transport.

## C. Use of Polar Cells

Pancreatic acini consisting of groups of 50–100 acinar cells maintained in their *in situ* polarized epithelial array were prepared by collagenase digestion using a modification of the method described by Bruzzone *et al.* (1985). With this preparation, normal cell–cell relationships and cell polarity are still maintained even over several hours of incubation *in vitro* at 37°C. Cells remain connected to each other by junctional complexes, including tight and gap junctions (Amsterdam *et al.*, 1978), and their apical margins delimit the beginning of the duct system or centroacinar lumen. Acini have been shown to be more responsive in releasing amylase on exposure to secretagogues such as carbamylcholine or cholecystokinin than are isolated pancreatic cells, presumably because of this preservation of cell coupling and maintenance of the apical structures required for regulated exocytosis (Hootman and Williams, 1987). An additional advantage of the acinar preparation is that the polarity of individual secretory cells can be clearly discerned in the confocal microscope. Nuclei that are basally located in the cell appear as darkened spheres, the fluorophore-lipid labeled Golgi is supranuclear, and the apices of the cells can be clearly seen delimiting the centroacinar lumen. Thus, in this preparation and with the enhanced spatial resolution offered by the confocal microscope, it is possible to clearly delineate the basal-to-apical axis of individual cells, which is critical for defining the axis over which fluorescent emission is measured.

## II. Analysis of Post-Golgi Lipid Transport

### A. NBD-Ceramide

In preliminary experiments, acini were labeled with NBD-ceramide on the stage of the confocal laser scanning microscope at 23°C and were imaged every 30 sec to determine the optimal time for labeled ceramide probe to accumulate in the Golgi against nonspecific background labeling. Within 30 sec to 1 min there was identifiable staining of the Golgi as indicated by a reticulated perinuclear staining and by 2 min of labeling, NBD-ceramide was specifically concentrated in Golgi cisternae (data not shown). Based on these preliminary experiments, culture dishes containing acini that had been allowed to settle on coverslips (see Section III) were labeled for up to 10 min with 5 $\mu M$ NBD-ceramide in the presence of 10% serum in a 37°C incubator. After this time, acini were rinsed in culture medium free of the probe and containing 10% serum and were chased for periods from 1 to 6 hr in a 37°C incubator. At each time point, replicate dishes were removed from the incubator, the coverslips containing the acini were placed in a flow-through perfusion chamber, and the preparations were imaged on a Bio-Rad (Cambridge, MA) MRC-600 CLSM equipped with the argon laser and the fluorescein filter cube. We are using a Zeiss Axiovert 10 inverted microscope, with a Zeiss ×63/NA 1.4 Plan-Apo objective. Images are downloaded to a Pinnacle Micro Reo 650 external optical disk and image analysis is accomplished with an Iris 4D/240GTX Silicon Graphics workstation. Photographs are taken on a matrix color graphic recorder (model 6564; Agfa, Orangeburg, NY).

After 1 hr of chase at 37°C (Fig. 1A), the majority of the fluorescent ceramide was contained within the perinuclear Golgi cisternae with relatively small amounts of label localized to the apical zones of the cell. By 1.5 hr of

---

**Fig. 1** Time course of lipid movement through pancreatic acinar cells stained with NBD-ceramide [chases of 1, 1.5, 2, 2.5, 3, 4, 5, and 6 hr correspond to (A–H), respectively]. Culture dishes were labeled for 10 min with NBD-ceramide in the presence of serum and at 1–6 hr dishes were removed from the incubator and fluorescently labeled cells were imaged with the CLSM. After 1 hr of chase (A) fluorescent probe accumulated specifically and in high concentration in well-defined perinuclear Golgi cisternae (open arrows) and little lipid was localized in the apical region near the lumen [large white arrows in (A–F)]. After 1.5 hr of chase (B) lipid began to move and was seen to spread from the trans face of the Golgi (arrows). The apical region, however, still remained relatively free of label. Lipid began to fill the apical region of cells after 2 hr of chase (C) and by 3–4 hr (E and F) the lumen was often obscured by secretory product. Structures reminiscent of condensing vacuoles (arrowheads) were most apparent after 1.5–3 hr of chase (B–E). Structures (small white arrows), later identified immunohistochemically as zymogen granules, began to accumulate apically within 2 hr of chase and continued until 6 hr. By 5 and 6 hr of chase (G and H) ringlike structures (short black arrows) that are produced by fluorescent lipid surrounding the nonfluorescent zymogen granules were seen emerging from the apical margin of the cells. By 6 hr there is an obvious decrease in the number of these structures remaining in the cytoplasm. Bar = 25 $\mu$m.

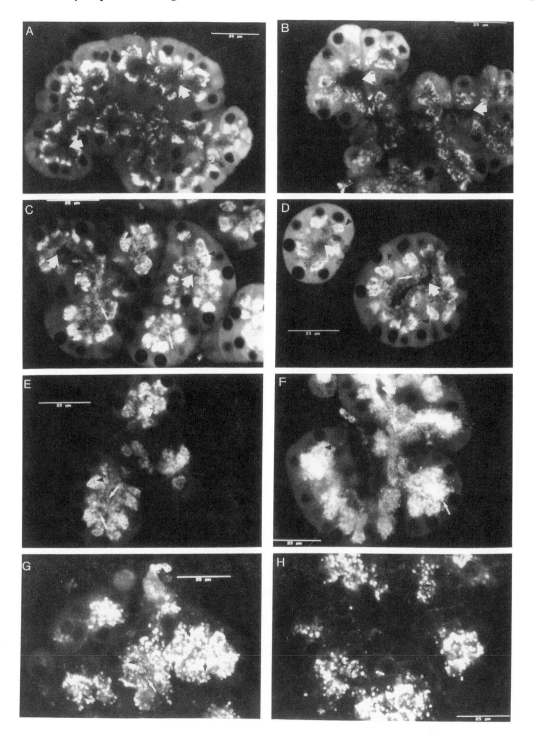

chase, the fluorescent lipid analog began to mobilize from the trans face of the Golgi, giving this organelle a vesicular appearance (Fig. 1B). By 2 hr of chase, the apical regions of the acinar cells contained label (Fig. 1C). By 3–4 hr of chase, the apical regions of the cells became so filled with spherical profiles that represent zymogen granule membranes that the centroacinar lumen was often obscured (Fig. 1E and F). With NBD-ceramide, it was possible to image minute details of the Golgi apparatus and post-Golgi secretory compartments, including condensing vacuoles and early and late zymogen granules (Fig. 1C–H). Condensing vacuoles were most apparent after 1.5–3 hr of chase. Fluorescently labeled zymogen granule membranes became evident in the apical cytoplasm by 2 hr of chase and label continued to accumulate in these structures for up to 5–6 hr of chase, the maximum time of observation in our studies. At 5–6 hr of chase, labeling of zymogen granule membranes resulted in ringlike profiles ~0.5–1.0 $\mu$m in diameter that surrounded the nonfluorescent zymogen granule content. Further identification of these profiles as representing zymogen granules was obtained by using immunohisto-chemistry for their content of stored amylase and by their accumulation of acridine orange into their slightly acidic intracellular environment (Fig. 4) (De Lisle and Williams, 1987). By 6 hr of chase, we observed a decrease in the number of fluorescently labeled granules in the apical cytoplasm (Fig. 1H).

To quantify the spatial and temporal movement of labeled lipid probe over the Golgi-to-secretory granule pathway, we carried out microspectro-photometry of profiles of acinar cells normalized for length at varying times of chase. For this purpose, images of fluorescent lipid-labeled cells were displayed on the computer screen and cells whose basal-to-apical axis could be identified were measured. Our criterion for basal-to-apical axis was the ability to visualize in the same cell a ''negative'' spherical profile representing the nucleus (basal pole) and a defined centroacinar lumen delimited by the apices of several acinar cells (see Fig. 2). With this criterion, it was possible to generate an average basal-to-apical fluorescence intensity profile for labeled acinar cells at each time point ($n$ =25 cells for each time). Figure 2 contrasts the fluorescence profile from the 2-hr chase with that of the 5-hr chase to illustrate the sensitivity of the method. Graphs are plotted after the ASCII files generated from the Bio-Rad length morphometry program were manipulated by a macro program written for SYSTAT (program written by P. G. Thomas, Department of Cell Biology, Yale University, New Haven, CT). With the morphometry programs it was possible to correlate the location of intracellular structures such as the nucleus and the Golgi apparatus with fluorescence intensity values. Analyzing cells from the various time points make it possible to quantify the transport of fluorescent lipid analogs from the post-Golgi compartment to the apical zone of the cells during normal resting intracellular transport.

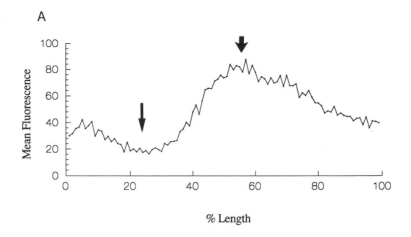

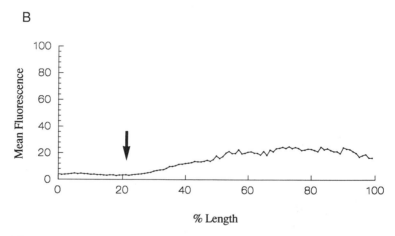

**Fig. 2** A fluorescence intensity profile for the normalized length of pancreatic acinar cells stained with NBD-ceramide and chased for 2 hr (A) and 5 hr (B). This graph is generated from ASCII files obtained from 25 cells analyzed with the length morphometry program on the Bio-Rad CLSM. Data are analyzed and plotted by SYSTAT on a MacIICI computer. The long black arrow indicates the position of the nucleus (from morphology) and the short black arrow indicates the position of the Golgi apparatus. The overall level of fluorescence intensity in cells decreases by 5 hr of chase (B).

## B. BODIPY-Ceramide

A kinetic study was also made with cells labeled with BODIPY-ceramide (Fig. 3). With BODIPY, the overall fluorescence was less even compared to the results with NBD-ceramide labeling. With BODIPY, the labeling in one cell often was of low intensity compared to its neighbor, which was brightly stained (Fig. 3).

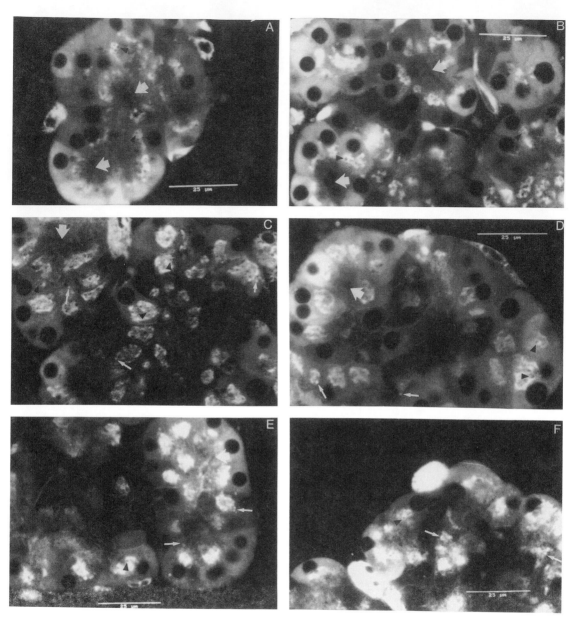

**Fig. 3** Time course of lipid movement through pancreatic cells labeled with BODIPY-ceramide [chases of 1, 1.5, 2, 2.5, 3, and 4 hr correspond to Fig. 1 (A–F), respectively]. The overall fluorescence of an acinus labeled with BODIPY-ceramide is less even (one cell is extremely dark next to a cell that is nearly saturated) and cytoplasm is stained more diffusely than in cells labeled with NBD-ceramide. In addition, there are differences in fluorescence localization with time. At 1 hr of chase there is still a zone free of fluorescence near the lumen (large white arrows); however, the lipid is not contained in a tight perinuclear Golgi apparatus. Instead, there are profiles of condensing vacuoles (arrowheads) evident from 1 to 4 hr of chase (A–F). Structures (white arrows) identified as zymogen granules (see Fig. 4) are seen from 2 to 4 hr of chase (C–F), a time course that matches the NBD-ceramide time course (Fig. 1). Bar = 25 $\mu$m.

Careful analysis of images acquired with the BODIPY probe also showed subtle differences in the kinetics and topology of staining with this fluoroprobe. For example, in the time course shown in Fig. 1, the condensing vacuoles were rarely seen to be labeled until 1.5 hr of chase, using NBD-ceramide, and reached peak levels at 2.5–3 hr of chase. In contrast, profiles of condensing vacuoles are evident in BODIPY-ceramide-labeled cells even at the 1-hr time point (Fig. 3A). Perhaps this is due to the increase in fluorescence yield with BODIPY-ceramide, allowing detection at an earlier time point, or perhaps there are actual differences in the site of insertion of the fluoroprobe into the lipid bilayer of the acinar cell membranes.

## C. Specific Immunohistochemistry

A specific antibody for amylase was used (Fig. 4) to stain the granule population in the apical cytoplasm of the pancreatic acinar cells in order to validate our assumption that the fluorescent lipid labels were marking the membranes of zymogen granules (Fig. 4A) (anti-amylase, gift of F. Gorelick, Yale University). Acridine orange, which stains acidic compartments, also stains this population of granules (Fig. 4B). These experiments thus confirm that the granule population followed in the NBD- and BODIPY-ceramide time courses were in fact zymogen granules.

## D. Inhibition of Lipid Transport into Post–Golgi Compartments

We used techniques known to perturb normal lipid transport in order to show that patterns of fluorescent lipid appearing in zymogen granule membrane derived from labeled membranes that originated in the Golgi . The transport of newly synthesized fluorescent sphingolipids from the Golgi to the plasma membrane has been shown to be inhibited in other nonpolar cells in the presence of the ionophore monensin (Lipsky and Pagano, 1985a). Fluorescent ceramide labeling of zymogen granules was completely blocked in pancreatic acinar cells by incubation with 1 $\mu M$ monensin following loading into the Golgi at 37°C. With this compound, the fluorescent NBD- and BODIPY-ceramide remained within the confines of the perinuclear Golgi even after 6 hr of chase at 37°C (data not shown). This directly contrasted to the patterns of lipid mobilization we have previously described, using these labels (Figs. 1 and 3). A temperature block of lipid movement through the pancreatic acinar cells was also used to perturb normal lipid transport mechanisms (Fig. 5). In these experiments, cells were labeled at 16 or 20°C with either the NBD- or BODIPY-ceramide lipid analogs and were chased for 1.5 hr at the same temperatures. The initial fluorescence labeling pattern obtained with NBD-ceramide was similar at both 16 and 20°C and did not change over the chase period at the same temperature. This temperature block produces a

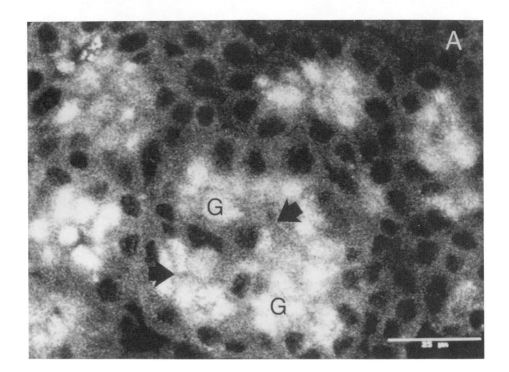

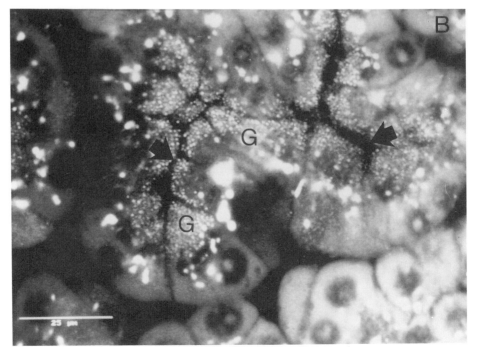

perinuclear Golgi pattern that is different from those collected from cells labeled for 10 min at 37°C, where the images correspond to the reticulate, interconnected images of the trans-Golgi network (see Fig. 1B for comparison).
Irrespective of the label, loading at 16 and 20°C prevents mobilization of lipid
into post-Golgi compartments. The pattern of BODIPY-ceramide loaded and
chased at 16°C is more vesicular than images collected from 20°C samples and
may indicate fluoroprobe loading into an earlier Golgi compartment.

## III. Methods

### A. Preparation of Pancreatic Acini

Pancreatic acini are isolated by an enzyme digestion procedure that maintains them in their *in situ* array for use in fluorescent imaging studies. The
following is a detailed description of our procedure, modified from that of
Bruzzone *et al.* (1985).

*Materials*
Complete dissociation medium (adjust pH to 7.4)

HEPES, 25 m$M$
NaCl, 125 m$M$
KCl, 4.5 m$M$
CaCl$_2$, 2.0 m$M$
MgCl$_2$, 1.2 m$M$
Glucose, 5.0 m$M$
Soybean trypsin inhibitor, 0.01%
Bovine serum albumin (BSA) (fraction V), 0.1%
Purified collagenase (CLSPA; Worthington Biochemical Corporation, Free-
    hold NJ): Store in dissociation buffer at −20°C in 200-$\mu$l aliquots at a
    concentration of 2000 U/ml. Use 200 $\mu$l/5.0 ml of dissociation medium

*Note:* All glassware should be freshly siliconized with Prosil-21 (PCR, Inc.,
Gainesville, FL).

---

**Fig. 4**  Specific immunohistochemical identification of zymogen granules. (A) Specific antibody to
amylase stains a granule population (G) that is located in the apical cytoplasm close to the acinar
lumen (large black arrow). Acridine orange, which stains acidic compartments, also stains this
population of granules (G) in the apical cytoplasm (B). The large fluorescent particles may be
lysosomes. Bar = 25 $\mu$m.

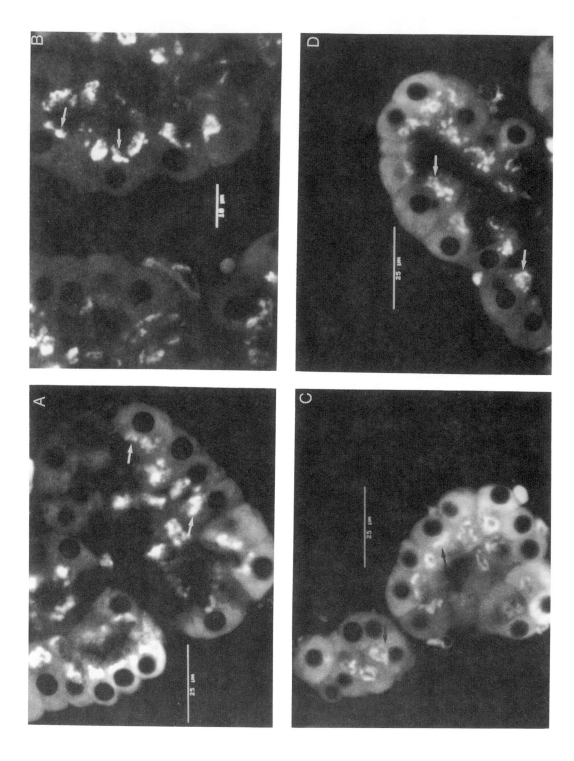

*Procedures*

1. The pancreas from a juvenile male rat approximately 70–100 g in weight is dissected free of associated fat and connective tissue. The gland is placed in ice-cold buffer solution containing 25 m$M$ HEPES, 5.0 m$M$ glucose, 4.5 m$M$ KCl, 1.2 m$M$ MgCl$_2$, 2.0 m$M$ CaCl$_2$, 125 m$M$ NaCl, 0.1% BSA, and 0.01% soybean trypsin inhibitor at pH 7.4.

2. The tissue is minced into 0.5-mm cubes and placed into a 25-ml Erlenmeyer flask in 5.0 ml of buffer as in step 1 but also containing 20 U of collagenase/ml (Worthington Biochemicals).

3. Shake the flask in a 37°C water bath at 120 oscillations/min for 5 min.

4. Transfer to a 15-ml Corex centrifuge tube Shake manually for a maximum of 10 min or until the tissue begins to fall apart into small clumps of acini. Rewarm the tube to 37°C as necessary.

5. Filter the tissue suspension once through a single layer of J&J Kling gauze, followed by filtration through Nytex (200-$\mu$m pore size). Rinse the filter with complete buffer to a final volume of ~20 ml.

6. Allow large clumps of undissociated tissue to settle for 20 sec, decant the supernatant, and from the supernatant allow acini to settle for 3–5 min. Aspirate off the supernatant containing small acini and cell debris and gently resuspend the loose pellet of acini with buffer containing 25 m$M$ HEPES, 5.0 m$M$ glucose, 4.5 m$M$ KCl, 1.2 m$M$ MgCl$_2$, 2.0 m$M$ CaCl$_2$, 125 m$M$ NaCl, 0.1% BSA, and 0.01% soybean trypsin inhibitor at pH 7.4 (1–2 ml).

## B. Protocol for Settling Pancreatic Acinar Cells onto Coverslips

1. After isolation, pancreatic acini are allowed to settle into a loose pellet in the bottom of a 15.0-ml polypropylene centrifuge tube (Corning, Corning, NY). The buffer covering acini is aspirated off and the acini are resuspended in buffer and allowed to settle again.

2. Fluorescent lipid labeling of acini: Aspirate off the buffer and resuspend the cells in 40 $\mu M$ NBD-ceramide or 40 $\mu M$ BODIPY-ceramide [from a 4 m$M$ stock solution in dimethylsulfoxide (DMSO) stored in the dark at −20°C] in complete Dulbecco's modified Eagle's medium (DMEM) containing penicillin/

---

**Fig. 5**  Temperature block of lipid movement through pancreatic acinar cells. Cells were labeled for 30 min with either NBD-ceramide (A and B) or BODIPY-ceramide (C and D) and were chased for 1.5 hr at 16°C (A and C) and 20°C (B and D). The fluorescence pattern obtained with the NBD-ceramide is similar at both temperatures. The fluorescence was localized in trans Golgi (Pagano, 1990a,b) and lipid was mobilized from the Golgi cisternae toward the apical margin (see white arrows). The pattern seen for BODIPY-ceramide at 20°C (D) is similar to the pattern seen for NBD-ceramide at 16 and 20°C (A and B). In contrast, BODIPY-ceramide at 16°C specifically accumulated (black arrows) in a tight pattern reminiscent of an earlier Golgi compartment (C). Bar = 25 $\mu$m.

streptomycin 25 m$M$ glucose, 10% fetal calf serum, and a final DMSO concentration of 1%. Cells are labeled for 10 min in the fluorescent analogs at 37°C in a $CO_2$/air incubator.

3. Resuspend the loose pellet of acini into complete saline containing penicillin/streptomycin. Always use siliconized pipettes (Prosil-21; PCR, Inc.) because acini are extremely sticky. Pipette 200–250 $\mu$l of cell suspension onto the center of precleaned glass coverslips placed in 35-mm plastic petri dishes. Cells are allowed to settle directly onto glass in the absence of protein in the 37°C $CO_2$/air incubator for 1 hr.

4. After 1 hr in the incubator, 1.0 ml of complete DMEM medium is added to the culture dishes and acini are returned to the $CO_2$ incubator. When cells are needed for recordings they are loaded into a perfusion chamber and are placed on a heated microscope stage (Sage air curtain; Sage Instrument Inc., White Plains, NY) as soon as possible after removal from the incubator.

To clean coverslips: Coverslips (22 × 22 mm) are placed in a covered jar secured to a rotating stage (agitated at 80–100 rpm for 5 min) and are cleaned by two rinses in 25% Radiac detergent (Atomic Products Corp., Shirley, NY), two rinses in 70% ethanol, and four rinses through 95% ethanol. Coverslips are stored in the last ethanol rinse and are flamed just before use. If longer recordings are desired coverslips should be ultraviolet (UV) sterilized for 30 min prior to use and sterile techniques should be implemented.

### C. Immunofluorescence with Anti-amylase

1. Resuspend isolated acini in complete buffer containing penicillin/steptomycin.

2. Allow acini to settle; aspirate off all but 2.0 ml of buffer. Settle 250 $\mu$l of cell suspension onto precleaned coverslips. Return the coverslips to the incubator for 1–2.5 hr in order to let the acini firmly adhere.

3. Aspirate off the medium and add 1–2 ml of 3% paraformaldehyde in phosphate-buffered saline (PBS) (50 m$M$ sodium phosphate–140 m$M$ NaCl, pH 7.4).

4. Fix the cells at room temperature for 1 hr.

5. Aspirate off the fixative and wash with 0.1 $M$ Tris (pH 7.4) for 2 min. Rinse on a rotary shaker (50–75 rpm); repeat rinse.

6. Aspirate off rinse and replace with 0.1% Triton X-100–0.1 $M$ Tris for 4 min on a rotary shaker.

7. Wash in 0.1 $M$ Tris–0.1% Triton X-100: three rinses (2 min each) on a rotary shaker.

8. Aspirate the supernatant and replace with 1% BSA–0.1 $M$ Tris–0.1% Triton X-100 for 15 min.

9. Dilute primary antibody, anti-amylase (polyclonal gift from F. Gorelick), 1 : 100 in 1% BSA–0.1 $M$ Tris–0.1% Triton X-100.

10. Place the coverslips and primary antibody into a moist chamber for overnight incubation in a 4°C refrigerator.

11. Rinse three times (2 min each) with 1% BSA–0.1 $M$ Tris–0.1% Triton X-100.

12. Dilute secondary antibody, goat anti-rabbit (rhodaminated, Vector Laboratories, Burlingame, CA), 1 : 100 in 1% BSA–0.1 $M$ Tris–0.1% Triton X-100; use 500 $\mu$l/coverslip. Cover with aluminum foil and incubate at room temperature for 1 hr.

13. Rinse three times (2 min each) in 0.1 $M$ Tris.

14. Mount in 1 drop of Aqua-Polymount (Polysciences, Warrington, PA) and seal with nail polish.

## D. Cold-Temperature Block of Lipid Transport

1. Place a 16 and 20°C water bath in a 4°C cold room in order to stabilize temperatures to close tolerances.

2. Float a plastic box in the water bath.

3. Place a moist paper towel in the bottom of the plastic box and place the culture dishes (coverslip preparations of cells inside) on top of the toweling. This keeps the temperature of the culture dish constant.

4. Load all dyes at 16 and 20°C, rinse, and then replace with culture medium that has been maintained at the same temperature.

5. Load the coverslip containing cells into the perfusion chamber immediately before viewing. The perfusion chamber should not be cold or it will fog up as it is viewed on the confocal microscope. View the coverslip for no more than 3–5 min, as lipid will begin to mobilize after this time. The entire procedure from start to finish should take 5 min and several images of the sample can be collected within these time constraints.

## E. Perfusion Chambers

We are currently using two versions of a perfusion chamber that was designed by S. Smith and P. Forscher (Forscher *et al.*, 1987). A description of these two chambers (Fig. 6), now available from the Yale University Medical School Machine Shop, follows.

### 1. Chamber A

This is a flow-through perfusion chamber that allows rapid exchange of solutions. The major principle behind this design is that a sandwich of coverslips

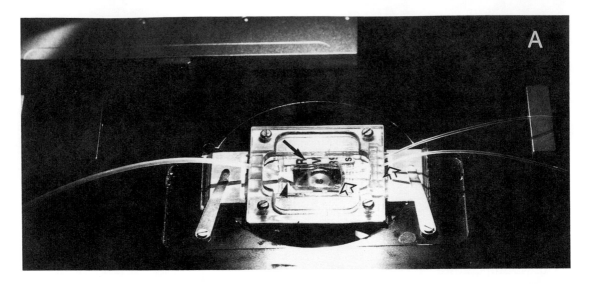

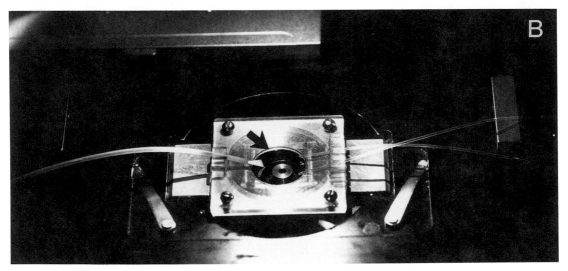

**Fig. 6**  (A) Flow-through perfusion chamber. A sandwich is made of glass coverslips separated by a spacer cut from a plastic ruler (arrow). The suction from the room vacuum attaches to a triangle of filter paper (arrowhead) on the opposite side from where the tubing delivering perfusate (open arrows) enters. (B) Open chamber. This chamber is not ideal for rapid superfusion experiments because it is open and it is not easy to regulate the volume of perfusate. This chamber is appropriate for thick specimens. A bead of vacuum grease is placed around the underside of the chamber top (arrow), insuring a leak-proof seal with a coverslip forming the bottom of the chamber. Thick specimens need to be held in place to prevent movement into the path of the laser. We use gauze glued to a ring of thick platinum wire to restrain specimens.

makes it possible to exchange a small volume of superfusate (a roughly 250- to 275-$\mu$l volume) rapidly (within tenths of a second).

1. With a diamond scribe, score a line 3–5 mm from the right-hand edge of a 22 × 22 mm No. 1 glass coverslip and break it.

2. Holding the coverslip in the same orientation, place a thin bead of silicone vacuum grease on the top and bottom edge (the short edges).

3. Cut a 2- to 3-mm wide by 20-mm long strip from a plastic ruler and place it on top of the bead of vacuum grease.

4. Run another bead of vacuum grease on top of the spacer.

5. Invert this assembly and lower it into the culture dish containing the coverslip with cells. Gently press this assembly down onto the coverslip and produce a sandwich that consists of cells on the bottom, a layer of medium, and the shortened coverslip on top.

6. Place the coverslip sandwich into the perfusion chamber and screw down the retaining screws at the four corners.

7. Insert tubing for perfusion and insert a triangle of filter paper in the tubing at the other end, which connects to a side arm flask hooked up to the room vacuum.

## 2. Chamber B

1. Place a bead of silicone vacuum grease around the underside of the chamber cover.

2. Gently press the cover (right side up) onto the coverslip containing the cells.

3. Fill the resulting reservoir with culture medium and screw the cover (with the coverslip attached) down onto the chamber base.

4. This chamber does not have a cover, so manipulations of the coverslip are possible.

## IV. Future Prospects

A strength of the procedures developed here is the ability to actually quantify the fluorescence of labeled lipids as they are transported through the post-Golgi secretory compartments. This paves the way for careful kinetic analysis of stimulated secretion. It is also possible to use a fluorescent light source to photoconvert fluorescent markers to an electron-dense diaminobenzidine (DAB) product that can be used for electron microscopy (Sandell and Masland, 1988; Pagano et al., 1991). Both NBD- and BODIPY-ceramide lend themselves to this technique (Pagano et al., 1991). Minute differences in the location of labeled lipids should be resolvable by coupling the increased resolution of the electron microscope with the sensitivity of the DAB reaction product.

# References

Amsterdam, A., and Jamieson, J. D. (1974a). *J. Cell Biol.* **63**, 1057–1073.

Amsterdam, A., and Jamieson, J. D. (1974b). *J. Cell Biol.* **63**, 1037–1056.

Amsterdam, A., Solomon, T. E., and Jamieson, J. D. (1978). *Methods Cell Biol.* **20**, 361–378.

Bruzzone, R., Halban, P. A., Gjinovci, A., and Trimble, E. R. (1985). *Biochem. J.* **226**, 621–624.

Chattopadahyay, A. (1990). *Chem. Phys. Lipids* **53**, 1–15.

Cooper, M. S., Cornell-Bell, A. H., Chernjavsky, A., Dani, J. W., and Smith, S. J. (1990). *Cell* **61**, 135–145.

De Lisle, R. C., and Williams, J. A. (1987). *Am. J. Physiol.* **253**, G711-G719.

Forscher, P., Kaczmarek, L. K., Buchanan, J., and Smith, S. J. (1987). *J. Neurosci.* **7**, 3600–3612.

Hootman, S. R., and Williams, J. A. (1987). *In* "Physiology of the Gastrointestinal Tract" (L. R. Johnson, ed.), pp. 1129–1146. Raven, New York.

Inoué, S. (1990). *In* "Handbook of Biological Confocal Microscopy" (J. B. Pawley, ed.), Rev. Ed., pp. 1–14. Plenum, New York.

Jamieson, J. D., and Palade, G. E. (1971). *J. Cell Biol.* **50**, 135–158.

Kobayashi, T. T., and Pagano, R. E. (1989). *J. Biol. Chem.* **264**, 5966–5973.

Lipsky, N. G., and Pagano, R. E. (1985a). *J. Cell Biol.* **100**, 27–34.

Lipsky, N. G., and Pagano, R. E. (1985b). *Science* **228**, 745–747.

Pagano, R. E. (1989). *Methods Cell Biol.* **30**, 75–85.

Pagano, R. E. (1990a). *Curr. Opinion Cell Biol.* **2**, 652–663.

Pagano, R. E. (1990b). *Biochem. Soc. Trans.* **18**, 361–366.

Pagano, R. E., and Sleight, R. G. (1985). *Science* **229**, 1051–1057.

Pagano, R. E., Martin, O. C., Kang, H. C., and Haugland, R. P. (1991). *J. Cell Biol.* **113**, 1267–1279.

Palade, G. E. (1975). *Science* **189**, 347–356.

Pawley, J. B. (1990). *In* "Handbook of Biological Confocal Microscopy" (J. B. Pawley, ed.), Rev. Ed., pp. 15–26. Plenum, New York.

Sandell, J. H., and Masland, R. H. (1988). *Histochem. Cytochem.* **36**, 555–559.

Van Meer, G. (1989). *Annu. Rev. Cell Biol.* **5**, 247–275.

Van Meer, G., Stelzer, E. H. K., Wijnaendts-van-Resandt, W., and Simons, K. (1987). *J. Cell Biol.* **105**, 1623–1635.

Van't Hof, W., and Van Meer, G. (1990). *J. Cell Biol.* **111**, 977–986.

Webb, R. H., and Dorey, C. K. (1990). *In* "Handbook of Biological Confocal Microscopy" (J. B. Pawley, ed.), Rev. Ed., pp. 41–51. Plenum, New York.

# CHAPTER 9

# Confocal Immunofluorescence Microscopy of Microtubules in Amphibian Oocytes and Eggs

## David L. Gard

Department of Biology
University of Utah
Salt Lake City, Utah 84112

# I. Introduction

Superposition of fluorescence from outside of the focal plane, and the resulting loss of image contrast and detail, presents one of the major obstacles to immunofluorescence microscopy of large cells such as amphibian oocytes and eggs. Until recently, this obstacle could be avoided only by laborious sectioning techniques or computerized deconvolution to remove image contributions from outside the focal plane (Agard *et al.*, 1989). The advent and increasing availability of confocal microscopes has dramatically facilitated immunofluorescence microscopy of microtubule organization in large cells. The optical sectioning capabilities afforded by confocal microscopy eliminate the out-of-focus fluorescence that degrades conventional epifluorescence images of large cells (see Fig. 1) (White *et al.*, 1987), and allow the rapid collection of images without the inconvenience of physical sectioning or complicated computerized deconvolution. The following discussion draws from our experiences with confocal immunofluorescence microscopy to examine microtubule organization in amphibian oocytes (stage I through maturation), eggs, and early embryos (Gard, 1991, 1992; Schroeder and Gard, 1992). Although the discussion is restricted to microscopy of amphibian oocytes and eggs, the goal is to provide a practical guide to immunofluorescence and confocal laser scanning microscopy (CLSM) of microtubules, and many of the techniques should prove useful for other large cells or complex tissues. Related techniques for whole-mount or histological preparation of amphibian oocytes and embryos have been discussed by Klymkowsky and Hanken (1991) and Kelly *et al.* (1991).

# II. Antitubulin Immunofluorescence Microscopy

## A. Fixation

Many different fixation procedures have been used previously for cytochemical, immunocytochemical, and ultrastructural examination of cytoskeletal organization in amphibian oocytes, eggs, and early embryos (Brachet *et al.*, 1970; Chu and Klymkowsky, 1989; Dent and Klymkowsky, 1989; Elinson and Rowning, 1988; Heidemann and Kirschner, 1975; Huchon *et al.*, 1981; Jessus *et al.*, 1986; Karsenti *et al.*, 1984; Palacek *et al.*, 1985). However, as we examined microtubule organization in *Xenopus* embryos and oocytes at an increasingly finer scale, we found that the procedures previously used did not adequately preserve microtubule structure and organization.

For example, we initially used immunofluorescence microscopy to describe the organization of microtubules and microtubule organizing centers (MTOCs) in blastula-stage *Xenopus* embryos fixed in 100% methanol (Gard *et al.*, 1990). When examined at the low magnifications imposed by sample size and conventional epifluorescence techniques, spindles and cytoplasmic asters were readily apparent in methanol-fixed blastomeres. However, on examination at higher

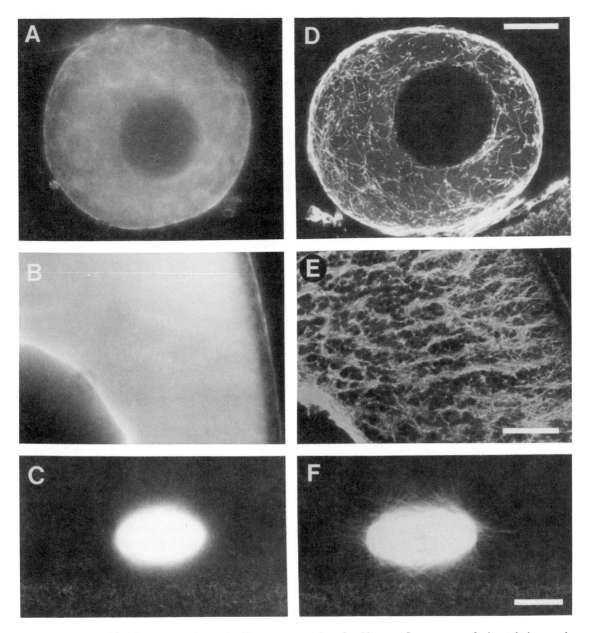

**Fig. 1** A comparison of epifluorescence and confocal immunofluorescence of microtubule organization in *Xenopus* oocytes. (A–C) Immunofluorescence of microtubules in (A) stage I, (B) stage VI, and (C) prometaphase I *Xenopus* oocytes, using standard epifluorescence optics. Fluorescence from outside the focal plane severely degrades the images, lowering contrast and obscuring details of the microtubule organization. (D–E) Single optical sections of similar samples [(C) and (F) are images of the same spindle] obtained by CLSM provide a dramatically improved view of microtubules in all three samples. (A–C) were photographed on a Zeiss axiophot with a ×63 NA 1.4 Plan-Apochromatic objective. (D–F) were obtained with a Bio-Rad MRC-600 fitted to a Nikon Optiphot and a ×60 NA 1.4 Plan-Apochromatic objective. Scale bar = 25 $\mu$m in (D) and (E), 10 $\mu$m in (F).

magnification and resolution by CLSM, microtubules of the interphase asters appeared fragmented and collapsed into bundles (D. L. Gard, unpublished observations), indicating that microtubule preservation was not optimal in methanol-fixed cells. In subsequent investigations of microtubule organization in *Xenopus* oocytes (stages I–VI), we have compared the preservation of microtubules in oocytes fixed by several different protocols. The results of these comparisons are summarized below.

Cytoplasmic microtubules in oocytes fixed with 100% methanol or acetone (at −20°C or room temperature) usually appeared severely fragmented (see Fig. 2), confirming results obtained previously with methanol-fixed embryos. Microtubule fragmentation was most evident in the cell interior, whereas microtubules in the cortex of stage VI oocytes or early embryos were often preserved to a greater degree (Elinson and Rowning, 1988; Houliston and Elinson, 1991). Addition of dimethylsulfoxide (DMSO) (Dent's fixative; Dent and Klymkowsky, 1989), taxol (up to 1 $\mu M$), or formaldehyde (3.7%) during methanol fixation had minimal effect on microtubule preservation. Fixation with methanol–acetic acid (10%) or Carnoy's solution (ethanol–chloroform–acetic acid; Clark, 1981) proved the least satisfactory, preserving few cytoplasmic microtubules. In addition, the mitochondrial mass of stage I oocytes fixed with methanol–acetic acid or Carnoy's solution exhibited a bright, diffuse staining with antitubulin antibodies.

In addition to the poor preservation of microtubules, several other problems were often encountered with cells fixed in methanol. Significant shrinkage and distortion of oocytes was observed commonly after fixation in methanol or other alcohol-based fixatives. Oocytes fixed in alcohol-based fixatives were also quite fragile, and tended to break apart during subsequent processing for immunofluorescence. This was particularly true of large ooctyes and unfertilized eggs, in which the cortical cytoplasm often broke away from the deeper cytoplasmic layer.

Despite the above-mentioned drawbacks, fixation in methanol or methanol–DMSO (Dent's fixative) has proved useful for whole-mount immunocytochemistry of microtubules and intermediate filaments in oocytes and early embryos (Chu and Klymkowsky, 1989; Dent and Klymkowsky, 1989; Klymkowsky *et al.*, 1987). In addition, meiotic and mitotic spindles remained relatively intact after methanol fixation, allowing dual-fluorescence visualization of microtubules (with anti-tubulin) and chromosomes (with propidium iodide) during meiotic maturation (Gard, 1992; see also Section II,H).

Preservation of oocyte microtubules by formaldehyde, in the absence of microtubule-stabilizing agents, was inconsistent. Microtubules in smaller (stage I) oocytes often exhibited discontinuities suggestive of incomplete fixation, whereas few cytoplasmic microtubules were preserved in larger (stage VI) oocytes. Inclusion of glycerol (30%) as a microtubule-stabilizing agent during formaldehyde fixation improved microtubule preservation in stage VI oocytes. However, severe osmotic distortion of the oocytes, resulting from the high

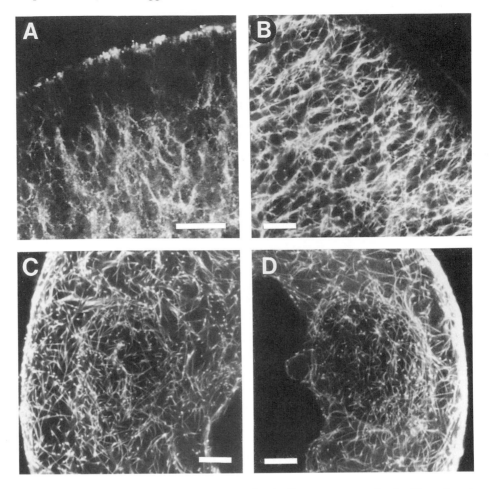

**Fig. 2** A comparison of microtubule preservation in *Xenopus* oocytes fixed with methanol, formaldehyde–taxol, or formaldehyde–glutaraldehyde–taxol. (A) A stage VI oocyte fixed with 100% methanol. Note the poor preservation of microtubules. (B) A stage VI oocyte fixed with formaldehyde–glutaraldehyde–taxol. (C) A stage I oocyte fixed with formaldehyde–taxol. (D) A stage I oocyte fixed with formaldehyde–glutaraldehyde–taxol. Scale bar = 25 μm in (A) and (B), 10 μm in (C) and (D).

glycerol concentration, limited the effectiveness of this protocol. Addition of taxol [0.1–1.0 $\mu M$ FT fix (see Gard, 1991)] also improved microtubule preservation by formaldehyde in stage VI oocytes, without the distortion associated with glycerol-containing fixatives. Preservation of microtubules in oocytes fixed with formaldehyde–taxol was substantially improved by postfixation in methanol (see subsequent text).

The most consistent preservation of individual microtubules throughout oogenesis and early embryogenesis was obtained with combinations of formaldehyde and glutaraldehyde. We have compared glutaraldehyde concentrations ranging from less than 0.1 to 2%. Our current protocol (see Table I) uses a modification of Karnovsky's fixative (Karnovsky, 1965) containing 3.7% formaldehyde, 0.25% glutaraldehyde, and 0.5 $\mu M$ taxol in a modified microtubule assembly buffer (FGT fix; Gard, 1991, 1992). This protocol provides a compromise between the improved microtubule preservation and the increased autofluorescence and poor penetration properties associated with higher glutaraldehyde concentrations (see below; see also Cross and Williams, 1991, for a discussion of the effects of glutaraldehyde fixation on microtubule structure). Although taxol is normally included during fixation, identical results have been obtained in the absence of taxol (FG fix; Gard, 1991, 1992; Schroeder and Gard, 1992).

**Table I**
**Antitubulin Immunofluorescence for Confocal Microscopy**[a]

1. Samples should be as free of extraneous tissue or extracellular material as possible. Oocytes are isolated by collagenase digestion followed by manual removal of residual follicle material (Gard, 1991). Eggs and early embryos are dejellied with 2% cysteine (pH 8.0) or 5 m$M$ dithiothreitol (in 30 m$M$ Tris-HCl, pH 8.5)
2. Fix oocytes for 2–8 hr in ~1 ml of FGT or FG fix (see Section IV) at room temperature
3. Postfix in 100% methanol overnight. Samples can be stored in methanol indefinitely at room temperature or −20°C.
4. Bleach with peroxide–methanol (Dent and Klymkowsky, 1989) for 24–72 hr at room temperature (optional) Exposure to fluorescent room lights or sunlight appears to speed the bleaching process
5. Rehydrate in PBS (several changes at room temperature)
6. Use a sharp scalpel blade to bisect the oocytes or eggs (optional)
7. Incubate in 100 m$M$ NaBH$_4$ (in PBS; no detergents) for 4–6 hr at room temperature, or overnight at 4°C. Do not cap tubes
8. Carefully remove NaBH$_4$, and wash samples with TBSN for 60–90 min at room temperature (three or four washes, ~ 1 ml each)
9. Incubate samples 16–36 hr at 4°C in 75–150 $\mu$l of primary antibody diluted in TBSN plus 2% BSA, with gentle rotation
10. Wash in TBSN for 30–48 hr at 4°C, changing buffer at 8- to 12-hr intervals
11. Incubate 75–150 $\mu$l of secondary antibody diluted in TBSN plus 2% BSA for 16–36 hr at 4°C (with gentle rotation)
12. Wash with TBSN, as in step 9
13. Dehydrate in 100% methanol: three or four changes over 60–90 min at room temperature (graded series of methanol can be used if shrinkage or distortion is excessive). Samples can be stored indefinitely in methanol
14. Remove methanol, and add ~1 ml of BA:BB clearing solution. *Do not mix.* Methanol-dehydrated oocytes will float. Tap tubes on bench to break surface tension. Oocytes will clear as they sink through BA:BB (takes 5–10 min). Remove clearing solution and replace with fresh BA:BB[b]
15. Mount in BA:BB (see above)

[a] All incubations and washes can be performed in 1.5-ml microcentrifuge tubes (about 5–15 oocytes per tube).

[b] If samples retain a milky appearance, they may not have been adequately dehydrated. Poorly dehydrated samples can be salvaged by repeating the dehydration and clearing. Borohydride reduction can be eliminated and incubation times can be shortened for FT or methanol-fixed samples.

Fixation in glutaraldehyde introduced a number of secondary problems. First, glutaraldehyde fixation is incompatible with some antibodies and staining procedures. None of the commercial tubulin antibodies we have used (see Table VI in Section IV) have suffered from this difficulty. However, other antisera should be tested for their compatibility with glutaraldehyde fixation (methanol or formaldehyde fixation can be used with antibodies incompatible with glutaraldehyde). Second, glutaraldehyde-fixed samples must be treated with sodium borohydride to eliminate unreacted aldehydes and diminish background autofluorescence (Weber *et al.*, 1978). Finally, penetration of antibodies into glutaraldehyde-fixed oocytes was substantially slower than into methanol- or formaldehyde-fixed samples (see Section II,D).

In our protocol, the primary fixation with formaldehyde–taxol or formaldehyde–glutaraldehyde–taxol is followed by postfixation in 100% methanol (at −20°C or room temperature). We initially included this postfixation as an intermediate step prior to bleaching with peroxide–methanol (Dent and Klymkowsky, 1989; see subsequent text). However, we have subsequently found that postfixation in methanol significantly improved microtubule preservation in oocytes fixed with formaldehyde–taxol (A. D. Roeder and D. L. Gard, unpublished observations) (microtubule preservation in oocytes fixed with glutaraldehyde-containing fixatives was not dependent on postfixation). As an added advantage, oocytes can be stored in methanol for extended periods without noticeable deterioration.

## B. Bleaching

A dense layer of pigment in the animal hemisphere of amphibian oocytes and eggs conceals underlying cytoplasmic structures. The dark pigments found in amphibian oocytes and eggs can be bleached with hydrogen peroxide and methanol as described by Dent and Klymkowsky (1989). Microtubule organization and reactivity with anti-tubulin antibodies appear unaffected by extended bleaching (as much as 72 hr). Exposure to fluorescent room lights or natural sunlight appears to speed the bleaching process.

## C. Borohydride Reduction of Unreacted Aldehydes

Cells fixed with glutaraldehyde should be treated with sodium borohydride to eliminate unreacted aldehydes and reduce background fluorescence (Weber *et al.*, 1978). We have used concentrations of $NaBH_4$ ranging from 50 to 200 m$M$ (in phosphate-buffered saline (PBS) without noticing any detrimental effect on microtubule structure, organization, or antibody reactivity. $NaBH_4$ should be used in buffers lacking detergents to prevent foaming, and containers should be left uncapped during borohydride treatment to prevent pressure build-up.

## D. Antibody Incubations

Preparation of oocytes and eggs for immunofluorescence microscopy is similar in most respects to that for other cell or tissue samples, with two exceptions: (1) oocytes are not attached to a substrate (such as a coverslip or microscope slide), and (2) the large size of oocytes and eggs requires that antibody incubations and intermediate washes be lengthened considerably.

The large size of oocytes prevents them from being easily attached to a solid substrate. Oocytes, ovaries from small frogs, or small pieces of adult ovary are therefore processed *en bloc* in 1.5-ml microcentrifuge tubes. The entire process of preparing oocytes for immunofluorescence, from fixation through clearing, can be accomplished in a single microcentrifuge tube. As many as 15–20 stage VI oocytes (1.2-mm diameter) can be processed per tube, using 75–150 $\mu$l of diluted antibodies. During antibody incubations or intermediate washes, samples are gently rotated (1–3 rpm) on a tissue infiltrator (Ted Pella, Redding, CA) or other laboratory rotary mixer.

The penetration of antibodies into formaldehyde–glutaraldehyde-fixed oocytes is limited to 75–100 $\mu$m in an overnight incubation (12–16 hr at 4°C; penetration was somewhat faster in methanol- or formaldehyde-fixed oocytes). We often bisect large cells (stage VI *Xenopus* oocytes and unfertilized eggs) to facilitate penetration of antibodies. Even after bisection, incubations in primary and secondary antibodies range from 16–48 hr (at 4°C). The duration of intermediate washes also must be increased, resulting in intermediate rinses ranging from 32 to 48 hr (at 4°C; with several changes of buffer).

In our experience, nonspecific staining of oocyte cytoplasm by monoclonal anti-tubulin antibodies has been slight, and we have not found it necessary to preblock samples prior to incubation with primary antibodies. Bovine serum albumin and nonionic detergent [Nonidet P-40 (NP-40) or Triton X-100] are included in both primary and secondary antibody solutions, and fluorescent secondary antibodies are routinely preadsorbed with rat liver acetone powder (Sigma, St. Louis, MO; Karr and Alberts, 1986) to minimize nonspecific interactions.

## E. Fluorochromes for Single- and Dual-Label Confocal Immunofluorescence Microscopy

The choice of fluorochromes for laser scanning confocal microscopy is limited by the emmision lines of commonly available lasers. The argon ion lasers found on many first-generation laser scanning microscopes provide strong emmision lines at 488 and 514 nm. Although fluoresceins ($\lambda_{ex}$ 490 nm; Haugland, 1991; Tsien and Waggoner, 1989) are excited more efficiently by argon ion lasers, both fluorescein- and rhodamine-conjugated secondary antisera have proved useful for CLSM. In large part, the poor efficiency with which rhodamines ($\lambda_{ex}$ 540–575 nm; Haugland, 1991; Tsien and Waggoner, 1989) are excited by argon ion lasers is countered by their greater resistance to photobleaching. For this reason, we prefer rhodamine-labeled secondary antibodies for most applications.

Dual-label immunofluorescence has, in practice, proved more problematic. The emmision maxima of fluoresceins and rhodamines are too close to allow efficient separation by commonly used dichroic interference filters. Texas Red (Molecular Probes, Eugene, OR), which has an emission maximum near 615 nm, can be more easily separated from fluorescein emission. However, Texas Red ($\lambda_{ex}$ 591) is poorly excited (<10%) by the 488- and 514-nm emission lines of argon ion lasers. The availability of laser scanning confocal microscopes equipped with argon-krypton lasers, providing a strong emission line at 568 nm, facilitates dual immunofluorescence with fluorescein and Texas Red as fluorochromes. Finally, new fluorochromes are currently under development (by Molecular Probes and other vendors), with application in laser scanning microscopy a key feature in their design.

## F. Clearing

Accumulation of yolk during oogenesis renders *Xenopus* oocytes (stages II–VI), eggs, and early embryos completely opaque. To circumvent the obvious difficulties associated with microscopy of nontransparent samples, previous investigations of cytoskeletal organization during late oogenesis and early embryogenesis in amphibians resorted to involved embedding and sectioning techniques (Huchon *et al.*, 1981; Palecek *et al.*, 1985; Jessus *et al.*, 1986; see Kelly *et al.*, 1991, for a discussion of histological methods), or restricted views to the immediate cortical regions of the cell (Elinson and Rowning, 1988; Houliston and Elinson, 1991; see Huchon *et al.*, 1988, for isolation of oocyte cortices). The development of a procedure using benzyl alcohol and benzylbenzoate (BA:BB) to clear *Xenopus* eggs (Murray and Kirschner, as cited in Dent and Klymkowsky, 1989) has greatly facilitated application of immunofluorescence and other microscopic techniques to the study of amphibian oogenesis and early development. BA:BB renders *Xenopus* oocytes, eggs, and early embryos nearly transparent, and has also been found useful for a wide variety of animal, plant, and fungal tissues (references cited in Klymkowsky and Hanken, 1991; Kropf *et al.*, 1990).

Despite its usefulness as a clearing agent, BA:BB has several disadvantages. BA:BB is immiscible with aqueous solutions, limiting its use to samples that can be dehydrated in methanol, ethanol, or acetone prior to clearing. Both benzyl alcohol and benzyl benzoate are natural products. However, BA:BB clearing solution should be considered toxic (Klymkowsky and Hanken, 1991; see also Section IV), and appropriate caution should be used when mounting and handling samples prepared with BA:BB. Caution is also advised while examining samples mounted in BA:BB. Although many laboratory plastics are resistant to BA:BB (a notable exception being computer keyboards), care should be taken to avoid costly damage to microscopes or other equipment. Additional drawbacks to the use of BA:BB as a clearing agent, discussed in greater detail by Klymkowsky and Hanken (1991), include the brittleness of BA:BB-cleared samples and the solubility of many histochemical stains in BA:BB.

## G. Mounting Oocytes for Confocal Microscopy

Most high-power objectives have working distances that allow complete optical sectioning of oocytes up to 125 $\mu$m in diameter. For this reason, small oocytes or intact ovaries from small frogs can be dehydrated, cleared, and mounted in BA:BB between a standard glass slide and coverslip. Alternatively, small transparent oocytes can be mounted directly in an aqueous mounting medium, skipping the dehydration and clearing steps. In both cases, sufficient pressure is applied to seat the coverslip without destroying the oocytes, and excess mounting solution is aspirated before sealing the coverslip with fingernail polish.

The limited working distance (less than 200 $\mu$m) of the high-numerical aperture objectives needed to resolve microtubules (see Section III,B) limits examination of the interior of larger oocytes or eggs. To circumvent this limitation, we manually bisect larger oocytes and eggs with a fine scalpel blade, and then collect optical sections from below the knife-damaged region (Gard, 1991, 1992; Schroeder and Gard, 1992). Bisected oocytes and eggs are normally mounted in BA:BB in 0.5-mm deep depression slides, with either their cortical or cut face toward the coverslip (allowing cortical graze or cross-sectioning, respectively). Alternatively, intact stage VI oocytes or eggs are mounted in machined aluminum chamber slides with coverslips cemented to each face, allowing examination of the opposing cortical surfaces. Both depression slides and aluminum slides can be cleaned with acetone and reused.

Samples mounted in BA:BB and sealed with several coats of clear fingernail polish can be kept in the dark at room temperature for extended periods without appreciable fading (see cautionary notes in Section IV). Fingernail polishes or other sealants should be tested for their compatibility with BA:BB before use (clear Sally Hansen's ''Hard-As-Nails,'' available from many cosmetic suppliers, works well as a sealing agent).

## H. Dual-Fluorescence Microscopy of Microtubules and Chromosomes

The commonly used DNA stains Hoechst 33258 ($\lambda_{ex/em}$ 343/480; Tsien and Waggoner, 1989; Haugland, 1991) and diamidinophenylindole (DAPI; $\lambda_{ex/em}$ 345/455; Tsien and Waggoner, 1989; Haugland, 1991) are incompatible with the argon ion or krypton–argon lasers commonly available on CLSM systems. We have obtained good results with the DNA intercalating dye propidium iodide (PI) ($\lambda_{ex/em}$ 530/615; Arndt-Jovin and Jovin, 1989) as a chromatin stain for dual-fluorescence CLSM (Color Plate 14; Table II). Propidium iodide, which is

**Table II**
**Dual–Fluorescence Microscopy of Microtubules and Chromosomes**

1. Fix oocytes overnight in 100% methanol (see discussion of methanol fixation)
2. Rehydrate in TBSN (no BSA)
3. Use a sharp scalpel blade to bisect oocytes (optional)
4. Incubate for 16–24 hr in primary antibody diluted in TBSN plus 2% BSA (4°C with gentle rotation)
5. Wash for 16–36 hr in TBSN at 4°C (with gentle rotation), changing buffer every 8–12 hr
6. Incubate for 16–24 hr in secondary antibody diluted in TBSN plus 2% BSA (4°C with gentle rotation)
7. Wash in TBSN as in step 5
8. Stain oocytes with propidium iodide (5–10 $\mu$g/ml) dissolved in 100% methanol (two changes for 15–20 min each)
9. Wash twice with 100% methanol (two changes for 30 min each)
10. Clear and mount in BA:BB[a]

[a] Alternatively, add PI to the last TBSN wash, and dehydrate in methanol as described in Table I. High levels of apparent cross-channel fluorescence appear to result from nonspecific binding of PI to cellular structures (including microtubules). This might be caused by excessive PI concentration or staining time. Try decreasing the concentration (to 1 $\mu$g/ml) or staining time, or increasing the wash times.

similar in structure to ethidium, can be excited by the 514-nm emission line of argon ion lasers, and can be viewed with either the GHS (rhodamine) or dual-filter sets supplied with the Bio-Rad MRC-600 (Bio-Rad Microsciences, Cambridge, MA). In our experience, PI staining of chromatin was most effective in oocytes fixed with methanol alone (Gard, 1992; see also Section II,A). Similar results were obtained with ethidium homodimer (Molecular Probes). A number of new asymmetric cyanine DNA-specific dyes have been developed and marketed by Molecular Probes. Preliminary results with YO-PRO-1 ($\lambda_{ex/em}$ 491/509) and BO-PRO-3 ($\lambda_{ex/em}$ 575/599) indicate that these dyes may prove useful for laser scanning confocal microscopy of aldehyde-fixed specimens. A more complete discussion of nuclear stains for fluorescence and confocal microscopy can be found in Arndt-Jovin and Jovin (1989) and Summers (*et al.* [10], this volume).

## I. Minimizing Photobleaching of Fluorescent Samples

Fading or photobleaching of fluorescent samples during observation, a problem commonly associated with fluorescence microscopy, is also encountered with laser scanning microscopy. In practice, however, we have not found photobleaching to be any more severe during laser scanning confocal microscopy. This may be due, in part, to the scanning nature of the illumination. Mounting samples in BA:BB clearing solution appears to afford some protection against photobleaching, particularly when using rhodamine as a fluorochrome. In an extreme case, we have collected more than 600 scans from a rhodamine-labeled sample without undue fading (less than 50% loss of fluorescent intensity). The rapid fading of fluorescein-labeled samples can be reduced by inclusion of propyl gallate (Giloh and Sedat, 1982) in the BA:BB mounting solution (however, see comments in Section IV). Photobleaching of samples in aqueous solutions or other mounting agents can be reduced by including anti-fade agents such as *p*-phenylenediamine, 1,4-diazabicyclo(2.2.2)octane (DABCO; Johnson *et al.*, 1982), *N*-propyl gallate (Giloh and Sedat, 1982), or NaN$_3$ (see Rost, 1991, and references therein for a discussion of the applications and merits of different antifade agents).

## III. Confocal Microscopy of Microtubules

The following discussion is intended as a nontechnical guide to confocal laser scanning microscopy (CLSM) of microtubules in large cells and complex tissues, based on our experiences with a Bio-Rad MRC-600 CLSM (Gard, 1991, 1992; Schroeder and Gard, 1992). Readers using other commercially available CLSM microscopes should consult the manufacturer literature for descriptions of comparable hardware and software features.

### A. Choosing Objectives for Confocal Microscopy of Microtubules

We routinely use Plan-Apochromatic objectives ranging from ×10 (NA 0.45, for wide fields) to ×60 (NA 1.4, for high resolution) for confocal microscopy of microtubules in amphibian oocytes. Flat-field (plan) objectives eliminate the spatial distortion of optical sections that would result from a curved focal plane. A simple test for comparing the field flatness and optical section thickness afforded an objective is outlined in Table III. We also found that Plan-Apochromatic objectives from several manufacturers gave consistently brighter images than fluorite (fluor or neofluor) objectives of similar numerical aperture and magnification (from the same or different manufacturers).

### B. Numerical Aperture and Resolution of Microtubules

Despite having a diameter only 25 nm (substantially below the resolution limit of light microscopy) individual microtubules are detectable by immunofluorescence microscopy (Weber *et al.*, 1978; Sammak and Borisy, 1988). The apparent diameter ($D$) of a single microtubule detected by immunofluorescence in a laser scanning confocal microscope is a function of the diameter of the diffraction-limited Airy disk of the objective;

$$D = 1.22\lambda/\text{NA}$$

where $\lambda$ is the excitation wavelength and NA is the numerical aperture of the objective. Thus objectives with large numerical apertures (NA 1.3–1.4) provide the best resolution of microtubule detail. Our ×60 objective (NA 1.4) provides

**Table III**
**Assessing Field Flatness and Optical Section Thickness with an**
**Inclined Reflector**

1. Prepare an inclined reflective slide by cementing a coverslip (or half of a microscope slide) to a microscope slide at an angle of 5–15°. It is not necessary to know the angle of the inclined coverslip
2. Collect a confocal image of the inclined surface
3. The image produced by a flat-field lens should appear as a straight stripe (in a vertical or horizontal orientation on the display monitor, depending on the orientation of the inclined reflector relative to the direction of scanning). The image stripe represents the focal "plane" of the objective, and should be straight and even in width at all confocal apertures (stripe width varies as the confocal aperture is changed). Curvature of the stripe, or broadening at its edges, is an indication that the objective is not well corrected for flatness
4. The width of the image stripe is a function of thickness of the optical section. The apparent thickness of an optical section ($S$; in $\mu$m) can be determined by measuring the stripe thickness ($T$; full width at half-maximum height, in arbitrary units such as pixels) and the horizontal displacement of the stripe ($D$; in the same arbitrary units) produced by a known shift in stage position ($F$; focus change, in $\mu$m):

$$S = F \times T/D$$

Representative optical section thicknesses for four objectives (with numerical apertures from 0.25 to 1.4) are presented in Table V

images of individual microtubules with apparent diameters of approximately 0.4 $\mu$m, consistent with the theoretical limits of resolution of this objective.

Unfortunately, the shorter working distances (less than 200 $\mu$m) associated with high numerical apertures constrain examination of large cells such as oocytes. Longer working distances can be obtained by decreasing objective numerical aperture, at the expense of image resolution. As an example, we often use a ×40 NA Plan-Apochromatic objective (NA 1.0) when dictated by the need for greater working distance. However, images obtained with this objective are noticeably less "crisp" than those obtained with our ×60 (NA 1.4) objective. Objectives providing magnifications of ×10 (NA 0.45) and ×20 (NA 0.75) provide substantially greater working distances, and are useful for wide-field views of microtubule organization when resolution of individual microtubules is not required.

## C. Image Scale and Resolution

The resolution of individual microtubles provided by laser scanning confocal microscopy is also a function of the image magnification or image scale. This results from the pixelated nature of images obtained by digital imaging techniques, including CLSM (Inoúe, 1986). For optimum resolution and image accuracy, the image scale (magnification) during collection should provide a pixel size less than or equal to one-half of the theoretical limit of resolution imposed by the objective (a condition of the Nyquist theorem; Inoúe, 1986).

In practice, good microtubule images (with apparent diameters approximating the Airy disk diameter of 0.44 $\mu$m) were obtained with a $\times$60 NA 1.4 objective and an image scale providing pixel sizes from 0.18 to 0.09 $\mu$m/pixel (corresponding to zoom settings 1.5–3 on a Bio-Rad MRC-600). The resolution of wide-field views provided by lower zoom settings was limited by pixel size, resulting in microtubule images that did not appear smooth. Larger image scales revealed no additional detail, and increased the rate of photobleaching. Additional enlargement of images collected at optimum scan-zoom settings can be obtained by using postcollection zoom features found on most CLSM (the Alt-Z command of the SOM software provided with the MRC-600), without compromising image quality.

The optimum range of zoom settings should be determined for each objective. As an example, a comparison of the magnification, pixel scale, and resolution of four common objectives is shown in Table IV (pixel size can be directly accessed by using the "scale bar" feature of both CM and SOM software supplied with the Bio-Rad MRC-600). We collect most images with scan-zoom settings of 1.5–2, which provide the best compromise between wide fields of view, minimal photobleaching, and optimum resolution. Selected regions of these images are then enlarged by using the postcollection zoom (ALT-Z feature of the SOM software) for detailed examination or photography. In practice, wide-field images should be collected before moving to higher magnification objectives or increasing the zoom factor. Collection of high-magnification images first often leads to unsightly photobleached rectangles in any wide-field images subsequently collected.

**Table IV**
**Comparison of Resolution and Pixel Size[a] (Image Scale) for Different Objectives**

| Objective | | | Pixel size ($\mu$m)[b] | | | |
|---|---|---|---|---|---|---|
| M | NA | R ($\mu$m) | Zoom 1 | Zoom 1.5 | Zoom 2.0 | Zoom 3.0 |
| $\times$10 | 0.45 | 0.70 | 1.66 | 1.12 | 0.83 | 0.55 |
| $\times$20 | 0.75 | 0.31 | 0.83 | 0.55 | 0.42 | 0.28 |
| $\times$40 | 1.0 | 0.31 | 0.42 | 0.28 | 0.21 | 0.14 |
| $\times$60 | 1.4 | 0.22 | 0.28 | 0.18 | 0.14 | 0.09 |

[a] For optimum image accuracy, the pixel size should be equal to or less than one-half of the objective resolution. At lower magnifications, image resolution is limited by pixel size rather than by the microscope objective.

[b] Pixel size was calculated for full-screen images (768 $\times$ 512 pixels) collected with the given Plan-Apochromatic objectives, using a Bio-Rad MRC-600 fitted to a Nikon Optiphot ($\times$40 from Zeiss; all others from Nikon). M, Objective magnification; NA, objective numerical aperture; R, diffraction-limited resolution calculated from the Rayleigh criteria: $R = 0.61\lambda/NA$ ($\lambda = 514$ nm).

## D. Optical Sectioning of Whole-Mounted Samples

The suppression of fluorescence from outside of the focal plane, often referred to as "optical sectioning," is one of the primary advantages provided by confocal microscopy applied to large biological samples (White *et al.,* 1987). The apparent thickness of optical sections obtained by confocal microscopy is a function of both the numerical aperture of the objective and the confocal pinhole aperture. For practical purposes, the approximate thickness of optical sections can be determined empirically from images of an inclined reflecting surface (see Table III). Representative section thicknesses obtained with several different objectives are shown in Table V. We commonly use confocal apertures in the intermediate range, providing optical section thickness from 1 to 2 $\mu$m (with a ×60 NA 1.4 objective). Smaller apertures (thinner optical sections) result in dimmer images, requiring increased laser intensity or photomultiplier gain (and the inherent problems of photobleaching and image noise). Larger apertures provide thicker optical sections in which details appear less crisp.

## E. Factors Affecting Image Brightness

Many factors affect the brightness of a confocal image, including characteristics of the sample, the microscope objectives, the laser intensity, the confocal aperture, and the photomultiplier sensitivity. The relative brightness (*B*) obtainable with a given objective is a function of both numerical aperture (NA) and magnification factor (*M*) (Inoúe, 1986):

$$B = (\text{NA}/M)^2$$

Although a ×10 NA 0.45 objective provides a brighter image than a ×60 NA 1.4 objective, increasing brightness by decreasing objective magnification can also

**Table V**
**Representative Optical Sections from Selected Objectives**[a]

| Objective | | Section thickness ($\mu$m) at given aperture | | | |
|---|---|---|---|---|---|
| *M* | NA | Open | Two-thirds | One-third | Closed |
| ×10 | 0.45 | 38 | 25 | 13 | 7.0 |
| ×20 | 0.75 | 14 | 10 | 6.7 | 5.0 |
| ×40 | 1.0 | 6.1 | 4.2 | 2.6 | 1.4 |
| ×60 | 1.4 | 3.7 | 2.0 | 1.0 | 0.7 |

[a] Section thickness (full width at half-maximum) was determined for objectives with different numerical apertures as described in Table III, using a Bio-Rad MRC-600 fitted to a Nikon Optiphot. Section thicknesses for other objectives of similar numerical aperture will vary.

affect resolution. Low-magnification objectives normally have smaller numerical apertures, which limit resolution of microtubule detail.

Increasing image brightness by increasing illumination (laser intensity) comes at the expense of more rapid photobleaching. To minimize photobleaching during image collection, we typically use neutral-density (ND) filters to reduce laser intensity to 3–10% of maximum (ND 1–1.5, with a 25-mW laser). Inclusion of antifade agents in the mounting solution can also significantly reduce photobleaching (see above).

The confocal aperture controls image brightness by changing the volume of sample from which photons are collected. More photons are collected from a thicker optical section, resulting in a brighter image. Conversely, thin optical sections obtained by closing down the confocal aperture provide a dimmer image (all other factors being equal).

Image brightness also can be increased by adjusting the sensitivity (gain) of the photomultiplier or detector. However, increasing detector sensitivity also results in increased noise, and images that appear grainy. Photomultiplier noise can be significantly reduced by averaging or filtering successive scans of the sample (at the expense of increased photobleaching).

In practice, confocal aperture, laser intensity, and gain all interact to determine the brightness of the collected image. These parameters must be balanced empirically against each other, and against the inherent brightness and stability of the fluorescent sample. In our experience, the best images of microtubules were obtained by Kalman averaging 5–15 successive scans (1 sec/scan), using (1) moderate confocal apertures, providing optical sections 1–2 $\mu$m thick, (2) neutral-density filters reducing laser intensity to 3–10% of maximum, and (3) moderate gain settings (50–75% of maximum). When image brightness must be increased, adjustments are first made to the photomultiplier gain, followed by laser intensity and/or confocal aperture.

For best results, image brightness should be adjusted to make full use of the dynamic range of the instrument. Setting of the gain and black level to their optimum levels is facilitated by use of a false-color display that maps the zero intensity (black) and peak intensity (white) to contrasting colors such as green and red (the "setcol.cmd" program supplied with SOM operating software for the Bio-Rad MRC microscopes; Color plate 14A). We routinely use this program during image collection to ensure maximum use of the gray scale afforded by the instrument.

With intrinsically faint samples, it is often not possible to collect an image spanning the entire brightness range of the instrument (especially if thin optical sections are required). Although the framestores of the Bio-Rad MRC microscopes collect 16-bit images (corresponding to 1024 gray levels), in the normal operating (byte) mode images saved to disk are truncated to 8 bits (256 gray levels). Unless quantitative comparisons of fluorescence intensity are to be made, intrinsically faint images should be rescaled before saving them to disk, to make full use of the 256 gray levels available (using the base and scale commands of the MRC microscopes, combined into a command program N.CMD). Images that are to be analyzed quantitatively should not be rescaled before saving to disk, or should be saved in both raw and scaled versions.

## F. Dealing with Extreme Contrast

The extreme brightness differences between meiotic and mitotic spindles and surrounding astral or cytoplasmic microtubules make it difficult to capture both populations of microtubules in a single image. Detail of the astral microtubules is often lost if brightness is optimized for the central spindle (as in Fig. 3A). Conversely, increasing the photomultiplier sensitivity (gain) to reveal the peripheral or astral microtubules oversaturates details of the central spindle (as in Fig. 3B).

Two strategies can be used to deal with the extreme contrasts posed by meiotic and mitotic spindles. First, contrast can be altered after image collection by modifying the look-up tables (LUTs) used to map pixel intensity to display brightness. Application of a simple custom LUT (using the Bio-Rad LUT syntax: $0 = 0; 50 = 100; 150 = 200; 255 = 255$) to the data set displayed in Fig. 3A selectively expands the lower range of pixel intensities, significantly enhancing the appearance of the peripheral microtubules without oversaturating the central spindle (Fig. 3C).

In the second approach, images are collected by a nonlinear mapping of the photomultiplier output to pixel value. Nonlinear outputs are available through use of the enhance feature of the Bio-Rad MRC-600. The enhance control functions similarly to the gamma control of a scanning electron microscope. At its off (or 0) setting, the output of the photomultiplier is essentially linear. Positive enhance settings (+1 through +4) provide nonlinear outputs that expand the lower range of the gray scale and compress the upper range (the magnitude of the effect increases from +1 to +4). Negative enhance settings (−1 through −4) have the opposite effect, compressing the lower range of the gray scale while expanding the upper ranges.

Enhance settings that provide optimum contrast should be determined empirically. We find settings +1 to +3 most useful for imaging spindles (Fig. 3D; collected at enhance setting +2 on a Bio-Rad MRC-600). Negative enhance settings can be used to increase the contrast of phase and Nomarski DIC images obtained with transmitted light. The use of nonlinear mapping of the photomultiplier output prevents direct comparison of pixel brightness, and is not advised for images that require quantitative analysis.

## G. Processing CLSM Images

The digital nature of CLSM images allows application of a wide variety of image-processing techniques, both during and after image collection (Inoúe, 1986). In practice it is best to collect the best possible image and minimize the

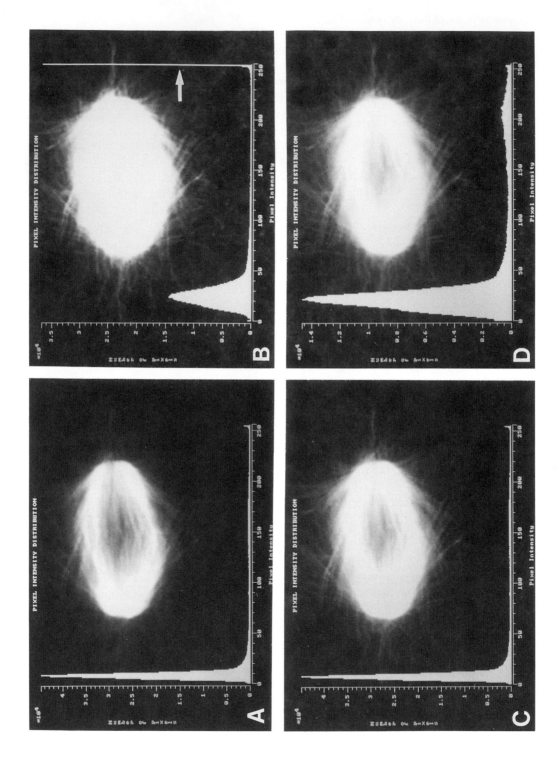

subsequent postcollection manipulation. Processing during image collection entails optimizing the magnification, optical section thickness, use of the gray scale, and contrast (using nonlinear outputs, if needed). In addition, photomultiplier noise can be minimized by averaging several successive images, using the Kalman or other averaging algorithms available with commercial confocal microscopes.

Postcollection image processing can include rescaling images to ensure maximum use of the gray scale prior to saving to disk, application of smoothing filters, edge-enhancement filters (the "crispening" filters accompanying the SOM software from Bio-Rad), image addition (projections, see following) or subtraction, or other transforms. Because such transformations change the relative pixel intensities, substantial image processing should be performed only after the unmodified data have been saved (to floppy, hard, or optical disk). In our laboratory, we limit postcollection processing of individual images to rescaling prior to saving an image, and minor contrast adjustment or image smoothing prior to photography.

## H. Serial Optical Sectioning

Attachment of a stepping motor to the stage focus (a feature available with most commercial confocal microscopes) allows automated collection of extensive series of optical sections (often referred to as $z$ series). We find that the optimal spacing for serial optical sections is equal to or slightly greater than the apparent thickness of the optical sections (1.0- to 1.5-$\mu$m spacing for a section thickness of 1.0 $\mu$m). This minimizes section overlap without creating large gaps between sections.

The ease with which large samples can be serially sectioned by CLSM often leads to collection of data sets containing large numbers of images, and inherent problems of data storage. For example, serial optical sectioning of an entire stage I *Xenopus* oocyte 100 $\mu$m in diameter requires 50–70 optical sections,

---

**Fig. 3** Effects of scaling and nonlinear output on image contrast. (A) A prometaphase spindle (also shown in Figs. 1C and D and Color Plate 14), collected with gain and black levels optimized for details in the central spindle. The overlying histogram of pixel intensities reveals that the majority of pixel values falls below 20. (B) The same spindle, collected with the gain setting increased to highlight microtubules of the peripheral spindle. Oversaturation of the central spindle is evident in both the image and in the excessive number of pixels with peak intensity in the overlying histogram (arrow).(C) The same data set as in A [compare the pixel intensity distribution in (A) and (C)], displayed with a custom LUT that selectively expands the lower range of lower pixel brightness (Bio-Rad LUT syntax: 0 = 0, 50 = 100, 150 = 200, 255 = 255). Peripheral microtubules are more apparent, without loss of detail in the central region of the spindle. (D) The same spindle, collected by nonlinear photomultiplier output (enhance +2 on the Bio-Rad MRC-600). Note the enhanced detail in the peripheral microtubules without oversaturation of the central spindle, and the expansion of the lower range of pixel intensities in the histogram. All images were photographed and printed under identical conditions.

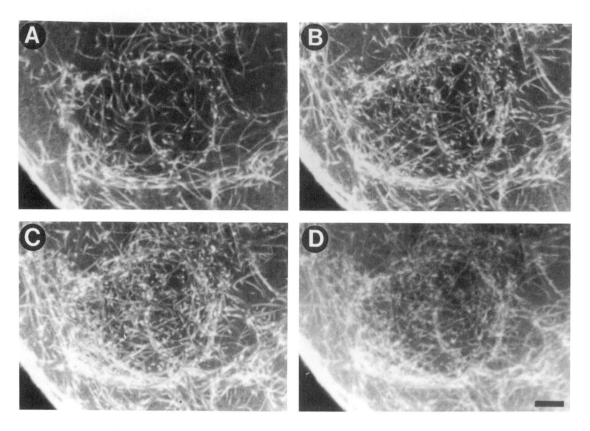

**Fig. 4**  Projection of serial optical sections provides increased depth of focus. (A–D) The distribution of microtubules surrounding the mitochondrial mass of a stage I *Xenopus* oocyte. (A) A single optical section (~1 μm thick). (B and C) Projections of two (B) or three (C) adjacent optical sections (using a maximum brightness projection algorithm) reveal increasingly greater numbers of microtubules in the mitochondrial mass. (D) Projection of two optical sections [as in (B)], using a linear summation algorithm. Note the decreased contrast apparent when using the linear summation projection algorithm [compare to (B)]. Images were photographed and printed under identical conditions. Scale bar = 10 μm.

resulting in a data set requiring up to 24 Mbytes of disk space. For this reason, we limit most series of optical sections to 10–12 images (see following), often finding it more useful to collect a limited number of optical sections evenly spaced through the sample rather than an extensive set of serial sections. Alternatively, large series of serial optical sections can be stored as projections (see following). However, the spatial information lost during image projection cannot be recovered.

Images providing an extended depth of focus can be obtained by projecting adjacent serial sections. We find that projection algorithms displaying the maximum pixel brightness from each of the projected sections provide better contrast between microtubules and the surrounding cytoplasm (a comparison of linear summation and maximum brightness projection algorithms is shown in Fig. 4).

In theory, the depth of focus obtainable through projection of serial optical sections is limited only by the working distance of the objective and characteristics of the sample, such as transparency and depth of antibody penetration. However, in practice, projection of an excessive number of images often results in a confused image, decreasing the ability to follow individual microtubules (Fig. 4). The optimum number of sections to project is best determined empirically.

Several options exist for presenting the three-dimensional spatial information inherent in a series of optical sections of microtubules. Perhaps the simplest presentation is as a series of individual optical sections. Alternatively, most commercially available CLSM systems provide software for construction of stereo pairs (or stereo anaglyphs) from data sets containing a series of optical sections. Impressive video sequences can be created by transferring large series of serial optical sections to analog optical memory disks, for replay at standard video rates. Finally, more complicated three-dimensional reconstruction of the image can be accomplished with commercially available software packages.

## IV. Recipes and Reagents

Unless noted otherwise, reagents were from Sigma Chemical Corporation (St. Louis, MO). We have used the antitubulin antibodies listed in Table VI with good results.

Fix buffer:
80 m$M$ potassium piperazine-$N,N'$-bis(2-ethanesulfonic acid) (pH 6.8)
1 m$M$ MgCl$_2$
5 m$M$ ethylene glycol-bis ($\beta$-aminoethyl ether)-$N,N,N',N'$-tetraacetic acid (EGTA)
0.2% Triton X-100
Formaldehyde–glutaraldehyde fix with taxol (FGT-fix):
3.7% formaldehyde (from 37 or 18% stock)
0.25% glutaraldehyde (from a 50% stock)
0.5 $\mu M$ taxol (from a 100 $\mu M$ stock)

Mix in fix buffer. Use immediately (within 1 hr). Formaldehyde can be analytical grade (Mallinkrodt, Paris, KY) or electron microscopy (EM) grade (methanol free; Ted Pella, Inc., Redding, CA). Glutaraldehyde is EM grade (stored as a 50% stock at 4°C; Ted Pella, Inc.). We have not tested glutaraldehyde from other sources. Taxol is from a 100 $\mu M$ stock in DMSO, stored at −20°C (from National Cancer Institute; commercially available from CalBiochem, La Jolla, CA). FG-fix is the identical formulation without taxol. FT-fix is the identical formulation without glutaraldehyde.

Peroxide–methanol bleach (After Dent and Klymkowsky, 1989):
1 part hydrogen peroxide (30%): 2 parts 100% methanol (100%)

Peroxide is an excellent bleaching agent for oocyte pigments, clothing, and skin. Use caution to avoid damage to clothing or painful chemical "burns."

Phosphate-buffered saline (PBS):
128 m$M$ NaCl
2 m$M$ KCl
8 m$M$ Na$_2$HPO$_4$
2 m$M$ KH$_2$PO$_4$ (pH 7.2)

Tris-buffered saline with NP-40 (TBSN):
155 m$M$ NaCl
10 m$M$ Tris-HCl (pH 7.4)
0.1% NP-40 (Triton X-100 can be substituted for NP-40.)

Tris-buffered saline (without detergent) can be substituted for PBS during NaBH$_4$ reduction.

Benzyl alcohol–benzyl benzoate clearing solution (BA:BB) (from Murray and Kirschner, as cited by Dent and Klymkowsky, 1989):
1 part benzyl alcohol:2 parts benzyl benzoate
propyl gallate (50 mg/ml; optional)

Propyl gallate reduces photobleaching of fluorescein-labeled samples. The slight brownish color imparted to BA:BB by propyl gallate does not affect clearing. However, somewhat paradoxically, extended storage in propyl gallate causes samples to fade. For this reason, long-term storage of samples in BA:BB with propyl gallate is not advised.

**Table VI**
**Antitubulin Antibodies**

| Antibody | Antigen | Species | Source[a] | Reference |
|---|---|---|---|---|
| DM1A | $\alpha$-Tb | Mouse | ICN | Blose et al. (1984) |
| DM1B | $\beta$-Tb | Mouse | ICN | Blose et al. (1984) |
| 6-11B-1 | $\alpha$-Tb[b] | Mouse | NCA[c] | Piperno et al. (1987) |
| Tub-1A2 | $\alpha$-Tb[d] | Mouse | Sigma | Kreis (1987) |

[a] Vendors: ICN Immunologicals (Lisle, IL); Sigma Chemical Corporation (St. Louis, MO); fluorescein- and rhodamine-conjugated secondary antibodies were obtained from Organon Teknika-Cappel (Malvern, PA).
[b] Specific for acetylated $\alpha$-tubulin. Preferentially stains nondynamic microtubules.
[c] NCA, Not commercially available.
[d] Specific for tyrosinated $\alpha$-tubulin. Stains dynamic microtubules.

Benzyl alcohol and BB are natural products found in flower oils (BA) and balsams (BA and BB). Both are mildly aromatic, and are used in the perfume and confection industries. The $LD_{50}$ values for ingestion of BA and BB in mice are 3.1 and 1.4 g/kg, respectively (Merck index). However, both are skin irritants, and caution should be used to avoid contact (especially with the eyes).

Most laboratory plasticwares (microcentrifuge tubes, etc.) are compatible with BA:BB, notable exceptions being cellulose acetate and the plastic used in computer keyboards. We have heard rumors of microscope objectives being destroyed ("unglued") by careless use of BA:BB. Although we have not had any severe mishaps, caution is advised when mounting and examining samples prepared with BA:BB, to avoid costly damage to microscopes and other equipment.

Glycerol mounting solution:
10 m$M$ Tris-HCl (pH 8.0)
10 to 100 m$M$ NaN$_3$ in 90% glycerol

NaN$_3$ provides some protection against photobleaching. Other antifade agents include phenylenediamine, DABCO, or propyl gallate.

## Acknowledgments

The author would like to thank M. Schroeder, A. Roeder, B. Error, A. Friend, and D. Affleck, all of whom have contributed to the work described. Special thanks are due Dr. Ed King for his assistance with the confocal microscope facility. The work described has been supported by a grant from the National Institute of General Medical Studies. Acquisition of the confocal microscope was made possible by an award from the University of Utah.

## References

Agard, D. A., Hiraoka, Y., Shaw, P., and Sedat, J. W. (1989). *Methods Cell Biol.* **30**, 353–377.
Arndt-Jovin, D. J., and Jovin, T. M. (1989). *Methods Cell Biol.* **30**, 417–448.
Blose, S. H., Meltzer, D. I., and Feramisco, J. R. (1984). *J. Cell Biol.* **98**, 847–858.
Brachet, J., Hanocq, F., and Van Gansen, P. (1970). *Dev. Biol.* **21**, 157–195.
Chu, D. T. W., and Klymkowsky, M. W. (1989). *Dev. Biol.* **136**, 104–117.
Clark, G. (1981). *In* "Staining Procedures" (G. Clark, ed.), pp. 1–26. Williams & Wilkins, Baltimore.
Cross, A. R., and Williams, R. C., Jr. (1991). *Cell Motil. Cytoskeleton* **20**, 272–278.
Dent, J., and Klymkowsky, M. W. (1989). *In* "The Cell Biology of Development" (H. Schatten and G. Schatten, eds.), pp. 63–103. Academic Press, San Diego.
Elinson, R., and Rowning, B. (1988). *Dev. Biol.* **128**, 185–197.
Gard, D. L. (1991). *Dev. Biol.* **143**, 346–362.
Gard, D. L. (1992). *Dev. Biol.* **151**, 516–530.
Gard, D. L., Hafezi, S., Zhang, T., and Doxsey, S. J. (1990). *J. Cell Biol.* **110**, 2033–2042.
Giloh, H., and Sedat, J. W. (1982). *Science* **217**, 1252–1255.
Haugland, R. P. (1991). "Handbook of Fluorescent Probes and Research Chemicals." Molecular Probes, Inc., Eugene, Oregon.

Heidemann, S. R., and Kirschner, M. W. (1975). *J. Cell Biol.* **67,** 105–117.

Houliston, E., and Elinson, R. (1991). *Development* **112,** 107–117.

Huchon, D., Crozet, N., Cantenot, N., and Ozon, R. (1981). *Reprod. Nutr. Dev.* **21,** 135–148.

Huchon, D., Jessus, C., Thibier, C., and Ozon, R. (1988). *Cell Tissue Res.* **154,** 415–420.

Inoúe, S. (1986). "Video Microscopy." Plenum, New York.

Jessus, C., Huchon, D., and Ozon, R. (1986). *Biol. Cell.* **56,** 113–120.

Johnson, G. D., Davidson, R. S., McNamee, K. C., Russell, G., Goodwin, D., and Holborow, E. J. (1982). *J. Immunol. Methods.* **26,** 231–242.

Karnovsky, M. J. (1965). *J. Cell Biol.* **27,** 131a.

Karr, T. L., and Alberts, B. M. (1986). *J. Cell Biol.* **102,** 1494–1509.

Karsenti, E., Newport, J., Hubble, R., and Kirschner, M. (1984). *J. Cell Biol.* **98,** 1730–1745.

Kelly, G. M., Eib, D. W., and Moon, R. T. (1991). *Methods Cell Biol.* **36,** 389–417.

Klymkowsky, M., and Hanken, J. (1991). *Methods Cell Biol.* **36,** 419–441.

Klymkowsky, M. W., Maynell, L. A., and Polson, A. G. (1987). *Development* **100,** 543–557.

Kreis, T. E. (1987). *EMBO J.* **6,** 2597–2606.

Kropf, D. L., Maddock, A., and Gard, D. L. (1990). *J. Cell Sci.* **97,** 545–552.

Palecek, J., Habrova, V., Nedvidek, J., and Romanovsky, A. (1985). *J. Embryol. Exp. Morphol* **87,** 75–86.

Piperno, G., LeDizet, M., and Chang, X.-J. (1987). *J. Cell Biol.* **104,** 289–302.

Rost, F. W. D. (1991). "Quantitative Fluorescence Microscopy." pp. 115–127. Cambridge Univ. Press, Cambridge, England.

Sammak, P. J., and Borisy, G. G. (1988). *Cell Motil. Cytoskeleton* **10,** 237–245.

Schroeder, M. M., and Gard, D. L. (1992). *Development* **114,** 699–709.

Tsien, R. W., and Waggoner, A. (1989). "The Handbook of Biological Confocal Microscopy" (J. B. Pawley, ed.), pp. 153–161. IMR Press, Madison, Wisconsin.

Weber, K., Rathke, P. C., and Osborne, M. (1978). *Proc. Natl. Acad. Sci. U.S.A.* **75,** 1820–1824.

White, J. G., Amos, W. B., and Fordham, M. (1987). *J. Cell Biol.* **105,** 41–48.

# CHAPTER 10

# Applications of Confocal Microscopy to Studies of Sea Urchin Embryogenesis

## Robert G. Summers,* Stephen A. Stricker,† and R. Andrew Cameron‡

\* Department of Anatomy and Cell Biology
State University of New York at Buffalo
Buffalo, New York 14214

† Department of Biology
University of New Mexico
Albuquerque, New Mexico 87131

‡ Division of Biology
California Institute of Technology
Pasadena, California 91125

METHODS IN CELL BIOLOGY, VOL. 38

## I. Introduction

The principles, advantages, and some of the general applications of confocal microscopy are presented by Wright *et al.* ([1] in this volume). The primary benefit of the confocal microscope derives from its ability to obtain optical sections from which out-of-focus information has been removed by the confocal aperture. The background rejection of the confocal aperture is only one consideration, however. Specimen preparation is an equally important factor that determines whether or not sections of sufficient resolution and contrast can be successfully obtained from deep within a thick specimen (see Cheng and Summers, 1990). Once confocal images of adequate quality are collected from the interior of an entire specimen or from a limited area of interest within that sample, the optical sections are stored individually in a digital form on the host computer. Subsequently, these data sets can be transformed into three-dimensional, stereoscopic, or extended-focus views that allow an entire specimen to be viewed in focus (Boyde, 1990).

The ability to obtain volumetric renderings of confocal images is particularly important to the embryologist who is interested in spatial relationships of cells, organelles, or molecules during development. In addition, confocal microscopy can also be used for time-resolved studies of living specimens. In fact, when the temporal and spatial resolution capabilities of confocal microscopy are combined, "four-dimensional" images of biological specimens can be produced (with the fourth dimension being time).

In this article, techniques are outlined for performing laser scanning confocal microscopy on fixed or living sea urchin embryos. Following a brief description of the methodology required for microscopic analyses in general (e.g., gamete collection, culturing methods, microinjection, and sample preparation), specific applications of confocal microscopy are presented in three parts. In the first section, protocols are described for using confocal microscopy and three-dimensional visualizations to investigate nuclear divisions in embryos that were fixed during cleavage. The second part, which covers some uses of confocal microscopy on living specimens, describes time-lapse analyses of calcium dynamics, four-dimensional studies of embryogenesis, and supravital staining of nuclei as visualized by confocal microscopy employing the two-photon excitation technique. Finally, the third section provides methods for investigating the relationship between cell lineage and patterns of gene expression.

Although the methods described in this article directly pertain to sea urchin embryos, many of the techniques can be adapted for use on other cellular and developmental systems. It should also be noted that in a few instances (e.g., with regard to microinjection methodology, confocal microscope set-up, and three-dimensional reconstructions), more than one protocol is included in cases in which slightly different techniques are employed in the laboratories of the contributing authors. However, neither the description of a single protocol nor the inclusion of several alternative methods is meant to imply that the specific protocols listed in the article are the only techniques that will work. Instead, these techniques are simply examples of methods that have been tested on sea urchin embryos and proved to be useful.

## II. General Methods

### A. Animals, Gametes, and Culturing Methods

Adult specimens of several species of sea urchins including *Arbacia punctulata, Lytechinus pictus, Lytechinus variegatus,* and *Strongylocentrotus purpuratus* can be purchased from biological supply houses [e.g., Gulf Specimens Co., Inc. (Panacea, FL) or Marinus, Inc. (Long Beach, CA)]. For many of the analyses illustrated in this article, *L. pictus* was chosen, because gravid females produce relatively clear eggs, and adults tend to be hardy enough to survive for long periods in closed, aerated aquaria containing artificial seawater (e.g., "Instant Ocean", Aquarium Systems Inc., Mentor, OH). The reproductive season of these *L. pictus* in the field occurs from spring until early fall. In the laboratory, however, ripe specimens that are kept under a constant temperature and light regime (13–18°C; 12 hr dark : 12 hr light) remain gravid beyond the end of the natural breeding season, especially if the animals are fed. Thus gametes can be obtained for experiments and observations throughout much of the year. Gametes of *S. purpuratus* are obtainable in quantities sufficient for biochemistry and the molecular biology of development is much better understood for this species than for the other species listed. Under appropriate conditions these animals will also provide gametes all year long (Leahy, 1986). Although less clear than the *Lytechinus* species because of large amounts of yolk and pigment, these embryos are useful when the microscopic observations are to be correlated with spatially restricted gene activity during development.

Prior to the collection of gametes, the sex of *L. pictus* adults can often be determined by external examinations, because females tend to have proportionately larger gonopores than do the males. The shedding of gametes is induced either by mild electrical shock (Lutz and Inoué, 1986) or by the injection of 1–2 ml of 0.55 $M$ KCl through the peristomial membrane that surrounds the mouth region. Sperm is collected "dry" on petri dishes, whereas eggs are shed into beakers filled with filtered seawater (FSW), according to standard methods (Hinegardner, 1967; Leahy, 1986; Strathmann, 1987). After washing several times in filtered sea water, eggs remain viable for several hours provided they are kept cool (13–18°C) and in a monolayer. Undiluted sperm, on the other hand, can be used for at least 2 days if kept in a refrigerator.

To obtain embryos, washed eggs are inseminated with a freshly prepared sea-water solution of diluted sperm (Strathmann, 1987).

Zygotes are then washed 5 min after insemination with filtered sea water to remove excess sperm. Only batches of embryos with better than 95% fertilization envelope elevation and less than 5% abnormal first cleavage (polyspermy) should be used. Monolayers of embryos can then be cultured at the following temperatures: *L variegatus* (25°C), *L. pictus* (18°C), *S. purpuratus* (15°C), according to protocols outlined by Strathmann (1987).

## B. Microinjection

### 1. Microinjection of Calcium Indicators

A variety of fluorescent calcium indicators that are suitable for confocal laser scanning microscopy (e.g., fluo-3, calcium green, fura-red) can be obtained from Molecular Probes, Inc. (Eugene, OR). These dyes are available in either the cell-impermeant form that must somehow be introduced into the cell (e.g., via microinjection or electroporation), or in the acetoxymethyl (AM) ester derivative form that can diffuse across most cell membranes. Once loaded into the cell, the AM ester is cleaved by esterases, and the dye is thus trapped within the cell (Tsien, 1989). In the case of *L. pictus* calcium-sensitive dyes are microinjected into the eggs, because simple incubation in the AM esters does not produce a utilizable signal.

In dealing with any of the fluorescent calcium indicators, care should be taken to minimize exposure of the dyes to light. Stock solutions ranging from 4 to 10 m$M$ are made by dissolving the powdered dye in an injection buffer consisting of 10 m$M$ N-2-hydroxyethylpiperazine-$N'$-2-ethanesulfonic acid (HEPES) and 100 m$M$ potassium aspartate, pH 7.2. After centrifuging the dye stocks at full speed in a microcentrifuge for 5 min to sediment particulate material, aliquots of 5–10 $\mu$l are distributed to plastic tubes and subsequently frozen. Following thawing, each tube can be used for several injections and stored in the refrigerator for at least a few days.

To perform microinjections, freshly spawned eggs that had been washed at least 5 times to remove the jelly coat are attached to specimen dishes that had been coated with protamine sulfate (grade II; Sigma Chemical Co., St. Louis, MO). Specimen dishes can be prepared in advance by using a heated brass cork borer of appropriate diameter (e.g., 20 mm) to punch out a hole in the bottom portion of a 60-mm plastic petri dish while twisting the dish around the borer to punch out a hole. A No. 1 coverslip is then glued over the hole, using epoxy-type glues (e.g., Elmer's Super-Fast), which appear to be less toxic than the cyanoacrylate "super glues."

To affix the eggs for microinjection, the coverslip of the specimen dish is coated with a freshly made, 10- to 20-mg/ml solution of protamine sulfate in distilled water. Coating is achieved by covering the coverslip with the protamine sulfate solution for 1–5 min. The protamine sulfate is then thoroughly aspirated, leaving only a thin film of the fluid over the coverslip. Before the protamine sulfate has completely dried, approximately 0.5 ml of washed eggs in sea water is pipetted on the coverslip and allowed to settle without agitation for 3–5 min. The eggs are then fully covered with 15–20 ml of sea water that is gradually introduced at the edges of the dish to minimize disturbances to the specimens.

Microinjections are most easily accomplished on an inverted microscope, using a high-precision micromanipulator to position the injection pipette. The actual delivery of the dye into the eggs can be performed with a hydraulic-based system (e.g., Hiramoto, 1974; Kishimoto, 1986) or a high-pressure "picospritzer," which is commercially available from several companies (e.g., Eppendorf, Hamburg; Narishige, Tokyo). The analyses of calcium dynamics described in this article were carried out with a Zeiss Axiovert 10 (Carl Zeiss Inc., Thornwood, NY) inverted microscope that was interfaced with an Eppendorf 5170/5242 pressure injection system. To prepare injection pipettes, capillary tubing (e.g., 1.2-mm o.d./0.6-mm i.d. borosilicate glass with filament from Sutter Instruments, San Rafael, CA) is acid cleaned in aqua regia (82 ml of HCl, 18 ml of $HNO_3$) before being pulled on a Narishige PB-7 vertical puller. The pulled pipettes are then backloaded with approximately 1–3 $\mu$l of the dye solution, using a micropipetter (Gilson Pipetteman P-20, Rainin Instrument Co., Woburn, MA) that is attached to a drawn-out plastic tip ("microloaders"; Eppendorf). The dye-loaded injection pipette is then carefully positioned with the micromanipulator on the coverslip, and a small portion of the pipette tip is broken by tapping the microscope so that the pipette can be used for microinjections. Penetration of the injection pipette into the egg can be aided by tapping the microscope as the pipette indents the oolemma, or by initiating the injection just before moving the pipette into the cell, so that the pressure of the flowing dye helps to pierce the cell. Eggs that have been freshly spawned (i.e., within 1–2 hr) are easiest to microinject. Occasionally, however, during times early or late in the breeding season even freshly spawned eggs are recalcitrant to injection, and thus must simply be discarded in favor of eggs from another female.

Once the cells have been penetrated, the dye is injected with the minimum pressure required to deliver the fluid into the cytoplasm (typically 100–300 hPa, but these values are dependent on the size of the micropipette opening). Successful delivery can be monitored by observing the "clearing" of the cytoplasm as fluid enters the cell. With a picospritzer, it is difficult to determine the volume that is actually injected into the cell, although it is estimated that the optimal amount of dye to be delivered is on the order of 1–2% of the cell volume (for a more quantitative method of determining injection volumes by the "double oil drop" technique, see Hiramoto, 1974). To optimize viability during microinjections, care should be taken to keep the eggs cool (e.g., 15°C), and to avoid illuminating the eggs with short-wavelength light (i.e., the eggs should not be constantly checked by fluorescence microscopy to see if the dye has entered the cell).

## 2. Microinjection of Lineage Tracers and Nucleic Acids

The strategy for the injection of lineage tracers and nucleic acids is similar to that used for calcium indicators. It is based on methods published by McMahon *et al.* (1985) and Colin and Hille (1982). Because the observation of treated embryos will occur later, after hatching, an optically clear substrate is not required and unfertilized eggs are electrostatically affixed to plastic dishes. The affixed eggs may be fertilized and injected immediately or incubated to the proper stage, placed under a microscope, and then injected. The mode of injection differs depending on the task at hand: pressure injection is used for DNA, RNA, and fluorescent lineage tracer solutions into eggs, zygotes, and two-cell embryos whereas iontophoretic injection is required for the smaller cells of later embryonic stages.

Methods for injection of lineage tracers were previously reported (Cameron *et al.*, 1987, 1989, 1990). The eggs of the purple sea urchin, *S. purpuratus,* possess a more tenacious jelly coat than those of *L. pictus.* A brief wash in sea water titrated to pH 5.0 [2 $\mu$l of 0.5 *M* citric acid per milliliter of FSW brings it to pH 5.0] removes the coat. To prepare eggs in batches, the previously settled eggs are suspended in 100 ml of acid seawater for 4 min with occasional swirling. The seawater is returned to pH 8 by the addition of 1.5 ml of 1 *M* Tris-HCl, pH 8.0. The eggs are allowed to settle and washed several times with filtered seawater. Then a number of eggs that will not form more than a monolayer are placed in a dish. These eggs can be transferred to coated dishes and fertilized throughout the day of injection. Enough eggs for a few dishes (300–500) can be dejellied by brief exposure to acid seawater followed by transfer to coated dishes. The time of exposure to acid seawater is thus brief and can be controlled to achieve optimum sticking. The jelly coat contains components that aid in activating the sperm. If the jelly is removed too vigorously, fertilization may be difficult. With caution, unfertilized eggs can be injected with a minimum of activation. Much of the gene transfer work has utilized this method (McMahon *et al.,* 1985). However, freshly fertilized eggs are easier to inject because the operator does not have to be overly cautious to avoid activation. Because the cortex of the sea urchin egg stiffens and the extracellular coats harden following fertilization (Vacquier, 1981), the zygotes of *S. purpuratus* become difficult to inject by 30 min after fertilization. The eggs are fertilized with a freshly diluted sperm suspension and the embryos allowed to develop to the desired stage for injection, if necessary. The number of eggs fixed to an individual plate varies with the goal. An operator injecting zygotes with free-flowing needles can conveniently work with as many as 200–300 per dish, whereas injection of later cleavage stage embryos in blastomeres of specific embryonic regions is limited to 10–20 embryos per dish before the injection period exceeds the cleavage stage (about 1 hr at 16°C).

With the exocytosis of the cortical granules at fertilization, the vitelline layer rises off the egg surface and, in combination with components of the cortical granules, forms the fertilization envelope. Closer to the egg surface a second extracellular layer, the hyaline layer, forms from other components of the cortical granules. A peroxidase that cross-links the components of the nascent fertilization envelope is secreted into the newly formed perivitelline space (Foerder and Shapiro, 1977). Extensive discussions of techniques to dissolve extracellular coats are published (McClay, 1986; Harris, 1986; Weidman and Kay, 1986). Fully hardened fertilization envelopes are tough and can even prevent penetration of the egg or break the tips of fine injection microneedles. The hardening of this layer can be inhibited by the addition of 1 m$M$ 1,2,3-aminotriazole (ATA) in FSW (Showman and Foerder, 1979). Therefore all seawaters used for the incubation of embryos contain 1 m$M$ ATA. For the first 5–10 min after fertilization the hyaline layer remains relatively soft. Later it, too, can interfere with the impalement of the zygote or blastomeres for either pressure or iontophoretic injection. To soften the hyaline layer, which is composed of a calcium-gelable protein (Kane, 1970), the embryos are rinsed three times with calcium- and magnesium-free seawater (CMFSW) just before injection. Following injection, calcium and magnesium ion concentrations are returned to those of artificial seawater, the dish is then washed several times with 0.45 $\mu$m FSW containing penicillin (20 units/liter) and streptomycin (50 mg/liter) and the embryos are incubated in the dark at 16°C until the desired stage is reached.

Injection solutions should approximate the internal milieu to the extent that they do not interfere with normal cell function. A potassium concentration of 200 m$M$ seems to provide a minimum condition that does not disturb sea urchin embryogenesis. DNA reporter gene solutions also contain 20–40% glycerol to minimize the physical shearing that is anticipated to occur when the solution is ejected from the small orifice under pressure. RNA solutions have been effectively injected as water solutions but these molecules are usually much shorter in length than DNA molecules. Usually each egg is injected with 1000–1500 copies of a reporter gene construct along with carrier DNA (5-fold mass excess of *Hin*dIII-digested sea urchin genomic DNA). Reporter gene injection solutions are prepared the day they are used. Biologically inert fluorescent molecules that are large enough to remain confined by the cell membrane, yet are not sequestered in subcellular compartments, are the ideal markers for tracing cell lineages during development. Dextran, a poly-D-glucose that is aminated and that can be conjugated with a variety of fluorochromes, has been used extensively as a cell lineage tracer (reviewed by Luby-Phelps, 1989). In addition, the presence of lysine residues renders the molecule more efficiently retained during fixation. A number of dextrans of various molecular sizes and with various fluorochromes are available through Pharmacia (Piscataway, NJ) and Molecular Probes. We use an $M_r$ 10,000 dextran with one to three fluorochromes per molecule from Molecular Probes. We have used both fluorscein- and tetramethyl rhodamine-conjugated dextrans in double-labeling experiments. The rhodamine dextran is preferable because tissue autofluorescence is least at the rhodamine excitation wavelength. Lineage tracer solutions are made up in water at 50–100 mg/ml and frozen at −20°C in aliquots, although repeated freeze-thawing does not seem to harm the solutions. Thawed labeling solutions are spun in a microfuge to pellet any solids that might clog the injection micropipette. Injection micropipettes for pressure injection are pulled from 1-mm o.d.

glass capillary tubes with filament (''Omega Dot''; Frederick Haer and Co.). The micropipettes have been successfully formed by a single pull on a variety of horizontal and vertical pipette pullers. They should be several millimeters long, flexible, and closed at the end. Just before injection begins, the micropipettes are opened under the injection microscope by breaking against a scratch in the culture dish or on a fire-polished glass rod. An inverted Leitz microscope or a Zeiss Standard 16 modified to a fixed stage configuration is routinely used for microinjections. We also employ a thermoelectric cold stage set to 16°C for the injection of *S. purpuratus* embryos, although some species (e.g., *L. pictus*) can be handled at room temperature. The injection micropipette is manipulated with a Leitz micromanipulator and the pressure is provided by an oil-filled syringe with a screw adjustment. A hydraulic axial manipulator (Narashige) has been used for blastomere injection. More recently, we have employed an electronically actuated pressure valve (Picospritzer II; General Valve Corp., Fairfield, NJ) for both fluorescent tracers and nucleic acids. However, this device increases the time per injection and thus decreases the throughput compared to the free-flowing micropipette. Single blastomeres or contiguous pairs of blastomeres from cleavage-stage embryos have been injected iontophoretically with fluorescent lineage tracers from thin-walled aluminosilicate glass microelectrodes possessing tip resistances in the range of 10–50 M$\Omega$. We routinely use 1.2 × 0.90 mm filament glass, 4 in. long (A-M Systems, Everett, WA). The micropipettes are pulled on a programmable Flaming/Brown micropipette puller (model P-80/PC; Sutter Instrument Co.). A two-step program that pulls a micropipette with a wide shoulder and a short tip to facilitate delivery of the viscous dextran solution works best. The electrodes are filled at the tip with lysinated rhodamine dextran in water (LRD) (50 mg /ml) or lysinated fluorescein dextran in water (LFD) (50 mg/ml) and backfilled with 1.2 $M$ LiCl. Impalement of the cell is verified by the measurement of a resting potential. Fluorescent dextran is ejected with positive current pulses.

## C. Sample Preparation

The capability of producing clear optical sections of thick specimens is of particular use when studying sea urchin embryos, which range generally from 65 to 150 $\mu$m in thickness. In the simplest cast, embryos can be stained with supravital dyes and observed in the living state. For observations of living embryos in which only optical clarity is important, species with the most translucent cytoplasm (e.g., *Lytechinus* spp.) are best when compared with those with larger amounts of yolk or pigment (e.g., *Strongylocentrotus* spp.) because both excitation and emission light is scattered and/or absorbed by these organelles. The techniques for introducing vital dyes into the embryos by microinjection are included in Section II,B and the results of confocal microscopic imaging of supravitally stained embryos are described in Section IV.

Embryos may be fixed before staining. The simplest approach is to fix in one of the aldehydes (e.g., formaldehyde) and stain. A significant drawback is that residual aldehydes are themselves autofluorescent, and may produce nonspecific background autofluorescence. An example of a rapid method for staining fixed embryos is described in Section III,A. An alternative is a nonaldehyde fixative (e.g., Carnoy's; Section III,A), in which nonspecific fluorescence is not a problem, but the nonaldehyde fixatives generally do not preserve structure as well as the aldehydes.

The highest signal from fixed and stained thick specimens is obtained by dehydrating and clearing them in clearing agents with a refractive index that most closely matches that of the oil immersion optics ($n \approx 1.5$). Clearing agents replace intracellular water ($n \approx 1.3$) within the specimens and thus minimize reflection, refraction, and scattering of light at interfaces of subcellular components in hydrated fixed or living cells and tissues. Some clearing agents that have been employed successfully are glycerol ($n^{20} = 1.47$), methyl salicylate ($n^{20} = 1.53$), and benzyl benzoate ($n^{20} = 1.57$). Embryos may be mounted in the clearing agents and the coverslip sealed to prevent evaporation [wax or nail polish for glycerol or ultraviolet (UV)-polymerizable acrylic for esters]. $z$-Axis distortion or elongation, which interferes with volumetric reconstruction, is minimized by selecting a clearing agent with a refractive index that most closely matches the oil immersion optical path. According to P. Hertzler (personal communication), stained specimens can be stored in methyl salicylate for 6 months or more with little or no fading of the fluorophore and photobleaching seems to be reduced in specimens mounted in methyl salicylate when compared to glycerol.

Because of the short working distances of the high-numerical aperture (NA) lenses used for most confocal applications and the thickness of the sea urchin embryo, No. 0 coverslips (nominal thickness, 75–125 $\mu$m) can be used. Coverslips must be supported to prevent distortion of both living and fixed embryos. Glass coverslip fragments, glass spheres, or human hair can be used as supports. For example, plutei of *S. purpuratus* are just captured and prevented from movement when No. 0 coverslip fragments are used as spacers.

## III. Patterns of Karyokinesis in Fixed Specimens

The use of DNA stains in conjunction with confocal optical microscopy is particularly useful in the determination of cell arrangements and numbers and in the analysis of the patterns of karyokinesis that transform the single-celled zygote into a multicellular embryo (Summers and Cheng, 1989). Of particular benefit are the three-dimensional, "extended focus" (Boyde, 1990) views that allow the nuclei from an entire embryo or a selected region of the embryo to be viewed in focus simultaneously. Three-dimensional studies have been aided by volumetric visualization and analysis software that operates on stacks of serial optical sections obtained with the confocal microscope.

## A. Staining of Nuclei and Chromosomes

Nuclear staining facilitates the counting of cells and helps to determine anatomical features as well as the proper staging of embryos. A rapid method for obtaining uniform nuclear staining is discussed below (Cameron *et al.*, 1991).

Embryos are fixed for 1 hr in 1% formaldehyde in filtered sea water and then washed several times with filtered sea water. These fixed embryos are stained for about 10 min with propidium iodide (0.5 mg/ml) diluted from a stock solution with filtered sea water, then rinsed with filtered sea water and mounted in sea water for observation. Color Plates 26 and 27 are images of plutei prepared from propidium iodide-stained specimens. Because propidium iodide is extracted by alcohol during dehydration, these specimens cannot be dehydrated and cleared.

An alternative for nuclear and chromosomal staining is the Feulgen reaction, which is highly specific for DNA and can be utilized to stain blastomere nuclei of fixed embryos for observations of karyokinesis. A colorless form of the dye, pararosaniline sulfate (a Schiff reagent) is converted to a colored (magenta) form on covalent bonding to vicinal aldehydes within the tissue being stained. These aldehydes are produced specifically in DNA by hydrolysis of deoxypentose sugars with HCl in advance of staining with Schiff reagent. Time and conditions for hydrolysis, staining, and bleaching vary with the tissue being stained and fixation protocol. The method presented here will work for all three species listed in Section II,A, and is modified from Nislow and Morrill (1988). Although for our purposes the reaction was used qualitatively, it can also be used for quantitative DNA measurements. An excellent discussion of the chemistry and quantitative application of the Feulgen reaction has been authored by Schulte (1991). The Feulgen stain is particularly resistant to photobleaching when specimens are dehydrated, cleared, and mounted as described below. It should also be noted that the absorbance maximum of the DNA-bound basic fuchsin Schiff reagent is $\approx 550$ nm (Kasten, 1958; Ploem, 1967) and it is excitable with the 514-nm line of the argon ion laser (and also by the 529- and 568-nm lines of the argon and krypton–argon lasers, respectively).

For the Feulgen reaction for DNA, $\sim 0.25$ ml of packed embryos was removed from cultures at appropriate times following insemination and fixed for 24 hr in Carnoy's solution (3 : 1, ethanol : glacial acetic acid; see Summers *et al.*, 1991, for details). Removal of the fertilization envelope is discouraged because its presence does not interfere with Feulgen staining and denuded embryos tend to stick together by their hyaline layers and clump during processing. The use of a nonaldehyde fixative eliminates the possibility of fixative-derived residual aldehyde groups within embryos and hence alleviates the necessity for aldehyde blockers to eliminate nonspecific (background) staining. With sea urchin embryos, the nuclear staining results obtained with Carnoy's fixative are comparable to those from aldehyde-containing fixatives. If aldehyde-containing fixatives are essential, an aldehyde blocking protocol should precede the hydrolysis and staining protocols. For example, sodium borohydride (0.5% in an appropriate buffer) is used to block aldehydes following fixation.

Following fixation, embryos are washed twice in distilled water (5 min each wash), rinsed in ice-cold 1 N HCl for 3 min, and placed into hot (60°C) 1 N HCl for 8 min with gentle agitation to ensure complete hydrolysis. Following hydrolysis, the embryos are washed three times (2 min each wash) in ice-cold 1 N HCl and in distilled water three times (5 min each). Samples are placed into Schiff reagent at room temperature [prepared from basic fuchsin (after DeTomasi, 1936, as cited in Pearse, 1961) for 90 min in the dark. After staining, the embryos are washed for 15 min in sodium metabisulfite bleach (see Pearse, 1961), washed three times in distilled water (5 min/wash), dehydrated through a graded ethanol series (30–100%), cleared with two changes of methyl salicylate, and mounted on microscope slides in methyl salicylate (Section II,C above and Summers *et al.,* 1991). Embryos to be studied were selected with conventional wide-field microscopy, using transmitted illumination with white incandescent light. This permits us to choose embryos for confocal microscopy without prior exposure to the laser light source. An example of an optical section stained with pararosaniline–Schiff is shown in Fig. 2.

An alternative Schiff-type reagent can be prepared from acriflavine-HCl (Kasten *et al.,* 1959; Van Ingen *et al.,* 1979). This dye has a maximum absorbance of ~460 nm when bound to DNA and is excitable with the 488-nm line of the argon ion laser. For this method, embryos were fixed and DNA hydrolyzed as above. The embryos are then stained with acriflavine-Schiff reagent strictly according to Culling and Vassar (1961). An example of an optical section stained in this manner is shown in Fig. 1. The acriflavine-Schiff reagent is slightly less useful than pararosaniline-Schiff reagent for the following reasons: (1) embryonic nuclei and chromosomes are stained pale yellow and are less visible with transmitted white light, and (2) acriflavine is more susceptible to photobleaching.

## B. Confocal Microscopy of Feulgen–Stained Specimens

Feulgen-stained embryos can be observed with the Bio-Rad (Richmond, CA) MRC-600 confocal microscope. A Nikon ×40 Fluor, NA 1.3 objective lens and the green (GHS) filter set is used for basic fuchsin-Schiff reagent. In all cases, the 25-mW argon ion laser is set to maximum power (''H'') and the preamplifer gain set to maximum (''10''). The 568-nm line of the krypton–argon laser can also be used. The amount of excitation light is adjusted by placing neutral-density filters in the excitation light path to obtain an adequate emitted signal from the embryos and minimize exposure to laser light (photobleaching and specimen damage). The rationale for always using the maximum laser power is that the light feedback control in the laser may not function as well at the lower

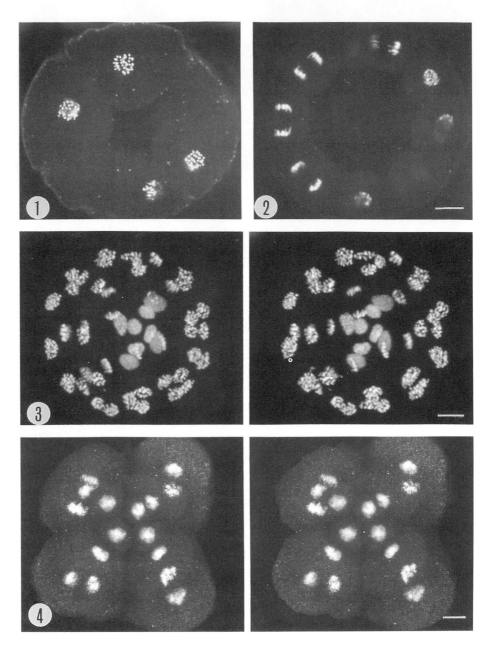

**Fig. 1** Single optical section of a fourth cleavage embryo of *L. pictus* stained with the acriflavine Schiff-type reagent for DNA, using the Feulgen procedure. This optical section was taken from 30 $\mu$m from within the 95-$\mu$m thick embryo. Contrast has been adjusted so that both chromosomes and cell outlines can be seen. Bar = 10 $\mu$m.

**Fig. 2** Single optical section of a seventh cleavage embryo of *L. variegatus* stained with the Feulgen reaction for DNA. This section, obtained from 50 $\mu$m deep within the embryo, is 1 of 83 serial sections. Bar = 10 $\mu$m.

setting. The maximum gain setting is always used because the photomultiplier is the least noisy part of the collection system and it is important to minimize the amount of laser light reaching the specimen while still obtaining a usable emitted signal. The confocal (detector) pinhole is set at "2" divisions of openness (a measured diameter of 2 mm; 3.8 optical units), which provides appropriate spatial filtration (background rejection) and maximum throughput of emitted light for sections of 1 $\mu$m (Sandison et al., 1993).

Serial optical sections ($z$ series) are collected by Kalman averaging [12 accumulations (MRC-500) vs 3 accumulations (MRC-600)] at 1-$\mu$m increments through entire (intact) embryos. An example of such an optical section is shown in Fig. 2. Generally, a 512 $\times$ 512 pixel image size is selected rather than the 768 $\times$ 512 pixel image size to reduce computer storage space (262 vs 394 kbytes) with zoom setting adjusted to the maximum possible to fit the embryo into the 512 $\times$ 512 box. These settings provide the pixel resolution that equals or slightly exceeds the optical resolution obtainable with this system (number of pixels per micrometer). This will optimize image information content with a minimum of photobleaching. Acquiring higher pixel densities will only increase photobleaching without appreciably increasing information content. Stereo views are produced by the pixel offset method, using a maximum projection algorithm (Bio-Rad software), and are shown in Figs. 3 and 4. Individual sections or stereographs are photographed onto either Kodak (Rochester, NY) T-Max 100 or Kodak Technical Pan films, using an analog photorecord device (Polaroid Freeze Frame or Presentation Technologies Screen Star). Positive projection slides (rather than photonegatives) can be obtained directly by inverting the contrast ramp and photographing with Technical Pan Film (medium contrast development at ASA 125). An analog photorecord device meets the framestore resolution capabilities of the image acquisition system and is less expensive for this application than the digital counterpart.

## C. Three-Dimensional Reconstructions with STERECON

We have extended the usefulness of the stereo views prepared from $z$ series of confocal optical sections (e.g., Color Plates 15–19) by using the three-dimensional imaging and image analysis program STERECON as developed by

---

**Fig. 3** Stereo pair of projection images of a sixth cleavage L. pictus embryo, vegetal polar view (micromeres facing the viewer) stained with the Feulgen reaction for DNA. Projections were prepared from 85 optical sections taken at 1-$\mu$m increments through the embryo. Pixel shift = +0.75, −0.75; bar = 10 $\mu$m.

**Fig. 4** Stereo pair of projection images of the living fourth cleavage L. pictus embryo stained with Hoechst 33342, vegetal polar view. Thirty-six optical sections were taken at 3-$\mu$m increments, using two-photon excitation microscopy. Pixel shift = 0, +0.75; bar = 10 $\mu$m.

the NIH Biological Microscopy and Image Reconstruction Resource (Albany, NY) (Marko *et al.*, 1988; Leith *et al.*, 1989). With STERECON, it is possible to create a precisely calibrated three-dimensional volumetric representation of a specimen from confocal optical sections and to move a drawing cursor in three dimensions within that volume—in this case a sea urchin embryo (Summers *et al.*, 1991). Contours of structures and lines interconnecting structures within the volume can be drawn and stored in an overlay data set while viewing both the volume and contours in three dimensions. Both linear and volumetric measurements and calculations can be performed on these data.

In our investigation, we were interested in determining the patterns of cleavage of blastomeres in the sea urchin embryo during the synchronous cleavage period (first through seventh cleavages) by calculating the angular relationships between the dividing nuclei in anaphase of each cleavage cycle and the polar (animal–vegetal) axis of the spherical embryo. It was possible to classify cleavages as meridional, latitudinal, or oblique and to determine the variability of any patterns that were discerned (see Summers *et al.*, 1993). Lines that interconnect the sets of chromosomes and that represent the nuclear division axis (which is exactly perpendicular to the future plane of cleavage) are created by two methods: (1) drawing a line between the visually determined centers of anaphase chromosomal masses while viewing them in three dimensions or (2) computing the centers of mass of each of the daughter sets of chromosomes and plotting a line between these centers of mass. From these data, the angles that nuclear divisions and cleavage furrows form with the polar axis of the embryo can be calculated; comparable data are produced by both methods. Color Plates 15 and 16 show an original data set and the resultant nuclear division axes. Color Plates 17 and 18 show the ability of the computer to detect chromosomes in optical sections. The boundaries of the chromosomes have been determined by intensity thresholding. When these boundaries are displayed from an entire series of optical sections, a faithful three-dimensional rendition of the data set is produced (Color Plate 19).

## IV. Confocal Microscopy of Living Specimens

It has become increasingly apparent that confocal microscopy is not only useful in investigations of fixed samples but can also be employed in studies of living specimens. By combining the confocal microscope with specific probes such as fluorescent dyes that are sensitive to changes in intracellular ion concentrations, many physiological processes can be monitored *in vivo*. Moreover, volumetric reconstructions of confocal data sets obtained from living specimens allow four-dimensional reconstructions (i.e., three-dimensional reconstructions over time) to be achieved. In this section, several specific applications of confocal microscopy to the study of living sea urchin embryos are presented to illustrate the potential of *in vivo* confocal microscopy. Additional examples involving living sea urchin embryos are also presented by Stricker *et al.* (1992) and in other articles in this volume ([1] and [7]).

## A. Time-Lapse Imaging of Calcium Dynamics

The confocal system used in studies of calcium dynamics consisted of a Bio-Rad MRC-600 laser scanning confocal unit interfaced with a Nikon Optiphot upright microscope (for a more detailed description of the instrument, see Stricker *et al.*, 1992, and [1] in this volume). To optimize cell viability, it is important to keep the laser illumination to the minimum required to obtain a utilizable signal. For most dye-loaded cells, sufficient illumination is achieved by setting the 25-mW argon ion laser of the confocal microscope to one-half power, and further attenuating the beam with a 1% transmittance neutral density filter. (*Note:* The one-half power setting is suitable for examinations of "fluorescein-like" dyes.) In addition, it is important that the specimen dish be cooled to 15–18°C. This can be accomplished with the aid of a thermoelectric cooling stage (e.g., KT controller; United Technology, Whitehouse Station, NJ). When using an upright type of optical microscope, observations are made by simply immersing a water immersion lens with a long working distance (e.g., Leitz ×25, NA 0.6; Zeiss ×40, NA 0.75) in the specimen dish.

To conduct time-lapse calcium imaging studies, one to several dye-loaded eggs are viewed at an optical plane near the equators of the eggs. The eggs are positioned in a 256 × 256 box to facilitate the handling of the large amounts of data that are generated in these studies. While setting up the time-lapse run, care should be taken to keep the illumination of these eggs to a minimum, as prolonged exposure to the laser beam seems to be toxic to these cells. To enhance the signal-to-noise ratio of the images obtained, each optical section is accumulated for two scans at normal scan rates (~1 sec/full scan).

Directly prior to the addition of several drops of diluted sperm to the specimen dish, a time-lapse recording set at 3- to 4-sec intervals is initiated for up to 15–20 min following insemination. Such time-lapse runs are accomplished with programs, available in the Bio-Rad software package, which allow an optical section to be acquired at the same position within the egg at the maximum frequency of every 3–4 sec (i.e., the time required for scanning the specimen and storing the data).

During the time-lapse runs, the data sets are written to the hard disk of the confocal microscope host compute and subsequently subjected to a pseudocolor conversion via the "geog" look-up table of Bio-Rad Corporation. In such pseudocolor representations of the images, blue colors are indicative of relatively low fluorescence intensities, whereas reds represent higher intensities. For hard copy output of the pseudocolored images, color prints can be obtained with a video printer, or from slides taken of the video monitor, using color slide film (see [1] for further details on hard copy output).

For volumetric reconstructions of confocal data sets, the time-lapse series of single optical sections through dye-loaded eggs can be transferred to a Silicon Graphics (Mountain View, CA) workstation (e.g., IRIS 4D-70GT), and three-dimensional renderings can be performed with the VoxelView software of Vital Images, Inc. (Fairfield, IA). Thus the circular optical sections of each egg are stacked together to form a cylinder that represents the optical section over time.

It should be noted that because the calcium indicators used with the confocal microscope tend to be nonratiometric dyes (Bright *et al.*, 1989), care must be taken in interpreting the images. For example, when comparing the fluorescent signals from two regions of a dye-loaded cell, a lower fluorescence in one region may not necessarily mean that the free calcium concentration is actually lower, because there may be confounding artifacts arising from differences in dye loading, path length, and/or cellular viscosity (Tsien and Peonie, 1986; Tsien, 1989). Nevertheless, as discussed by Stricker *et al.* (1992), normalized changes in the confocal signal calculated relative to prestimulation baseline levels can provide important information regarding the general trends in calcium dynamics. Examples of the kinds of confocal images that can be obtained by the methods described above are illustrated in Color Plates 20–22.

## B. Four-Dimensional Reconstructions of Embryogenesis

To obtain a fluorescent signal for *in vivo* confocal studies of embryogenesis, fertilized eggs of *L. pictus* can be stained with a 5- to 10-ng/ml solution of the vital membrane dye 3,3′-dihexyloxacarbocyanine iodide [DiOC$_6$(3)] (Molecular Probes, Inc.) for 2 min, before being washed twice in filtered sea water. Such treatments with DiOC$_6$(3) provide a generalized fluorescence throughout the egg cytoplasm, with a reduced signal emanating from the nuclear or spindle region of each stained cell. Other vital dyes tested (e.g., acridine orange, rhodamine 123, or thiazole orange) proved to be more toxic and/or were more prone to photobleaching than was DiOC$_6$(3).

For time-lapse confocal studies, the fertilized, DiOC$_6$(3)-labeled eggs are attached to a protamine sulfate-coated specimen dish such as is described in Section II,B, and immersed in 20 ml of filtered sea water maintained at 18°C. It is especially important to keep the embryos in relatively large volumes of sea water for these long-term examinations, and after several hours a few drops of distilled water may be added to compensate for any evaporative loss. Under these conditions, DiOC$_6$(3)-labeled embryos typically remain viable and cleave normally for at least 6 hr (i.e., to the morula/early blastula stage, prior to hatching).

Time-lapse serial *z* sections through developing embryos are collected by confocal microscopy, using a computer program (Bio-Rad Corp.) that steps the motor of the confocal system through the specimen at 5-$\mu$m intervals. The *z* series, which typically consists of 30 optical sections, is initiated 15–20 $\mu$m above the specimen and continued to 10–15 $\mu$m below the specimen to accommodate any shifting of the specimen or mechanical drift in the microscope during the course of a time-lapse run. Each optical section is averaged by accumulating three 256 × 256 scans at normal scan rates. Prior to recording, the gain and black level of the detector are set at compromise values to avoid saturation in the uppermost optical sections while detecting as much detail as possible in the lower sections.

Serial optical sections through the developing embryo can be stored at approximately 8-min intervals to the hard disk of the confocal microscope host computer and subsequently subjected to three-dimensional reconstructions by using the Vital Images volume-rendering software as described above (see also Section V,B). As is evident in the representative optical sections illustrated in Fig. 5 and Color Plate 15, a marked drop-off in the recorded signal typically

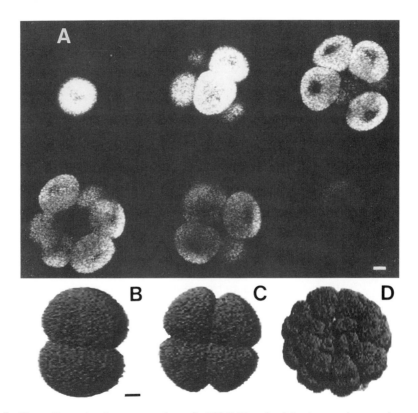

**Fig. 5** Three-dimensional reconstructions of a $DiOC_6(3)$-stained *L. pictus* embryo to show stages of cleavage. (A) Six representative optical sections of a serial $z$-section data set (the entire set consisted of 30 sections taken at 5-$\mu$m intervals) through an 8-cell embryo that was in the process of becoming a 16-cell embryo. The upper left-hand section occurred near the top of the embryo, whereas the lower right-hand section was collected near the bottom of the embryo. Note the falloff in fluorescence intensity in the lower region of the embryo. (B–D) Volumetric reconstructions of the serial $z$-section data sets obtained from time-lapse confocal imaging of a single living $DiOC_6(3)$-stained embryo. Scale bar = 10 $\mu$m.

occurs in the lowermost optical sections, owing to attenuation of the fluorescence by the overlying regions of the specimen. Nevertheless, relatively detailed three-dimensional images of whole embryos can be obtained and subsequently linked together to provide four-dimensional video sequences of development over time (data not shown).

## C. Supravital Staining of DNA and Two–Photon Excitation

Although useful information on the patterns of karyokinesis has been obtained from intact, fixed sea urchin embryos by confocal microscopy and computer graphic reconstructions (Summers *et al.*, 1991, and Section III of this chapter), a more dynamic view is often required. Additionally, investigations of nuclear divisions in living embryos help to confirm that the patterns observed in fixed specimens are not simply due to artifacts of fixation (shrinkage, swelling, and distortion). The goal of *in vivo* studies is to stain nuclei with a supravital DNA probe, and to obtain optical sections over an extended time period. From these time-lapse data, three-dimensional reconstructions may be prepared, and a single cell and its progeny can be tracked through multiple nuclear division cycles.

The most successful supravital staining of sea urchin embryonic nuclei has been accomplished by Hinkley and collaborators (Hinkley *et al.*, 1986, 1987), using the bisbenzimide (Hoeschst) dyes. These authors determined that the bisbenzimide dyes themselves have little or no toxic effect on development (Table 1 in Hinkley *et al.*, 1987). Unfortunately, however, these dyes require excitation with UV (~350 nm) light, which has deleterious effects on embryogenesis. In addition, UV light sources can pose difficulties for confocal microscopy by introducing problems of chromatic aberration and by requiring the use of special optics (lasers, mirrors, objective and ocular lenses, etc.).

One solution is to employ two-photon fluorophore excitation (Piston *et al.*, 1993) to obtain data from living embryos that have been stained with UV dyes. The two-photon effect is produced by the simultaneous absorption of two red photons from a highly focused laser, which stimulates visible fluorescence emission from a fluorophore that has a normal absorbance in the ultraviolet. With this technique, red (rather than UV) light is employed to excite a UV dye, with the premise that light of longer wavelengths is less damaging biologically. The localization of fluorophore excitation produces depth discrimination equivalent to the confocal pinhole (but without the attendant light loss) because the two-photon effect is limited to a thin focal volume ($z < 1$ $\mu$m for a high-numerical aperture objective) and falls off as $1/z^2$ above and below the focal plane. Specimen damage due to emitted photons is thus minimized. The use of red, instead of UV, light also allows the use of conventional optics in the scanning and imaging systems (Denk *et al.*, 1990).

For such studies, a Coherent (Palo Alto, CA) Satori dye laser can be used to generate 150-fsec pulses of 705 nm at a 76-MHz repetition rate. This pulse train is then fed to a Bio-Rad MRC-600 scan head that is optically coupled to the microscope and operated with the confocal pinhole completely open. To prepare samples, living embryos of *L. pictus* are stained with Hoechst 33342 (>0.5 μg/ml in seawater) for 0.5 hr before observation, washed in seawater, placed in 33-mm plastic petri dishes on a conrtrolled temperature microscope stage (Cloney *et al.*, 1970), and held at 18°C during observation. A water immersion lens (Zeiss Plan-Neofluor ×25, NA 0.8) and upright microscope are used to observe the stained embryos. The choice of sea urchin species is important, because *L. pictus* embryos could be sectioned throughout their entire depths, whereas the *S. purpuratus* could not, a difference presumably attributable to the absorption and scattering of light by the more highly pigmented cytoplasm in *S. purpuratus*. Vertical *z* series are routinely collected from embryos at 3-μm increments. A stereo pair of projection images from such a supravitally stained fourth cleavage embryo is shown in Fig. 4.

## V. Cell Lineage Analyses in Living and Fixed Specimens

A striking feature of embryonic development is the rapid segregation of the original egg cytoplasm into a large number of small cells with little or no increase in total mass. In all types of embryos there exist regular patterns of spatially restricted gene expression among these cells and in embryos with invariant cleavage, a correlation between cell lineage and gene expression patterns can be shown. The sea urchin embryo is made up of five tissue territories that are identifiable by a unique cell lineage history, an individual pattern of gene expression, and a specific combination of cell types (Davidson, 1990; Cameron and Davidson, 1991). The advances in video image-enhancing additions to epifluorescent microscopy, including laser scanning confocal microscopy, provide new tools for analysis of these three-dimensional patterns.

Methods of preparation and analysis of lineage tracing, using low light level fluorescence microscopy and laser scanning confocal microscopy, are described here. These methods have provided data leading to the concept of founder cell populations in sea urchin development and contributed new data for models of lineage-specific gene expression during sea urchin development. Because embryos are extremely sensitive to the prolonged exposure to excited fluorochromes, the shortest interval of radiation and the least concentration of indicators are recommended. These conditions result in low signals and high signal-to-noise ratios. To facilitate repeated observations during development and to screen treated embryos for subsequent analysis by confocal microscopy we routinely employ a low light level video-enhanced epifluorescent microscope system.

### A. Low Light Level Video Microscopy

Low light level images are collected from an Olympus BH-2 upright microscope fitted with differential interference optics and an epifluorescence illumination system. The images are recorded with a Hamamatsu C2400-08 silicon-intensified target (SIT) video camera and fed into an Imaging Technology series 151 image processor, which is controlled by an IBM-compatible AT 80386 computer. The output from the image processor goes to a Sony RGB video monitor. The computer also controls a Panasonic TQ-2028F optical disk recorder that receives output from the image processor. The Imaging Technology series 151 image processor can average images at video scanning rates to permit real-time signal averaging. This technology overcomes the inherent noise in SIT video cameras used at high gain settings. Thus low light level fluorescent images can be obtained repeatedly from live specimens over the course of embryonic development. As an example, a 72-hr pluteus of *S. purpuratus* observed with both transmitted and epifluorescent illumination is depicted in Color Plate 23. The embryo shown was injected at the 16-cell stage in 1 blastomere and allowed to develop to the pluteus stage. The particular labeled blastomere, NL1, contributes progeny to both the ciliated band of the oral hood and the aboral ectoderm.

Furthermore, the image processor contains at minimum four 8-bit image frame buffers, thus permitting the collection of individual images from different illuminations and the assembly of a composite pseudocolor 24-bit image. For example, two different fluorochromes and a bright-field image can be assembled into a three-color image from the single black-and-white video camera. In Color Plate 24, the bright-field image is represented in blue, the rhodamine image in red, and the fluorescein image in green. Cells arising from both groups overlap in the ciliated band and appear yellow (arrow). Also, a region contributed by only the fluorescein group is visible as a green gap in the yellow region (arrow).

Image-enhancing and filtering options are also available in the library of routines supplied with the Imaging Technology model 151 image processor. With the image-enhancing options, distracting background information can be removed before combining frames. Slight movements that occur between image collections can also be compensated. Crisping and smoothing operations are available to compensate for low signal-to-noise ratio images. A user interface to facilitate the use of these routines has been written (S. E. Fraser and G. Belford, Beckman Bioimaging Center, California Institute of Technology, Pasadena, CA).

## B. Confocal Microscopy and Three-Dimensional Reconstructions

The greatest amounts of three-dimensional information can be obtained from through-focus series obtained with the laser scanning confocal microscope. In addition to optically excluding out-of-focus fluorescence, which diminishes the sharpness of the fluorescent image, this instrument collects sets of images along the optical axis that can then be used to reconstruct the fluorescent information in three dimensions. The sea urchin embryo, at the end of embryogenesis, consists of 1800 cells, is approximately tetrahedral in shape, and measures about

150 × 100 $\mu$m. The ectoderm of about 1000 cells surrounds an optically transparent blastocoel containing the gut, coelomic pouches, and mesenchyme cells. A data set consisting of 20 optical sections along the $z$ axis carries all the detail necessary to make a three-dimensional reconstruction of this embryo. With a ×40 objective lens, the theoretical depth of field is about 1 $\mu$m and does not result in significant overlap between sections that are 5 $\mu$m apart (Young, 1989; Taylor and Salmon, 1989). We view samples previously selected and recorded on the low light level viewing system on the laser scanning microscope. Individual images of through-focus series are stored for later processing.

Once collected as a three-dimensional data set, images can be reconstructed as a projection of the three-dimensional data into a two-dimensional image (projection), as a stereo image, or as a three-rendered volume that can be rotated to give the three-dimensional effect. Examples of each are described below.

The region of the pluteus stage sea urchin embryo labeled with fluorescent cell tracer or fluorescent second antibody to reporter gene product usually occupies several sections of the volume containing the embryo. The best way to display this distribution of label in two dimensions is to create a projection of only the serial sections that contain the label and superimpose this projection image with the transmitted light image for interpretation. An embryo injected at the 16-cell stage in the aboral macromere is shown in Color Plate 25. The ectoderm labeling in the posterior apex, the labeled gut cells, and the labeled migratory cells that lie scattered through the blastocoel are all sharply in focus.

The simplest way to represent the three-dimensional information in a data set is with a stereo pair of images produced by the pixel offset method. A propidium iodide-stained embryo is displayed in Color Plate 26. Only the central portion of the series is shown without the ectoderm on either side. The cells of the gut and coelomic pouches are evident. These can be published as side-by-side pairs and projected for an audience as color (red–green or red–blue) anaglyphs or as polarized light stereo pairs (see [1] in this volume).

A number of commercially available three-dimensional rendering packages (e.g., VoxelView; Vital Images, Inc.) can be used to produce tilted or rotated views providing three-dimensional information that is difficult to view in any other manner. VoxelView treats the data sets passed to it as isotropic. That is, each voxel is considered to be equal in all dimensions. If the images are taken as 512 × 480 pixels to yield the maximum $xy$ dimensions and the embryo is 150 $\mu$m in length, the $z$ direction in each plane will be about 0.3 $\mu$m (150/512 = 0.3). The 20 $Z$ planes will comprise only about 6 $\mu$m in the reconstruction. The software permits interpolation between planes but anything in excess of two interpolated planes distorts the individual objects when viewed along the $z$ axis. That is, spheres become cylinders. Therefore the best to be done is a slightly distorted image in the $z$ direction. A photograph of a single frame from a three-dimensional animation is shown in Color Plate 27. The embryo in this case was labeled throughout with propidium iodide and the abanal half is rendered.

## VI. Conclusions

Modern methods in fluorescence microscopy coupled with computerized video hardware and newly developed reagents for cytology provide a robust suite of tools for analyzing developmental patterns. More recently, the advent of confocal microscopy and three-dimensional reconstruction methods have further enhanced the capabilities of researchers in various fields of developmental biology. In this article several applications of confocal microscopy to investigations of both fixed and living sea urchin embryos are illustrated to provide examples of some of the current capabilities of these techniques. Perhaps the greatest limitations of confocal microscopy at present are relatively slow acquisition rates (i.e., temporal resolution) and a somewhat limited choice of organelle- or molecule-specific probes that can be used in conjunction with the most widely used types of laser illumination systems. Both of these problems, however, are currently under intense technological investigation, suggesting that the already significant capabilities of confocal microscopy will be further enhanced in the near future.

### Acknowledgments

R.G.S. thanks Alan Stonebraker, David Piston, Michael Marko, Ardean Leith, and John B. Morrill for collaborative assistance. Technical assistance was provided by Thaddeus Szczesny and Edward Hurley. Project supported by NIH RR 06993 to R.G.S. and by NIH Biotechnological Resource Grants RR01219 to the NIH Biological Microscopy and Image Reconstruction Resource (Albany, NY) and RR04224 to the Developmental Resource for Biophysical Imaging and Opto-electronics at Cornell University (Ithaca, NY). S.A.S. gratefully acknowledges V. Centonze, P. DeVries, S. Paddock, and G. Schatten. R.A.C. wishes to thank E. H. Davidson and S. E. Fraser for their collaboration. The original research discussed here was supported by the NSF Program in Developmental Biology.

### References

Boyde, A. (1990). *In* "Handbook of Biological Confocal Microscopy" (J. Pawley, ed.), pp. 163–168. Plenum Press, New York.

Bright, G. R., Fisher, G. W., Rogowska, J., and Taylor, D. L. (1989). *Methods Cell Biol.* **30,** 157–192.

Cameron, R. A., and Davidson, E. H. (1991). *Trends Genet.* **7,** 212–218.

Cameron, R. A., Hough-Evans, B., Britten, R., and Davidson, E. H. (1987). *Genes Dev.* **1,** 75–84.

Cameron, R. A., Fraser, S. E., Britten, R. J., and Davidson, E. H. (1989). *Development* **106,** 641–647.

Cameron, R. A., Fraser, S. E., Britten, R. J., and Davidson, E. H. (1990). *Dev. Biol.* **137,** 77–85.

Cameron, R. A., Fraser, S. E., Britten, R. J., and Davidson, E. H. (1991). *Development* **113,** 1085–1091.

Cheng, P.-C., and Summers, R. G. (1990). *In* "Handbook of Biological Confocal Microscopy" (J. Pawley, ed.), pp. 179–195. Plenum Press, New York.

Cloney, R. A., Schaadt, J., and Durden, J. V. (1970). *Acta Zool.* (*Stockholm*) **51,** 95–98.

Colin, A., and Hille, M. B. (1982). *Am. Zool.* **22,** 900.

Culling, C., and Vassar, P. (1961). *Arch. Pathol.* **71,** 88–92.

Davidson, E. H. (1990). *Development* **108,** 365–389.

Denk, W., Strickler, J., and Webb, W. W. (1990). *Science* **2,** 73–76.

De Tomasi, J. A. (1936). *Stain Tech.* **11,** 137–144.

Foerder, C. A., and Shapiro, B. M. (1977). *Proc. Natl. Acad. Sci. U.S.A.* **74,** 4214–4218.

Harris, P. (1986). *Methods Cell Biol.* **27,** 243–263.

Hinegardner, R. (1967). *In* "Methods in Developmental Biology" (F. Wilt and N. Wessels, eds.), pp. 139–155. Thomas Crowell Co., New York.

Hinkley, R. E., Wright, B. D., and Lynn, J. W. (1986). *Dev. Biol.* **118,** 148–154.

Hinkley, R., Edelstein, R. N., and Ivonnet, P. I. (1987). *Dev. Growth Differ.* **29,** 211–220.

Hiramoto, Y. (1974). *Exp. Cell Res.* **87,** 403–406.

Kane, R. (1970). *J. Cell Biol.* **45,** 615–622.

Kasten, F. H. (1958). *Histochemie* **1,** 123–150.

Kasten, F. H., Burton, V., and Glover, P. (1959). *Nature (London)* **184,** 1797–1798.

Kishimoto, T. (1986). *Methods Cell Biol.* **27,** 379–394.

Leahy, P. S. (1986). *Methods Cell Biol.* **27,** 1–13.

Leith, A., Marko, M., and Parsons, D. (1989). *I.E.E.E. Comput. Graph. Appl.* **9,** 16–23.

Luby-Phelps, K. (1989). *Methods Cell Biol.* **29,** 59–74.

Lutz, D. A., and Inoué, S. (1986). *Methods Cell Biol.* **27,** 89–110.

McClay, D. R. (1986). *Methods Cell Biol.* **27,** 309–325.

McMahon, P., Flytzantis, C., Hough-Evans, B., Katula, K., Britten, R., and Davidson, E. (1985). *Dev. Biol.* **108,** 420–430.

Marko, M., Leith, A., and Parsons, D. (1988). *J. Electron Microsc. Tech.* **9,** 395–411.

Nislow, C., and Morrill, J. B. (1988). *Dev. Growth Differ.* **38,** 483–499.

Pearse, A. G. E. (1961). "Histochemistry: Theoretical and Applied," p. 823. Little, Brown & Co., Boston.

Piston, D. W., Summers, R. G., and Webb, W. W. (1993). *Biophys. J.* **64,** A110.

Ploem, J. S. von (1967). *Acta Histochem. (Jena) Suppl.* **7,** 339–343.

Sandison, D. R., Piston, D. W., and Webb, W. W. (1993). *In* "Three Dimensional Confocal Microscopy: Volume Investigation of Biological Specimens" (J. K. Stevens, L. R. Mills, and J. E. Trogadis, eds.). Academic Press, San Diego. In press.

Schulte, E. K. W. (1991). *Anal. Cell Pathol.* **3,** 167–182.

Showman, R. M., and Foerder, C. A. (1979). *Exp. Cell Res.* **120,** 253–355.

Strathman, M. F. (ed.) (1987). "Reproduction and Development of Marine Invertebrates of the Northern Pacific Coast." University of Washington Press, Seattle.

Stricker, S. A., Centonze, V. E., Paddock, S. W., and Schatten, G. (1992). *Dev. Biol.* **149,** 370–380.

Summers, R. G., and Cheng, P.-C. (1989). *In* "Proceedings of the 47th Annual Meeting of E.M.S.A" (G. W. Bailey, ed.), pp. 140–141. San Francisco Press, San Francisco.

Summers, R. G., Musial, C. E., Cheng, P.-C., Leith, A., and Marko, M. (1991). *J. Electron Microsc. Tech.* **18,** 24–30.

Summers, R. G., Morrill, J. B., Leith, A., Marko, M., Piston, D. W., and Stonebraker, A. T. (1993). *Dev. Growth Differ.* **35,** 41–57.

Taylor, D. L., and Salmon, E. D. (1989). *Methods Cell Biol.* **29,** 208–238.

Tsien, R. Y. (1989). *Methods Cell Biol.* **30,** 127–156.

Tsien, R. Y., and Poenie, M. (1986). *Trends Biochem. Sci.* **11,** 450–455.

Vacquier, V. D. (1981). *Dev. Biol.* **84,** 1–26.

Van Ingen, E. M., Tanke, H. J., and Ploem, J. S. (1979). *J. Histochem. Cytochem.* **27,** 80–83.

Weidman, P. J., and Kay, E. S. (1986). *Methods Cell Biol.* **27,** 111–138.

Young, I. T. (1989). *Methods Cell Biol.* **30,** 2–47.

**CHAPTER 11**

# Resolution of Subcellular Detail in Thick Tissue Sections: Immunohistochemical Preparation and Fluorescence Confocal Microscopy

**Irene L. Hale and Brian Matsumoto**

Department of Biological Sciences and
Neuroscience Research Institute
University of California, Santa Barbara
Santa Barbara, California 93106

# I. Introduction: Development of Fluorescence Microscopy Techniques for Resolution of Subcellular Detail

## A. Study of Cytoskeletal Organization in Cultured Cells

A question such as "how is the cytoskeleton organized?" can be answered adequately only by using high-resolution microscopy techniques that also provide three-dimensional information. Transmission electron microscopy (TEM) satisfies the first criterion, but is not convenient for three-dimensional analysis. Conversely, bright-field light microscopy, because of its shallow depth of field, can provide three-dimensional information conveniently by "optical sectioning" of thick specimens, but makes detection and resolution of small structures, such as individual cytoskeletal filaments, difficult. The theoretical limit of resolution of the light microscope is approximately 200 nm; however, much smaller structures can be visualized by enhancing their optical signal (Inoué, 1986). For example, the sensitivity and high contrast of fluorescence microscopy, coupled with the specificity of antibody labeling, have permitted the detection of individual cytoskeletal filaments even though their diameter is smaller than the limit of resolution. Osborn *et al.* (1978) compared immunofluorescence and TEM images of the same cultured cell and demonstrated that, under optimal conditions, single microtubules can be visualized by immunofluorescence microscopy. When measured by TEM, the diameter of these microtubules, which were labeled by indirect immunofluorescence (microtubule plus two IgG layers), was approximately 55 nm, much less than the limit of resolution of two point sources ($R$) by Rayleigh's criterion:

$$R = 1.22\lambda/2\text{NA} \qquad (1)$$

This value, which applies to lateral ($xy$) resolution, is approximately 230 nm for the wavelength of light ($\lambda = 520$ nm, i.e., fluorescein-conjugated antibody) and the objective lens numerical aperture (NA 1.4; 2NA applies to epiillumination) used in this study.

In this example, microtubules will have to be farther than 230 nm apart in the horizontal plane to be resolved. Axial ($z$) resolving power is lower than lateral resolving power. In the vertical dimension, two point sources must be two times farther than the Rayleigh limit apart, 460 nm in this example, to be resolved (see Inoué, 1986, for a discussion of resolution). Hence, immunofluorescence microscopy is a powerful tool for studying the cytoskeleton, enabling the cell biologist to observe both fine details and the three-dimensional structure of cytoskeletal arrays, as long as individual filaments are not too densely packed.

Historically, this level of detection and resolution has been attainable only with cultured cells. The main reason for this restriction is that monolayers of cells are an almost ideal optical pathway for fluorescence microscopy, whereas thicker tissue sections are not. For instance, in a monolayer, generally there are few fluorescent structures above or below the plane of focus, so that in-focus structures are seen against a dark background and the potential for high contrast with the fluorescent signal is realized. Another reason higher resolution images have been obtained with cultured cells is that the specimen preparation methods for monolayers are less damaging than many of those for intact tissues.

## B. Problems Encountered with Intact Tissues

The thickness of intact tissues presents several problems. The first two are related to the poor optical quality of tissue. It is not homogeneous with respect to optical properties such as refractive index and absorption, so light can be refracted, reflected, and scattered by structures between the plane of focus and the objective lens. One result is that light is attenuated as it passes through the tissue. Compounding this problem, when tissue is labeled with fluorescent probes, fluorochromes overlying the object of interest absorb some of the illuminating light. In addition, light from outside the plane of focus creates a high background signal in conventional fluorescence microscopy. Light spreads with distance along the vertical (optical) axis as a solid cone from fluorochromes in the focal plane, as well as from those outside it, which also are excited by the illuminating light. Autofluorescence can be another source of background. The resultant decrease in intensity of both exciting and emitted light and the increase in intensity of background light with thickness reduce sensitivity and contrast (Cheng and Summers, 1990; Inoué, 1990). This reduction in signal-to-noise ratio hinders detection of small objects and prevents discrimination of neighboring structures that, theoretically, should be resolved by a high numerical aperture lens. In short, the in-focus structures merge with the background.

The second problem is that objective lenses correct for spherical aberration only under specified conditions (Keller, 1990). These conditions include the refractive indices and dispersions of the components of the optical path between the object of interest and the objective, and the distance through these media that light traverses to reach the objective. Each component also must be optically homogeneous. Components may include immersion medium, coverglass, specimen mounting medium, and the tissue itself. For instance, the specified refractive index for oil immersion lenses is 1.51, which is the refractive index of immersion oil, coverglasses, and mounting media such as Permount. Focusing down into a thick, unembedded specimen introduces an increasingly thick layer of tissue, which, overall, has a refractive index closer, depending on the mounting medium, to that of water (1.33) or glycerol (1.47) and more importantly is not uniform in its optical properties. As the optical path is altered, correction for spherical aberration is lost. Consequently, resolution declines with depth (Keller, 1990; [3], this volume). The loss of correction also results in a decline in image intensity, in addition to the factors discussed above. A third problem is that lenses with a high numerical aperture for high-resolution work have short working distances, about 100–150 $\mu$m. A fourth problem is that antibodies and many other probes cannot penetrate far into tissues.

292 I. L. Hale and B. Matsumoto

The problems associated with thickness necessitate mechanical sectioning of tissues for both antibody labeling and imaging purposes. Although sectioning solves these problems, it can introduce others. First, to prepare tissues for sectioning, they often are embedded in paraffin or resin. Structural alteration, most noteably shrinkage, occurs with embedding procedures. When volume is decreased, structures are more tightly packed, reducing the ability to resolve them. Infiltration of paraffin and polymerization of some resins require temperatures hot enough to induce autofluorescence. Furthermore, embedding procedures may block antibody access to binding sites, alter antigen structure, or extract antigens, in turn decreasing fluorescence signal intensity. Therefore, pre- or nonembedding labeling methods often are preferable. Second, without some technique for removing the out-of-focus fluorescence signal, sections often need to be 5 $\mu$m thick or less for good contrast. Because some cells are larger and/or extend processes greater distances than this, serial sectioning may be required to view whole cells. Mechanical sectioning introduces artifacts and makes it difficult to gather three-dimensional information.

## C. Solutions to Problems with Intact Tissues

One of the goals of our research in retinal cell biology has been to observe cytoskeletal organization in the intact retina, rather than in enzymatically or mechanically dissociated cells (Nagle *et al.,* 1986; Vaughan and Fisher, 1987; Sale *et al.,* 1988), which previously had been the best preparation for resolving fine detail and at the same time obtaining three-dimensional information. Although individual, fluorescently labeled retinal cells can be imaged with good contrast, important information about the intact tissue is lost. In the intact retina it is possible to (1) see the orientation and distribution of cells within the retina, (2) compare cytoskeletal and other features among neighboring cells within a population, which is especially important for assessing responses to drug treatments and other manipulations, and (3) trace cell–cell contacts and synaptic connections. Another advantage is that cells remain whole, whereas during dissociation they can lose processes or, in the case of photoreceptors, break apart just distal to the nucleus. Additionally, the plasma membranes of the outer segment, the photosensitive compartment, and the inner segment, the metabolic compartment, remain as distinct domains. In rod photoreceptors these membranes can fuse during dissociation (Spencer *et al.,* 1988). We have been able to realize our goal by taking advantage of techniques that solve some of the problems outlined in Section I,B above. Gentle procedures for specimen preparation and techniques for removing the out-of-focus fluorescence signal have been equally important for maximizing resolution.

We initially developed a method combining preembedding labeling of thick-tissue sections with resin embedment and thin sectioning. Thick sectioning permits antibody labeling throughout the tissue, while mechanical thin sectioning physically removes much of the out-of-focus fluorescence. We sectioned retinal tissue for fluorescent probe labeling with a Vibratome (model 1000; Technical Products International, Polysciences, Warrington, PA), as an alternative to frozen sectioning. [See Priestley (1984) and Larsson (1988) for reviews of Vibratome methods. See also Baker and Reese [12], this volume.] The Vibratome cuts thick sections (>20 $\mu$m) of tissues with a transversely vibrating blade, so that soft tissues sustain minimal compression and can be supported with a noninfiltrating matrix, such as agarose. Vibratome sectioning produces minimal ultrastructural damage. It has been used successfully for TEM examination of immunolabeling, for example, with antibodies to neuropeptides and neurotransmitters and their synthesizing enzymes (reviewed in Priestley and Cuello, 1983), a Golgi apparatus enzyme (Novikoff *et al.*, 1983), and microtubules and microtubule-associated proteins in neurons (Matus *et al.*, 1981). It is even gentle enough for live retinal tissue (Mack and Fernald, 1991). We embedded labeled Vibratome sections in JB-4 (Polysciences), a hydrophilic resin, because it does not require tissue dehydration with organic solvents. JB-4 embedding seems to cause less extraction in general and, essential for our work, does not extract phalloidin, which is removed by alcohols. In addition, this resin exhibits low autofluorescence and can be polymerized on ice, to avoid tissue autofluorescence induced by heating. Sections 3–5 $\mu$m thick can be cut, providing adequate contrast for epifluorescence microscopy. Contrast can be enhanced further by using an objective lens with a diaphragm, which can be partially closed to reduce flare, and by using video image enhancement techniques.

Matsumoto *et al.* (1987) first employed these procedures to label actin with fluorescent phalloidin, a probe specific for filamentous actin, and to localize filaments in pseudopodia of the retinal pigment epithelium during phagocytosis of rod outer segment membranes. This combination of techniques has provided sufficient structural preservation and contrast to reveal domains of the actin (phalloidin labeling) and tubulin (antibody labeling) cytoskeletons in frog photoreceptors that are difficult to observe in other intact retinal preparations. Matsumoto (unpublished observations) (Fig. 1A) was able to detect the concentration of actin filaments in the ciliary stalk and resolve it from the nearby actin-filled, calycal processes. Vaughan *et al.* (1989) used this method to view the microtubule array in the ellipsoid region (shown in Fig. 2A and B), which is composed of a number of individual microtubules or small bundles that radiate from one of the basal bodies at the base of the ciliary stalk.

We have been able to substitute optical sectioning with the laser scanning confocal microscope (LSCM) (MRC-500; Bio-Rad, Cambridge, MA) for mechanical sectioning to generate the thin sections necessary for high contrast and resolution. In point scanning confocal microscopes such as this one, the illuminating light, a narrow laser beam, is scanned over the specimen and a pinhole aperture prevents light arising from outside the plane of focus from reaching the detector, a photomultiplier tube (reviewed in Brakenhoff *et al.*, 1989; White *et al.*, 1990; Inoué, 1990; [1], this volume) (see Fig. 4 in [1] for a light ray diagram). Although out-of-focus light cannot be eliminated completely, in practice the

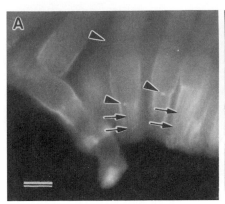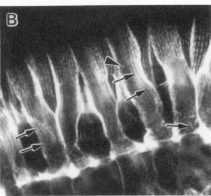

**Fig. 1** Comparison of epifluorescence and LSCM for viewing the actin cytoskeleton in photoreceptors. In both (A) and (B), 100-$\mu$m thick Vibratome sections of frog retina fixed in 0.1% glutaraldehyde–4% formaldehyde were labeled with rhodamine-conjugated phalloidin. Vibratome sections were cut parallel to the long axis of the photoreceptors. (A) An unenhanced epifluorescence image of a thin section (5 $\mu$m) cut from a Vibratome section embedded in JB-4 resin. (B) An LSCM image (single optical section, approximately 0.75 $\mu$m thick) of an unembedded thick section. The greater contrast with LSCM makes it easier to resolve actin cables and smaller bundles (arrows) in the photoreceptor inner segment. The actin network in the ciliary stalk (arrowheads) can be detected with both techniques. Scale bar = 10 $\mu$m.

fluorescence collected can be confined to an optical section as thin as 0.5–0.7 $\mu$m (objective lens NA 1.4) ( [1] and [9], this volume). This thickness is close to the axial resolution limit, for example, 0.46 $\mu$m for fluorescein emission (see Section I,A). Laser scanning confocal microscopy allows the shallow depth of field of the light microscope to be used effectively. The increased contrast acheived with the LSCM can be seen in Fig. 1; actin bundles in the photoreceptor inner segment that are indistinct in a 5-$\mu$m thick JB-4 section without image enhancement (A) are evident in an optical section 4 $\mu$m below the surface of a 100-$\mu$m thick Vibratome section (B). There are two other benefits of confocal microscopy to our work. First, resin or paraffin embedding is no longer necessary, and consequently structural alteration and autofluorescence caused by these procedures is eliminated (see Section II,B). Second, three-dimensional information can be gathered with ease. The combination of immunofluorescence and LSCM makes the goal of viewing cytoskeletal arrays and other subcellular detail in three dimensions in intact tissues not only theoretically possible for the cell biologist, but also feasible.

To take advantage of this potential, we have attempted to work out specimen preparation parameters, drawing on the preembedding Vibratome method, and confocal imaging parameters for resolution of subcellular detail in thick tissue sections. Of course, there is no single best tissue preparation and labeling method applicable to all probes or every antigen–antibody combination. In this article we present a convenient nonembedding method that requires no special equipment other than a Vibratome. This method is suitable for antigens that are not sensitive to aldehyde fixation and are not extracted by liquid-phase fixation or subsequent detergent permeabilization. With it we have successfully labeled a variety of antigens, including cytoskeletal, integral membrane, and soluble proteins, using antibodies as well as phalloidin and lectins. There are trade-offs between many of the parameters involved, so the challenge has been to achieve a collective compromise between them. These parameters and their impact on each other are discussed in Sections II and III. Detailed procedures are provided in Section V.

## II. Immunohistochemical Preparation of Thick Tissue Sections

### A. Fixation

Immunocytochemists always have been faced with a trade-off between the quality of tissue preservation and the retention of antigenicity. Preembedding techniques alleviate this problem, because they require only a relatively light fixation prior to antibody labeling, and because the dehydration and embedding procedures themselves can reduce antigenicity or extract antigens (Larsson, 1988). Preembedding immunocytochemistry introduces an additional trade-off, however, one between preservation and depth of penetration of antibodies and other probes into the tissue (Larsson, 1988; Priestley *et al.,* 1992). Both the quality of tissue preservation and the intensity of the fluorescent signal, partly determined by retention of antigenicity or of the antigen in the tissue, limit practical resolution in laser scanning confocal microscopy (LSCM), while the depth of probe penetration limits the three-dimensional information available. A knowledge of the properties of various fixative agents, with these trade-offs in mind, is helpful when choosing a fixative, but ultimately the choice must be made empirically for each antigen–antibody combination and each type of tissue. For several proteins we have found that an acceptable balance between these demands can be achieved with light aldehyde fixation. It may be desirable to include agents such as taxol ( [9], this volume) or ethylene glycol-bis ($\beta$-amino ethyl ether)-$N,N,N',N'$-tetraacetic acid (EGTA) (Osborn and Weber, 1982) to preserve microtubules optimally in some tissues. For complete discussions of other fixatives and conditions for particular immunocytochemical applications, the reader is referred to Osborn and Weber (1982) for microtubules, Priestley (1984) for neurotransmitters, enzyme markers, and neuropeptides, and Larsson (1988) and Priestley *et al.* (1992) for a general review.

Formaldehyde, alone or in combination with other agents, is a commonly used fixative for preembedding immunocytochemistry, because it is relatively mild and partially reversible (reviewed in Sternberger, 1979; Larsson, 1988). It forms stable methylene cross-bridges (reviewed in Puchtler and Meloan, 1985), but cross-links less extensively than glutaraldehyde. Thus it retains antigenicity well for many antigens and does not impede antibody penetration greatly. At the same time, formaldehyde is effective enough to preserve ultrastructure well, as observed when combined with ultracryotomy (Larsson, 1988). Its effectiveness is due partly to its rapid penetration. Cells are killed quickly enough to prevent autolytic damage (Pease, 1962). We have successfully used buffered 4% formaldehyde alone, pH 7.3 (granular paraformaldehyde; Electron Microscopy Sciences, Ft. Washington, PA) to fix retinal tissue for phalloidin staining (Molecular Probes, Eugene, OR) of filamentous actin (not shown) and for immunolabeling of cytoskeletal filaments [actin, not shown; tubulin, Fig. 2; glial fibrillary acidic protein (GFAP), Fig. 3; vimentin, not shown], integral membrane proteins (opsin, Fig. 4A–C; high molecular weight rim protein, not shown), and soluble proteins [cellular retinaldehyde-binding protein (CRALBP), Fig. 5; actin monomers, not shown]. (See Table I for a complete description of these primary antibodies.) In our studies this fixative provided the highest anti-tubulin labeling intensity, when compared to glutaraldehyde (0.1–1.0%), glutaraldehyde–formaldehyde combinations, or cold ($-10°C$) methanol. Labeling with actin, opsin, and rim protein antibodies was higher with formaldehyde alone than with glutaraldehyde–formaldehyde. Formaldehyde fixation retained CRALBP in the Müller cell, a type of glial cell, and the retinal

## Table I
## Primary Antibodies

**Anti-actin:** Recognizes nonmuscle actin. Polyclonal to chicken gizzard, dilution = 1/100 (Biomedical Technologies, Inc., Stoughton, MA)

**Anti-cellular retinaldehyde-binding protein (CRALBP):** Specific for the vitamin A carrier protein present in retinal pigment epithelium and Müller glial cells. Polyclonal to bovine, dilution = 1/400 (purified IgG) (Bunt-Milam and Saari, 1983)

**Anti-glial fibrillary acidic protein (GFAP):** Specific for an intermediate filament protein found in glial cells. Polyclonal to bovine, dilution = 1/400 (Dako, Carpinteria, CA)

**Anti-high molecular weight rim protein:** Recognizes an integral membrane protein restricted to the rims of the membranous disks that make up the photoreceptor outer segment. Polyclonal to frog, dilution = 1/200 (serum) (Papermaster et al., 1978)

**Anti-opsin (15–18):** Binds the photopigment of rod and the single-cone photoreceptors. Monoclonal to turtle opsin (surface loop between helices IV and V, lumenal/extracellular membrane face), dilution = 1/50 (hybridoma culture fluid) (Gaur et al., 1988)

**Anti-opsin (rho 4D2):** Binds the photopigment of rod photoreceptors. Monoclonal to bovine rhodopsin ($NH_2$ terminus, lumenal/extracellular membrane face), dilution = 1/50 (hybridoma culture medium) (Hicks and Molday, 1986)

**Anti-β-tubulin:** Recognizes the β subunit of tubulin. Monoclonal antibody, dilution = 1/1000 (ascites fluid) (Chu and Klymkowsky, 1989)

**Anti-vimentin:** Specific for an intermediate filament protein found in glial cells. Monoclonal to human, dilution = 1/400 (Dako, Carpinteria, CA)

pigment epithelium (Fig. 5A), and soluble actin in the photoreceptor. In addition, it preserved cytoskeletal filaments and the Golgi apparatus in the rod photoreceptor well. In fact, although overall cellular morphology was better preserved with glutaraldehyde–formaldehyde than formaldehyde alone, the appearance of the microtubule array in the ellipsoid region and of the Golgi apparatus was indistinguishable between the two fixatives (comparisons not shown; Figs. 2A and 4C, respectively, are examples of these structures). Microtubules were not disorganized, fragmented, or lost, and the Golgi apparatus was not collapsed or vesiculated. Formaldehyde alone is an excellent fixative for many antigen–antibody combinations, and is a good preliminary choice for testing this Vibratome technique.

We obtained the best preservation if tissues were fixed for about 8 hr or longer, and if they were stored in formaldehyde rather than buffer. Retinal tissues stored in buffer for longer than 1 week prior to labeling became soft and showed decreased fluorescence image sharpness. Formaldehyde fixation has been reported to be partially reversible by washing. Because formaldehyde forms stable cross-bridges, however, much of the fixative is not washed out by buffer. Perhaps storage in formaldehyde stabilizes cellular components that are not cross-linked but are more loosely bound by the fixative.

Because glutaraldehyde (a dialdehyde) is a more effective cross-linker than formaldehyde alone, it achieves superior preservation of cell shape (Sabatini *et al.*, 1963) and certain structures, for example, microtubules (Eckert and Snyder, 1978; Osborn and Weber, 1982), and better retention of soluble molecules, for example, neuropeptides (Larsson, 1988) and dyes. The cross-linking activity of glutaraldehyde, however, can reduce enzyme activity (Sabatini *et al.*, 1963), antigenicity, and antibody penetration (Priestley, 1984; Larsson, 1988; [9], this volume). We have observed reduced labeling with both anti-tubulin and anti-opsin, especially with glutaraldehyde concentrations of 0.5% or greater. For these reasons, many researchers use low concentrations (<0.5%) of this fixative in combination with formaldehyde. In our studies, a brief (<45 min) fixation in 0.1% glutaraldehyde (8% EM grade; Polysciences)–4% formaldehyde, pH 7.3, noticeably improved overall preservation, as judged by photoreceptor cell shape, photoreceptor outer segment membrane organization, and extraction visible by differential interference contrast. With formaldehyde fixation, photoreceptors sometimes appear stretched lengthwise, and the membraneous disks that make up the photosensitive outer segment become less tightly stacked (photoreceptor domains are marked in Fig. 4A). Even this light glutaraldehyde fixation, however, reduced antibody labeling intensity as much as threefold and the depth of tubulin antibody labeling, partly determined by the depth of antibody penetration, by 25–30% (see Section II,C,1). For some antibodies, for example, anti-tubulin, a decrease in labeling intensity is tolerable, because good image contrast can still be obtained (Fig. 2D and E). To allow comparisons of labeling intensity, the aperture size, illumination intensity, gain, and black level

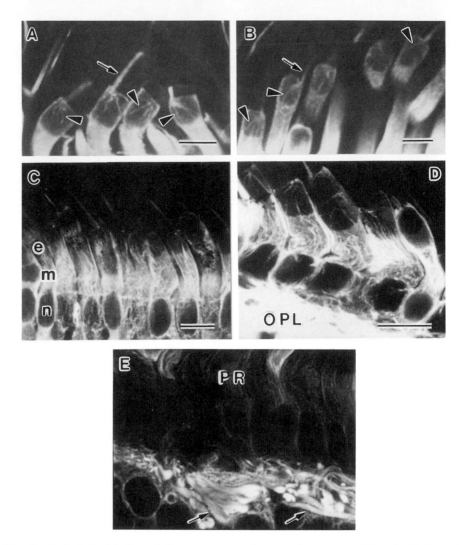

**Fig. 2** Antitubulin labeling of photoreceptors and neuronal processes. (A) and (B) show the microtubule array in the ellipsoid regions of longitudinally sectioned frog rod photoreceptors, which consists of a number of what are probably individual microtubules radiating from one of the basal bodies beneath the ciliary stalk. Laser scanning confocal microscopy (LSCM) provides sufficient contrast to visualize these microtubules in thick tissue sections. Arrows indicate the ciliary microtubules in the photoreceptor outer segment. These images also illustrate that detergent treatment does not damage these microtubules. This tissue was fixed in 4% formaldehyde alone. The length and number of microtubules (arrowheads) in the ellipsoid region appear to be the same in images of Vibratome sections labeled without [e.g., (A)] or with [e.g., (B)] detergent (1.0% Triton X-100) present throughout the antibody incubations (30 hr) and rinses. Scale bar = 10 $\mu$m. (C) and (D) demonstrate the ability of the LSCM to resolve the closely spaced microtubules in the myoid region (m) of frog photoreceptors. For orientation, the ellipsoid region (e) and nucleus (n) are also marked. Two optical sections (about 0.75 $\mu$m thick) were projected one on top of the other to generate these images. Extending the depth of field in this way allows structures such as microtubules to be followed for greater distances, as they pass in and out of two or more thin optical sections. (C) An

were held constant for all specimens and set such that the maximum intensity value for the brightest specimens overall or for the brightest structure(s) of interest did not exceed the upper limit of the intensity scale. The average pixel intensity over several areas containing the structure(s) of interest was then calculated for comparison.

Another problem with glutaraldehyde is that it produces both nonspecific labeling and/or autofluorescence, which can greatly reduce contrast. High background fluorescence in the plane of focus negates the gain in contrast achieved by the removal of out-of-focus fluorescence with LSCM. We have found that, fortunately, the level of background fluorescence is relatively low with light glutaraldehyde fixation. It should be emphasized that this is true only if a dilute (10% or less) stock solution sealed under nitrogen is used, the stock solution is stored frozen after opening, and the glutaradehyde is added to the fixative solution the same day it is used. Background fluorescence can be minimized further by (1) fixation on ice (not advisable for microtubules, which can be cold labile), (2) secondary fixation with paraformaldehyde alone, (3) thorough rinsing (Vaughn et al., 1981), and most effectively, by (4) reduction with sodium borohydride (Fisher Scientific, Pittsburg, PA) (Weber et al., 1978; Bacallao et al., 1990). Thus, if a light fixation with glutaraldehyde does not block access to or alter the antigenic determinant in question, preservation can be enhanced without too great of a decrease in signal-to-noise ratio.

Cold ($-10°C$) methanol, a precipitating fixative, preserves cytoskeletal components well, and because it extracts lipids it enhances antibody penetration (Osborn and Weber, 1982; Larsson, 1988). We have not adopted methanol fixation for retinal tissue for two reasons. First, retinas fixed in cold methanol alone are soft, making it difficult to handle and section them. Second, we obtained lower labeling intensity with this tissue, using anti-tubulin, when compared to retinal tissue fixed in formaldehyde alone. Because methanol is a precipitating fixative, the decreased labeling intensity may reflect blocking of antibody access to the antigenic determinant. We have not tried methanol as a secondary fixative, following formaldehyde.

---

image collected 15 $\mu$m below the surface of a thick Vibratome section. Image quality is still good at this depth, compared to (D), which was collected at the surface. Scale bar in (C) = 10 $\mu$m. (B), (D), and (E) demonstrate the extremely wide intensity range possible with fluorescently labeled tissue. In (B), labeling intensity in the myoid is sufficiently great that pixel intensities in this region are all near maximum when parameters are set to image preferentially the weak ellipsoid microtubule signal. In (D), the outer plexiform layer (OPL) is so bright that neuronal processes are obscured. (E) Beam intensity and gain had to be substantially reduced, to the point that the signal in the photoreceptors (PR) is almost undetectable, in order for individual horizontal cell processes (arrows) and other finer processes to be seen in the OPL. The power of LSCM to resolve fine detail in thick tissue sections is displayed once again by this single optical section (about 0.75 $\mu$m). (D) and (E) are neighboring fields at the same magnification. Scale bar in (D) = 10 $\mu$m.

## B. Vibratome Sectioning

Most tissues cannot be stained or viewed whole, and therefore must be sectioned. Thick sections for immunofluorescence LSCM can be obtained by sectioning resin- or paraffin-embedded tissue, by cryosectioning frozen tissue (the technique most widely used), or by sectioning unembedded tissue with the Vibratome. If resin is used for postembedding labeling, it must be possible to etch away the resin so that sections can be stained throughout their depth. To our knowledge, hydrophilic resins commonly used for postembedding immunocytochemistry, including LR White and Lowicryl, cannot be etched. We have adopted a nonembedding method for three reasons: superior structural preservation and contrast (allowing superior resolution) and convenience. Structural alteration with embedding techniques is caused by extraction and shrinkage. Shrinkage reduces resolution. If, when cell volume decreases, structures such as cytoskeletal filaments become packed too close together, they can no longer be resolved. We have measured an approximately 30% decrease in photoreceptor inner segment diameter (photoreceptor domains are marked in Fig. 4), which is about a 50% decrease in cross-sectional area, with paraffin and JB-4 embedment, compared to formaldehyde fixation with no embedment. Measurements were taken near the center of about 15 cells from 3 sections per treatment in 2 experiments. The ability to resolve structures also is affected by contrast, which depends on high labeling intensity and low background. We compared opsin antibody labeling [antibody (15–18); see Table I] of photoreceptor inner segments in formaldehyde-fixed retinas without (Vibratome sections) or with embedment. Labeling was more intense if the tissue was not embedded than after it was embedded in epoxy resin (etched sections). Labeling in unembedded and paraffin-embedded (dewaxed sections) (Paraplast X-tra; Ted Pella, Tustin, CA) retinas was comparable if Vibratome sections were not detergent permeabilized. When detergent was added to the antibody incubation solution, however, labeling intensity increased, for instance, about twofold for opsin immunolabeling with saponin treatment (see Section II,C,1; Fig. 4A and C). With tubulin, GFAP, and CRALBP antibodies, labeling intensity was reduced slightly after paraffin embedment. A much more serious problem with these embedding procedures is that they require heating to 55–60°C, which can induce autofluorescence. We have observed increases in background fluorescence great enough to begin obscuring small structures and fine detail. The importance of minimizing shrinkage and autofluorescence cannot be overemphasized.

Both freezing and Vibratome techniques can preserve cellular structure and antigenicity well. In the case of antigens that are extracted by liquid-phase fixation or are sensitive to certain fixatives, freeze-substitution or freeze-drying are the techniques of choice (see Larsson, 1988, for a discussion of these techniques). For other antigens, freezing and Vibratome techniques are convenient and probably equally effective, as long as ice crystal formation during freezing is prevented. We chose Vibratome sectioning because Vibratomes are relatively inexpensive and easy to use. The other sections in this article are applicable to either technique.

The Vibratome technique is convenient; it is straightforward and consists of only a few short steps. After fixation, tissue pieces first are immersed in an agarose or gelatin solution, for example, a 5% solution of low gelling temperature (37°C) agarose (type XI: Sigma, St. Louis, MO), which does not actually infiltrate the tissue, but simply gels around it to provide support. We use low gelling temperature agarose to prevent heat damage and a high level of tissue autofluorescence. Then the agarose is cut into blocks, each containing a tissue piece, and glued onto supports. The block and the Vibratome blade are submerged in a liquid bath in the boat of the Vibratome during sectioning. No further processing is necessary before sections are labeled with fluorescent probes. Sections between 25 and a few hundred microns can be cut; however, practical considerations limit section thickness. We have found that sections less than 40 $\mu$m thick can be too fragile to handle. Sections thicker than 40–50 $\mu$m may not useful if individual cells or populations of cells that occupy the entire thickness must be viewed, because antibody penetration is limited and because image intensity and resolution decline with depth. In this case, because high-resolution work is restricted to the upper 15–20 $\mu$m (see Section III,A), sections could be viewed from both surfaces.

## C. Labeling with Fluorochrome-Conjugated Probes

### 1. Penetration of Antibodies

To meet the goal of obtaining three-dimensional information, it must be possible for probes to penetrate some distance into thick sections. Limited penetration of antibodies and other probes into Vibratome sections is possible without permeabilization treatments; however, this may be insufficient for three-dimensional analysis. Penetration of 15 $\mu$m, that is, 1–1.5 hepatocytes, into sections of liver tissue has been reported by Novikoff *et al.* (1983) for unconjugated antibody followed by horseradish peroxidase-conjugated protein A. We have observed penetration of approximately 7 to 22 $\mu$m into retinal sections for unconjugated followed by fluorochrome-conjugated antibodies, depending on the antibody and tissue region (see, e.g., Figs. 5C and 6A). Note that these values actually are measurements of the depth of antibody labeling. Antibodies penetrate farther than this, but the level of binding depends on the concentration at a given depth in relation to antibody affinity and antigen concentration (Priestley *et al.*, 1992). Cell membranes can be permeabilized by several methods, including freeze-thawing and extracting lipids with organic solvents (dehydration-rehydration) or detergents (surfactants). [See Priestley (1984) and Larsson (1988) for reviews of permeabilization methods.] To enhance penetration and thoroughly rinse out unbound probe, we add detergent to all incubation and rinse buffers. We have not tried permeabilizing with detergent

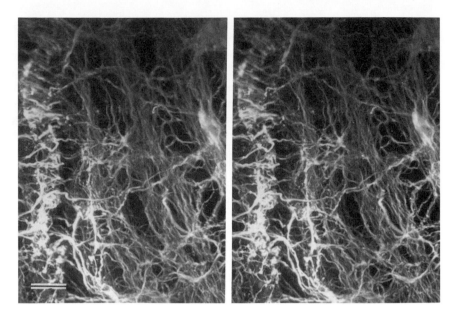

**Fig. 3**  Stereo pair of astrocytes labeled with an antibody to GFAP, a glial cell-specific intermediate filament protein. The tissue was fixed in 4% formaldehyde and permeabilized with 0.1% Triton
X-100. Laser scanning confocal microscopy images were collected at 0.5-$\mu$m increments through
12 $\mu$m near the vitreal suface of a whole mount of cat retina. The optical sections are parallel to the
vitreal surface, giving an *en face* view. To create the stereo pair, images were projected with a pixel
shift of −0.5 for the left and +0.5 for the right. This stereo pair shows the power of using LSCM to
optically section unembedded tissue for studying the distribution and orientation of cell processes in
three dimensions. The fine processes radiating from several astrocytes are distinct, and their
three-dimensional organization is easily traced. Several processes extend to contact a blood vessel
on the left. Scale bar = 20 $\mu$m.

before or at the same time as fixation, although extraction of unpolymerized
cytoskeletal subunits increases contrast and such procedures may further improve penetration (procedures reviewed in Osborn and Weber, 1982; Larsson,
1988). We have found that whereas probes as large as fluorochrome-conjugated
avidin ($m_r$ 66,000] penetrate at least 50 $\mu$m into tissue permeabilized with 0.1%
Triton X-100 (Sigma) (biotechnology reagent, electrophoresis grade; Fisher),
penetration of larger molecules, for example, antibodies (IgG; $m_r \sim$150,000), is
more restricted.

   We compared depth of antibody labeling in Vibratome-sectioned retinal tissue
without detergent and with L-$\alpha$-(palmitoyl)lysophosphatidylcholine [(palmitoyl)lysolecithin], a zwitterionic detergent (Sigma), Triton X-100, a nonionic detergent, and saponin, a sapogenin glycoside (Sigma). Zwitterionic and
nonionic detergents stabilize protein conformation when used to solubilize
membrane proteins. Lysolecithin, a natural component of cell membranes, has

been used for live cell work (Barak *et al.*, 1980). Saponin, which may selectively extract cholesterol, has been reported to be less extractive or damaging to membranes than Triton X-100 by the criterion of ultrastructural appearance (Ohtsuki *et al.*, 1978; Willingham and Yamada, 1979). We tested three concentrations of Triton X-100: 0.1, 0.2, and 1.0%. We used saponin and lysolecithin at 0.1%. The results of this comparison are compiled in Table II; percentage increases in immunolabeling depth, compared to no detergent treatment, are averages of values from several Vibratome sections in two experiments. Depth was measured from vertical ($xz$) scans through the sections, such as those in Fig. 6A–C. The depth of intense labeling was measured, although weak labeling extends farther. Sections were incubated in primary antibodies for 18–20 hr and in secondary antibodies for 12–14 hr. Depth was decreased with shorter incubation times, whereas it was not substantially increased with longer incubation times. Detergent was present during all incubations and rinses, unless otherwise stated. All incubations were performed at 4°C. For other details, see Section V,C. Sections of frog retina fixed in 4% formaldehyde or 0.1% glutaraldehyde–4% formaldehyde were used for anti-tubulin and sections of formaldehyde-fixed frog retina were used for anti-opsin, whereas sections of formaldehyde-fixed cat retina were used for anti-CRALBP.

Detergent permeabilization enhanced penetration of anti-$\beta$-tubulin, -CRALBP, and -opsin antibodies, with two exceptions. No increase was apparent with saponin treatment for anti-CRALBP or with lysolecithin for anti-opsin. Overall, saponin and lysolecithin were less effective than Triton X-100, presumably because they removed fewer membrane components. For the antibody to

**Table II**
**Increase in Depth of Immunolabeling with Detergent Permeabilization**

| | Percentage increase[a] | | | |
|---|---|---|---|---|
| | Antitubulin[b] | | Anti-CRALBP[c] | Anti-opsin |
| Detergent | Form.[d] | Glut.[d] | Form.[d] | Form.[d] |
| Triton X-100 (0.1%, 1- to 2-hr pretreatment) | 80 | 40 | NM[e] | NM |
| Triton X-100 (0.1%) | 100 | 55 | 40 | 125 |
| Triton X-100 (0.2%) | 170 | 60 | NM | NM |
| Triton X-100 (1.0%) | 200 | 140 | 45 | NM |
| Saponin (0.1%) | 75 | 15 | 0 | 80 |
| Lysophosphatidylcholine (0.1%) | 75 | 20 | NM | 0 |

[a] Increase over no detergent treatment.
[b] Depth in inner plexiform layer (mainly neuronal processes; see Fig. 2B).
[c] Depth in inner plexiform layer (Müller glial cells; see Fig. 6A).
[d] Fixation: Form, 4% formaldehyde; Glut., 0.1% glutaraldehyde–4% formaldehyde.
[e] NM, Not measured.

tubulin, labeling depth in the inner plexiform layer (Fig. 6A–C), which is composed mainly of neuronal processes, increased with Triton X-100 concentration. In formaldehyde-fixed tissue, the depth with 0.1% Trion X-100 was twice that with no detergent, and with a concentration of 1.0% was three times greater. A 1- to 2-hr pretreatment with 0.1% Triton X-100 was surprisingly effective; immunolabeling depth was increased almost as much as when detergent was present throughout antibody incubations. Brief detergent pretreatment may be useful if lengthy incubation in Triton X-100 extracts membrane components of interest. For antitubulin, depth of labeling in the inner plexiform layer in formaldehyde-fixed tissue ranged from approximately 7 $\mu$m without detergent to about 21 $\mu$m with 1.0% Triton X-100. Penetration is more restricted with fixation in 0.1% glutaraldehyde–4% formaldehyde. Without detergent, the depth of labeling was only slightly reduced; however, with 1.0% Triton X-100 it was limited to about 16 $\mu$m, a 25% reduction.

There were also differences in immunolabeling depth among tissue regions and among antibodies. For example, labeling with the antibody to tubulin extended deeper into the inner nuclear layer, which is composed mainly of cell bodies, than the inner plexiform layer, which is composed mainly of neurites; in formaldehyde-fixed tissue without detergent, labeling depths were approximately 22 $\mu$m (about three cell bodies) and 7 $\mu$m, respectively (Fig. 6A). In the inner nuclear layer, labeling depth was increased only slightly with detergent treatment. Glutaraldehyde–formaldehyde fixation reduced the depth of anti-tubulin labeling in the inner nuclear layer by approximately 30% for all treatments. Detergent treatment does not overcome the barrier to penetration presented by increased cross-linking with glutaraldehyde. Anti-CRALBP labeling extended deepest overall, even without detergent. The depth in the inner retina, where the Müller glial cells are located (shown in Fig. 5A), was about 20 $\mu$m with no detergent and about 29 $\mu$m with 1.0% Triton X-100 (Fig. 5C and E). In the retinal pigment epithelium (identified in Fig. 5A) it was lower, about 15 $\mu$m, and was not enhanced by detergent treatment. Anti-opsin labeling extended approximately 7 $\mu$m (about one cell diameter) into the photoreceptor layer with no detergent and 16 $\mu$m (about 2.5 cell diameters) with 0.1% Triton X-100. These variations indicate that factors other than detergent type and concentration, possibly including the type of antigen/organelle being labeled, structural features of the cell/tissue, and the degree of fixative cross-linking, as well as the concentration of the antigen and affinity of the antibody, affect antibody penetration.

In addition to the depth of antibody labeling, the intensity of labeling was also increased by detergent treatment for anti-tubulin and anti-opsin. The method of estimating intensity is described in Section II,A. Labeling of microtubules was increased uniformly in the plexiform and photoreceptor layers by the three detergents tested, up to about twofold with Triton X-100 (all concentrations), as shown in Fig. 6D and E. The effect of detergents on the intensity of labeling of the integral membrane protein, opsin, in rod photoreceptors was more complex.

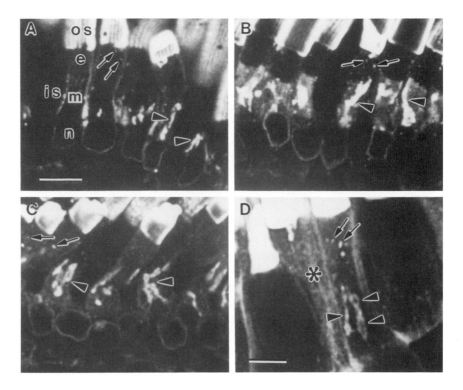

**Fig. 4**  Antibody and lectin (WGA) labeling of opsin, an integral membrane protein. The outer segment (os), inner segment (is), ellipsoid (e) and myoid (m) regions, and nucleus (n) are marked in (A) for orientation. Vibratome sections were cut parallel to the long axis of the photoreceptors. (A–C) Effects of detergents on anti-opsin (15–18) labeling intensity in formaldehyde-fixed frog rod photoreceptors. Antibody solutions contained either no detergent (A), 0.1% saponin (B), or 0.1% Triton X-100 (C). To allow comparisons of labeling intensity, the aperture size, neural density filter, gain, and black level were held constant and set such that the maximum intensity value for the brightest specimens was just below the upper limit of the scale. All images then were photographed and printed at the same exposure. Optical section thickness was about 1.0 $\mu$m. Labeling of the Golgi apparatus (arrowheads) and the area surrounding it, which probably is the endoplasmic reticulum (see Section II,C,1), was most intense with saponin (B). Labeling of vesicles in the ellipsoid region (small arrows) that may be post-Golgi transport vesicles was more intense with both detergents, as shown in (B) and (C). Scale bar = 10 $\mu$m. (D) Wheat germ agglutinin labeling of rod photoreceptor inner segment membranes is similar to that seen with anti-opsin, except for the absence of endoplasmic reticulum staining. Additionally, the extracellular matrix surrounding the photoreceptors is labeled as well, as seen between the photoreceptors and along the surface of the rod marked with an asterisk. This image is a projection of four optical sections so that the equivalent of an approximately 3-$\mu$m section through the cell is obtained. The advantage of such projections is that a greater portion of large organelles can be seen at the same time without the use of three-dimensional display techniques. Arrowheads indicate three segments of the Golgi that are at different depths. Scale bar = 5 $\mu$m.

The results for antibody (15–18) (see Table I) are as follows. Lysolecithin (0.1%) enhanced only Golgi apparatus labeling, when compared to no detergent (not shown). Saponin and Triton X-100 (both at 0.1%) altered opsin labeling intensity differentially for different membranous organelles. These two detergents increased labeling intensity for some organelles, while leaving others unchanged or reduced. Both enhanced labeling of the ellipsoid region vesicles and Golgi apparatus, saponin more so than Triton X-100 (Fig. 4A–C). Saponin treatment also dramatically enhanced labeling of what likely is the endoplasmic reticulum (Fig. 4B). This fairly uniform immunolabeling throughout the myoid region appeared identical to that seen with the lectin, concanavalin A, in this compartment (data not shown). This lectin recognizes $\alpha$-D-mannose and $\alpha$-D-glucose, which are components of the immature N-linked oligosaccharides added to secretory and membrane glycoproteins in the endoplasmic reticulum. Concanavalin A has been demonstrated to be a marker for this organelle in several cell types with high secretory activity (reviewed in Lis and Sharon, 1986). Opsin contains two N-linked oligosaccharides and is a major biosynthetic product of the photoreceptor. Hence, concanavalin A would be expected to label the endoplasmic reticulum of this cell (reviewed in Bok, 1985). Labeling of the endoplasmic reticulum with antibody (15–18) was difficult to detect with the other treaments (e.g., Fig. 4A and C). Thus, whereas saponin enhanced immunolabeling of endoplasmic reticulum membranes, Triton X-100 and lysolecithin did not. Detergent treatment previously has been shown to substantially improve immunolabeling of opsin (Hicks and Barnstable, 1987) and other membrane proteins (Pickel, 1981). Perhaps these detergents do so for antibody (15–18) by altering the membrane environment in such a way that antibody access or binding efficiency is improved, but only for particular, and different, organelles. On the other hand, treatment with saponin and Triton X-100 reduced inner segment plasma membrane labeling. Although no single treatment, including incubation in antibodies without detergent, was optimal, saponin provided the most comprehensive localization information for this monoclonal antibody to opsin.

Adding to the complexity, different results were obtained with another monoclonal antibody to opsin, rho 4D2 (see Table I) (data not shown). Faint endoplasmic reticulum labeling with this antibody was apparent without detergent treatment, and was increased to a lesser extent than that of other organelles by both Triton X-100 and saponin. In this case, Triton X-100 enhanced labeling of vesicles and Golgi slightly more than saponin. Variable effects of these detergents have been reported previously by Goldenthal et al. (1985), who observed reduced labeling of integral membrane proteins with Triton X-100 vs saponin treatment for some antibodies, but not others. Therefore it is worth the effort to test antibodies to membrane proteins without and with several detergents to obtain accurate assessments of protein presence and content in various membranous organelles. The choice of detergent for simultaneous labeling of a membrane protein and, for example, cytoskeletal elements should be based on this type of information.

We did not observe by fluorescence microscopy any damaging effects of the detergent treatments described here. At 0.1%, none of the detergents altered Golgi apparatus morphology in any obvious way, nor was there definitive evidence that they extracted opsin from photoreceptor membranes. Using the microtubules in the ellipsoid region of rods as test structures, we could not detect fragmentation or loss of microtubules in formaldehyde-fixed tissue, even at the highest Triton X-100 concentration (1.0%) (Fig. 2A and B). We had worried that membrane permeabilization might result in loss of soluble proteins from cells in formaldehyde-fixed tissue, but labeling intensity of CRALBP, a 33-kDa soluble protein, was not reduced by the detergent treatments we tested, including 1.0% Triton X-100 (compare Fig. 5C with Fig. 5D and E). Apparently, there is no trade-off between penetration and retention of structural integrity and integral membrane or soluble proteins at these concentrations.

The depth of immunolabeling can vary substantially depending on how long sections are incubated in antibody and how well the incubation solutions are stirred (see Section V,C), as well as with the factors discussed above. In addition, although sections are incubated free floating in antibody solutions, sometimes only one surface of the section is well stained (compare, e.g., Fig. 5C and D with Fig. 5E). For these reasons, we recommend performing an initial vertical ($xz$) scan to quickly assess penetration depth, and to determine whether the well-stained surface is facing the coverslip.

## 2. Fluorochromes

Signal intensity in LSCM varies not only with the binding efficiency of the probe, the abundance of the molecule being labeled, and any effect of tissue processing on these factors, but also with the fluorochrome used. There are a variety of fluorescent labels that can be conjugated to probes. The fluorescence intensity of a dye is determined by the product of the extinction coefficient, that is, probability of absorption, and the quantum yield, that is, probability of fluorescent emission, at a given wavelength. In addition, other properties such as absorption/emission maximum, emission lifetime, and photostability, together with the emission wavelengths of the laser, the wavelength selectivity of barrier filters, the wavelength sensitivity of the detector, and the environment of the fluorochrome, all determine the performance in LSCM of a given fluorochrome. The environment can be critical. Factors including the proximity to each other of dye molecules conjugated to a probe can have a dramatic effect on quantum yield. Environmental factors such as pH affect the photostability of some dyes. (See Tsien and Waggoner, 1990, and Brelje et al. [4], this volume, for reviews of fluorochromes and their properties.) For multiple-label imaging, the signals from two or more fluorochromes must be balanced to minimize crosstalk through barrier filters. (See Brelje et al. [4], this volume for a discussion of the parameters important in multiple-label confocal imaging.) Finally, contrast depends on the level of background fluorescence, and the molecules responsible for autofluorescence have characteristic absorption and emission spectra that

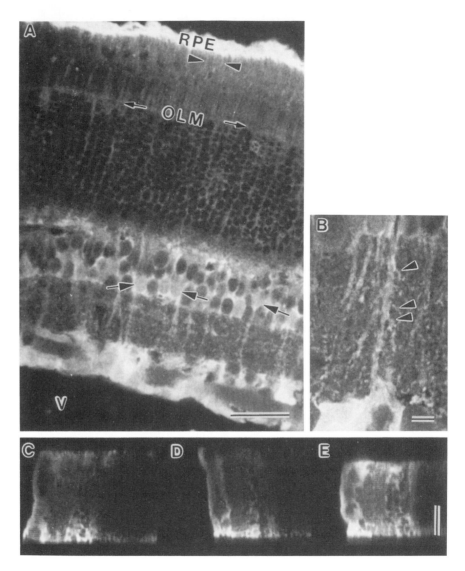

**Fig. 5** Antibody labeling of CRALBP, a soluble protein found in retinal pigment epithelium (RPE) and Müller glial cells. (A) Cat retinal tissue was fixed in 4% formaldehyde and permeabilized with 0.1% Triton X-100. The Vibratome section was cut parallel to the long axis of the photoreceptors. The position and orientation of these cell types within the cat retina, as well as their shape, are revealed in great detail, as CRALBP appears to be distributed throughout the entire cytoplasm. The RPE apposes the photoreceptors, and fine villous processes (arrowheads) can be seen projecting among the photoreceptor outer segments. Müller cells extend from just above the photoreceptor nuclei, where they form a barrier termed the outer limiting membrane (OLM, small arrows), to the vitreous (V), where they expand to form large end feet in the ganglion cell layer. Labeled Müller cell nuclei (large arrows) are present in the inner nuclear layer. Scale bar = 20 μm. (B) Müller cells also extend fine processes laterally. Several processes (arrowheads) can be traced as they branch from a

also must be considered. This section touches only briefly on this complex topic, and is intended to give an idea of the interplay among some of these elements.

Such interplay means that, in the end, the choice of fluorochrome(s) must be made empirically for each system. For example, features of the confocal system we use and the cell type we study present conflicting requirements. The Bio-Rad MRC-500 light source is an argon ion laser and the detector is a photomultiplier tube. Hence, fluorescein (FITC; absorption maximum = 490 nm, emission maximum = 520 nm) should be a better choice than rhodamine (TRITC; absorption maximum = 554 nm; emission maximum = 573 nm), because its absorption maximum is better matched to the emission wavelengths (488 and 514 nm) of the argon ion laser and its emission maximum is better matched to the spectral sensitivity of the photomultiplier tube, which is two to three times more sensitive to green light (see Fig. 12 of Majlof and Forsgren [3], this volume). Moreover, fluorescein has a higher quantum yield. In spite of this, we often have found it preferable to use rhodamine for immunolabeling of structures in the ellipsoid region of photoreceptors (photoreceptor domains are marked in Fig. 2), because there is strong autofluorescence from the mitochondria, which are concentrated in this region of the cell, that overlaps with and thus masks fluorescein emission. Although contrast is increased with rhodamine, we still have some difficulty detecting small structures, such as microtubules and transport vesicles, because of the low emission and detection of this dye in the MRC-500 confocal system. One solution to these problems is the krypton–argon ion laser used with the MRC-600. Its emission at 568 nm excites rhodamine more efficiently than the 514-nm line of the argon ion laser. A different type of solution is a sulfoindocyanine dye, CY3.18 (CY3), developed in Waggoner's laboratory (Southwick et al., 1990; Yu et al., 1992). It has an absorption/emission maximum similar to that of rhodamine, but a significantly greater extinction coefficient. More importantly, it was designed to interact less when several dye molecules are bound to a single antibody, as dye interactions usually reduce quantum yield substantially (Tsien and Waggoner, 1990). The CY3-conjugated secondary antibodies (available from Jackson ImmunoResearch, West Grove, PA) provide a signal intensity comparable to fluorescein in a region of the spectrum where autofluorescence intensity is low. These properties make CY3 especially useful for labeling molecules that comprise small structures, as

cell in this higher magnification image. For orientation, part of the end-foot region is visible in the lower left. Scale bar = 5 μm. (C–E) Comparison of anti-CRALBP penetration into formaldehyde-fixed cat retinal tissue with either no detergent (C), 0.1% saponin (D), or 1.0% Triton X-100 (E). Images are vertical scans through Vibratome sections approximately 100 μm thick, collected at constant intensity settings, as described for Fig. 4A–C. These images show the increase in immunolabeling depth obtained with Triton X-100, but not with saponin. They also show that labeling intensity is not changed by detergent treatment. [Note that only one surface of the sections in (C) and (D) is well stained, probably as a result of inadequate stirring during incubation in antibody solutions.] Scale bar (vertical) = 40 μm.

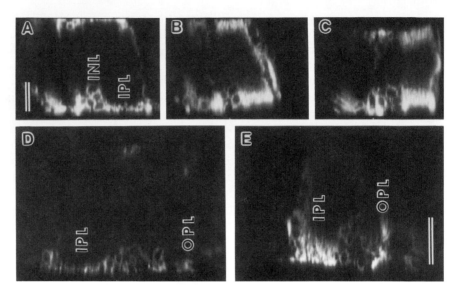

**Fig. 6** Increase in tubulin antibody penetration and labeling intensity with Triton X-100 treatment. Images are vertical (*xz*) scans through thick (75–100 $\mu$m) Vibratome sections of frog retina. (A–C) The increase in depth of immunolabeling in the inner plexiform layer (IPL) when sections are permeabilized with Triton X-100. The following treatments are shown: (A) no detergent; (B) 1–2 hr pretreatment with 0.1% Triton X-100; and (C) 1.0% Triton X-100 present during antibody incubations (30 hr) and rinses. (A) also shows the variation in depth among different regions of the frog retina, for example, between the inner nuclear layer (INL) and the inner plexiform layer (IPL), which is composed principally of neuronal processes. Scale bar (vertical) = 25 $\mu$m. (D and E) Comparison of antitubulin labeling intensity without detergent (D) or with 1.0% Triton X-100 (E). Intensity settings and photographic conditions were kept constant, as described for Fig. 4A–C. Labeling in the plexiform layers (IPL and OPL) was about twice as intense when Triton X-100 (1.0%) was present during antibody incubations. [Note that for (A), the gain was increased to match the intensity of (C).] Scale bar = 40 $\mu$m.

above, or are in low abundance, and for imaging at deeper optical planes within thick tissue sections (see Section III,A). However, the greater extinction coefficient of CY3 potentially limits its usefulness for imaging deep within tissue, because of self-shadowing. In addition, CY3 is more photostable than fluorescein.

Photostability is important, because multiple scans of each optical plane must be collected for averaging or integration, and multiple planes need to be imaged to gather three-dimensional information. In the latter case, as fluorochromes outside the plane of focus also receive some illumination, photobleaching can be a serious problem when many optical sections are collected. For fluorescein, the pH of the mounting medium greatly affects photostability. This dye is much more stable at or above pH 8 than it is at pH 7 ([4], this volume). Mounting in a solution containing an antioxidant, such as *n*-propyl gallate (Giloh and Sedat, 1982) or *p*-phenylenediamine (Johnson *et al.*, 1982), protects against bleaching and photodamage to the specimen. We have found that bleaching is noticeably decreased in a hydrophobic environment, for example, resin (embedded tissue) or glycerol. Therefore, we use a 5% solution of *n*-propyl gallate in 100% glycerol, which is diluted slightly by the buffer in the tissue sections. We also rinse fluorescein-labeled sections in pH 8 phosphate-buffered saline before mounting. These steps dramatically reduce photobleaching with our specimens.

## III. Confocal Imaging Parameters for Maximum Resolution

### A. Microscope

We have worked out these parameters using a Bio-Rad MRC-500 laser scanning confocal microscope with an argon ion laser light source and a photomultiplier tube detector. The same imaging parameters apply to other point scanning systems. The most critical variable for successful confocal imaging is alignment of the emitted beam with the pinhole aperture, which is achieved by adjusting the positions of the laser scanning mirrors. Even slight misalignment substantially reduces image intensity and contrast. For this reason, final alignment should be performed at the objective lens magnification and electronic zoom setting that will be used, because fine adjustments often are necessary after initial alignment with low-power lenses.

Three other imaging parameters are especially important to attaining the goal of maximizing contrast with LSCM, thereby maximizing detection and practical resolution. The first is the size of the pinhole aperture, which determines the extent to which out-of-focus light is excluded. Aperture size is variable in this system. At the minimum aperture size, the thickness of the optical section is minimized, approaching the axial resolution limit of the objective lens (see Section I,C). As the confocal aperture is opened, increasing levels of out-of-focus light obscure fine detail (See Section I,B). Table III in Gard ([9], this volume) provides information to determine the range of optical section thicknesses possible for several objective lens numerical apertures. The second imaging parameter is incident light intensity, which can be reduced by neutral density filters. Because the signal from fluorochromes saturates at a lower illumination intensity than autofluorescence, and scattered light signals do not saturate, keeping the illumination below the level of fluorochrome saturation maximizes contrast (Tsien and Waggoner, 1990). A compromise usually must be reached when setting these two parameters, such that neither is optimum by itself, but the combination produces the sharpest images. In general, we have obtained the best results by opening the aperture enough to allow the use of a neutral density filter that transmits 3% or less of the light. The third parameter is gain. We have found it preferable to set the gain somewhat below maximum to reduce electronic noise.

When these three parameters are adjusted for maximum contrast, the LSCM has minimum sensitivity. Remember that sensitivity is as important as contrast for detecting small structures. This trade-off creates the need for high labeling intensity and objective lenses with high light gathering capability and transmission (see Section III,B). In our experience, CY3-conjugated secondary antibodies give the highest signal. For tubulin primary and CY3-conjugated secondary antibodies, we have been able to use an NA 1.4 objective lens with a 1% transmission filter and with the aperture at minimum size. This was not possible with rhodamine or fluorescein. For this reason, CY3 noticeably improves our ability to resolve detail in the photoreceptor myoid region. Figure 2D is an image obtained with these parameters. A benefit of using a 3% or less transmission filter and a medium gain setting is that fewer scans per image are required when background signals (autofluorescence and scattering) and electronic noise are low, reducing photobleaching and saving time.

A fourth parameter affecting practical $xy$ resolution is the image scale, that is, pixel size, which is determined by the magnification of the objective lens and the electronic zoom setting. According to the Nyquist criterion, the zoom setting should be chosen to give a pixel size less than or equal to one-half the theoretical resolution of the objective (Inoué, 1986). If the pixel size is too large, the maximum resolution is not achieved (see [3], this volume); if it is too small, unnecessary photobleaching results.

The problem of exchanging sensitivity for contrast with LSCM is aggravated by a decline in image intensity with increasing depth into the specimen (see Section I,B). The decline in intensity with depth can be compensated for by increasing the gain or switching to a higher transmission neutral density filter at deeper optical planes. Increasing the number of scans accumulated for each image is then desirable, in order to compensate for the resultant increase in noise. Increasing the gain is helpful only up to the point at which electronic noise interferes with image contrast. Similarly, increasing illumination intensity is beneficial only until autofluorescence and scattering begin to obscure the primary signal, or until photobleaching becomes severe. For these reasons, Art (1990) suggests direct photon counting as a better solution for weak signals. A photon-counting circuit greatly reduces noise, so that weak signals are easier to detect above background. This option is available on the Bio-Rad MRC-600.

When collecting serial optical sections, termed $z$ series, expanding the intensity scale after each image is collected can help to maintain constant image intensity. This can be done with a pixel remap function. Pixel remapping is not effective if the intensity range across the scan area is broad; as long as the brightest areas remain at maximum value, the scale will not be adjusted. Note that remapped images no longer provide accurate quantitative intensity information. If sections are to be collected through a depth of more than 5–10 $\mu$m, adjacent series of several microns each may have to be collected, so that the gain can be adjusted. The effect of photobleaching in out-of-focus planes while other planes are being imaged can be minimized by collecting $z$ series beginning with the deepest optical section, as it has the lowest image intensity to start with.

An additional consideration is that fluorescence intensity usually is not even across the tissue section, because labeled structures are not uniformly distributed within the tissue or individual cells. The dynamic range of the photomultiplier tube can be too narrow to accommodate the wide range of fluorescence intensities. For this reason, we often find it necessary to set the illumination intensity, gain, and black level to bring out detail in a particular area of interest, even though other regions of the cell or tissue are obscured in that image. An example of this can be seen for anti-tubulin labeling in Fig. 2; compare the photoreceptor myoid region in Fig. 2B and D and the plexiform layer in Fig. 2D and E. When individual microtubules in the myoid region can be distinguished (Fig. 2D), microtubules in the ellipsoid region are difficult to detect. Likewise, when the beam intensity and gain are reduced so that neuronal processes in the plexiform layer can be distinguished (Fig. 2E), the weaker signal in the photoreceptors is almost below the threshold of detection. Conversely, when the beam intensity and gain are increased to lower the threshold so that labeling in the photoreceptors is easily detected, bright areas, such as the plexiform layers, become completely white, as in Fig. 2D. Remapping pixel intensities by modifying the look-up table (LUT) after image collection is a good solution if the intensity range is not too broad. A nonlinear intensity scale can be constructed to expand that portion of the range corresponding to the area of interest while other portions are contracted. In the tubulin labeling example, we expand the low to midportion of the range, corresponding to pixel intensities for the ellipsoid microtubules in Fig. 2C or the photoreceptors in Fig. 2D, and contract the upper end. In this way, the lower intensity values are increased, while the higher values are kept below maximum. In other words, we remap the linear scale to a plateauing curve (see also [9], this volume). If autofluorescence is present, a somewhat sigmoidal curve can be useful, to avoid raising the lowest values, which correspond to background fluorescence. This type of adjustment is more powerful if performed during collection. It is important, however, to compare images collected with and without adjustment to guard against information loss. The Bio-Rad MRC-600 has a nonlinear collection feature ([9], this volume).

We have encountered the following two difficulties with interpretation of confocal images of small structures. The first arises from the greater thickness of optical sections ($>0.5 \mu m$), compared to the size of the object. For example, thin structures, such as microtubules (antibody decorated, 55 nm), oriented perpendicular to the vertical axis are fainter than those that are parallel to it and thus span the depth of the optical section (van der Voort and Brakenhoff, 1990). Figure 1B illustrates a similar point for actin bundles. The actin cables that run under the photoreceptor inner segment and extend into the calycal processes appear fainter where the surface of the cell is perpendicular to the vertical axis than at the sides, where several cables are in line along the vertical axis and their signals are additive. The same is true of planar structures, such as the plasma membrane. The second difficulty is the result of out-of-focus light from the object being collected in adjacent optical sections. In $z$ series, the size of small structures can appear greater in the vertical dimension. We advise cutting both

longitudinal and cross sections of uniformly oriented cells, such as photoreceptors and epithelia, with the Vibratome to detect labeling of thin structures more
easily and to verify the shape of small structures. The concentration of actin
filaments in the photoreceptor ciliary stalk serves as an example. This actin
network appears as a small fluorescent spot (Fig. 1) in single optical sections of
either longitudinal- or cross-sectioned retinas. Yet it often can be followed
through two or even three adjacent optical sections, roughly 0.75 $\mu$m thick,
collected at 0.75-$\mu$m intervals.

Although image enhancement and the manipulation, display, and analysis of
three-dimensional images will not be discussed further here, what is done with
images after they are collected can be as important to obtaining accurate information as how they are collected. For discussions of these topics, the reader is
referred to Inoué (1986) and Chen *et al.* (1990) (see also [1] and [9], this volume).

## B. Lenses

Objective lens parameters and the ways in which they affect imaging in
confocal microscopy are discussed in detail by Keller (1990) and Majlof and
Forsgren ([3], this volume). In this section, we will touch only briefly on three
issues that have particular application to high-resolution imaging in thick tissue
sections. These issues are (1) the special importance of objective lens numerical
aperture to practical resolution in LSCM, (2) the trade-off that can be made
between correction and high lens transmission, and (3) ways to counteract the
loss of correction for spherical aberration with depth into thick tissue sections.
In microscopy in general, the highest resolution is possible by using lenses with
the best correction for aberrations and the greatest numerical aperture [Eq. (1)].
In LSCM, optical section thinness depends similarly on objective lens numerical
aperture and correction. Objective lenses also must be aligned with and matched
to the other optical components of the microscope. In fluorescence microscopy,
detection of small structures depends on how much light the objective can
gather and transmit. These factors are even more critical in LSCM, where light
is restricted by the pinhole aperture. The need for adequate correction for
aberrations now is counterbalanced by the need for high transmission (Keller,
1990). The fewer lens elements a lens has, the more light it will transmit, but
the less well corrected it will be. Lenses with the greatest numerical aperture
also provide the highest light-gathering capability. Image brightness in epifluorescence microscopy varies as

$$\text{Image brightness} = NA^4/\text{magnification}^2 \qquad (2)$$

Thus magnification becomes an additional consideration. Lower magnification
objectives are desirable.

We have been able to reach a good compromise by using high numerical
aperture, moderately to well-corrected immersion lenses of the lowest magnifi-

cation required. Immersion lenses, with their high numerical aperture, gather more light than dry lenses, and give a sharper image by reducing light scatter induced by an air–coverglass interface. It is worth sacrificing some correction to gain transmission with objectives over ×40. For example, although it is only partially corrected for spherical aberration at red wavelengths, we prefer a ×63/NA 1.3 Achromat (Fluoreszenz, oil; Leitz Wetzlar) vs a ×63/NA 1.4 Plan-Apochromat (oil; Nikon) for rhodamine- and CY3-conjugated probes for imaging below a few microns from the surface. Its greater transmission allows image collection deeper within the tissue section before image intensity decreases substantially (see Section I,B). In our experience, the loss in contrast from opening the pinhole aperture appeared to diminish image sharpness more than the effect of spherical aberration. Because the scan area can be restricted to the center of the field by means of an electronic zoom feature, use of Plan, or flat-field, objectives is not always critical. The electronic zoom feature also limits the need for a ×100 objective lens, which would give a dimmer image than lower magnification lenses of the same numerical aperture. For our studies, a ×40 NA 1.3 Apochromat (UVFl 40; Olympus) oil immersion lens provided the best images overall, because it combines a high numerical aperture, moderate magnification, and high transmission.

The shallow working distance (approximately 100–150 $\mu$m) of high-numerical aperture objectives is a limitation for work with thick tissue. With oil immersion lenses, however, the ability to resolve fine detail is lost well before the lens actually contacts the coverglass. In our experience, image quality deteriorates substantially below about 15 $\mu$m from the surface. We have implemented two partial solutions to counteract the decline in image intensity and resolution with depth caused by spherical aberration induced by the specimen (See Section I,B). The first is to mount the specimen directly on the coverglass if oil immersion lenses are used. This minimizes the space between the section and the coverglass to make the most of the limited depth into glycerol/tissue in which correction for spherical aberration is maintained. The second is to use a glycerol immersion lens (×40/0.9 NA, Plan-Neofluar, oil/glycerol/water; Zeiss) without a coverglass. With a glycerol immersion lens, the refractive index of a specimen mounted in glycerol is closer to that of the specified immersion medium. We found that image intensity was maintained at deeper focal planes with this glycerol lens than with a ×40/NA 1.4 oil immersion lens (see above); however, the image was noticeably less sharp. A better solution, then, would be a higher numerical aperture glycerol or water lens. This still is not a perfect solution, because biological material is optically inhomogeneous and therefore requires differing corrections for spherical aberration as one focuses into the tissue. Objectives with a correction collar can be adjusted, to a limited degree, to obtain sharp images at various depths within the specimen. Ideally, alterations in spherical aberration correction would be automatically and continuously applied as one focuses through the specimen. Unfortunately, such lenses are not currently available.

══════════  ## IV. Applications

### A. Retinal Cell Biology

We initially applied the Vibratome technique and LSCM to the study of cytoskeletal organization in cells in the vertebrate retina. This technique has considerably improved our ability to detect individual cytoskeletal filaments or small bundles, as well as fine cellular processes filled with filaments, in sections of intact retina at some depth below the surface of thick sections or whole mounts of the retina. For example, we have been able to obtain images of retinal astrocytes in the cat retina labeled with an antibody to the intermediate filament protein, GFAP, that show distinctly many fine processes radiating from the cells. Figure 3 is a stereo pair collected between 1 and 13 $\mu$m below the surface of a Vibratome section. This stereo pair demonstrates the power of collecting a series of high-contrast optical thin sections and creating a three-dimensional image from them. It is easy to trace even the most delicate GFAP-filled processes of these astrocytes in three dimensions. This figure also demonstrates the potential for gaining information both about identity, because GFAP is present specifically in glial cells, and morphology.

Previously, with JB-4 sections and video microscopy, it was not possible to distinguish the filamentous nature of microtubules in the photoreceptor myoid region. Tubulin labeling appeared nearly uniform. With the nonembedding procedure and LSCM, microtubule bundles in the myoid clearly can be resolved in images collected within the upper 15 $\mu$m of thick sections (Fig. 2C and D). This has enabled us to assess the effect of microtubule poisons on microtubules in this region, where the endoplasmic reticulum and Golgi apparatus are located, giving us further insight into our earlier studies on the role of microtubules in opsin transport (Vaughan *et al.*, 1989). A drug-sensitive population of microtubules is disassembled by colchicine, leaving uniform monomer labeling, while a relatively insensitive population remains near the nucleus (I. L. Hale and B. Matsumoto, unpublished observations). In addition, with this method we were able to resolve fine neuronal processes in the plexiform layers of the retina, as shown in Fig. 2E for processes in the outer plexiform layer labeled with anti-tubulin.

This method also has proved to be well suited for visualizing the distribution of integral membrane proteins and soluble proteins. The high contrast has allowed us to obtain images in which opsin-immunoreactive vesicles in the ellipsoid region of frog photoreceptors (Fig. 4B and C), which may be transport vesicles (Papermaster *et al.*, 1985), and the plasma membrane (Fig. 4A) are well defined (see also Matsumoto and Hale, 1993). In addition to antibodies, lectins, which specifically recognize carbohydrate residues, can be used with Vibratome sections. Wheat germ agglutinin (WGA) is specific for the terminal $N$-acetyl-$\beta$-D-glucosamine residues and $N$-acetyl-neuraminic acid residues found on mature N-linked oligosaccharides. Therefore, WGA labels the Golgi apparatus, transport vesicles, and plasma membrane (Lis and Sharon, 1986). In photoreceptors, this lectin labels the outer segment, along with these organelles (Fig. 4D), because the mature carbohydrate groups of opsin (and possibly other outer segment glycoconjugates) contain a terminal $N$-actyl-$\beta$-D-glucosamine residue (Wood and Napier-Marshall, 1985). The intense opsin immunolabeling in the myoid region thought to be Golgi labeling, for example, in Fig. 4C, at least partly colocalizes with WGA Golgi apparatus labeling, such as that seen in Fig. 4D. Optical sectioning has revealed important information about the morphology of the Golgi apparatus and the number and distribution of the putative transport vesicles.

Images of anti-CRALBP labeling demonstrate the usefulness of this method not only for soluble, but for cell-specific, antigens as well. CRALBP is a cytoplasmic vitamin A carrier. The locations of the CRALBP-positive cell types, retinal pigment epithelium and Müller glial cells, within the retina and their shapes can be seen in Fig. 5A. CRALBP is present in and allows tracing of fine lateral processes as they branch from the Müller cells (Fig. 5B).

## B. Drawbacks

The thick Vibratome section method has some drawbacks, as does any technique. These relate either to the tissue itself, to the confocal microscope system, or both. A relatively minor drawback is the impermanence of the tissue sections. They can be kept longer if stored in formaldehyde to prevent tissue degradation, but tissue autofluorescence gradually increases over time. We do not know of a way to forestall this, and have found that image quality is substantially reduced after 2 weeks. Another drawback is that when contrast is maximized in LSCM sensitivity is low, because the narrow pinhole aperture greatly restricts the amount of light reaching the detector. The lack of sensitivity poses a problem with weak fluorescent signals. A photon-counting circuit reduces noise, and therefore can improve detection of weak signals. The problem of the loss of spherical aberration correction with depth into the specimen currently restricts high-resolution imaging to approximately the upper 15–20 $\mu$m of thick sections. In addition, the limited penetration of antibodies into thick tissue sections also can restrict image collection to the upper 15 $\mu$m. For viewing large cells, sections twice the limiting thickness can be cut and the sections viewed from both surfaces. Antibody Fab fragments have the potential to solve the problem of antibody penetration. Changes in objective lens design to allow correction to be maintained through a range of depths could allow advantage to be taken of increases in antibody penetration. Perhaps the biggest drawback we have experienced arises from the limited dynamic range of the photomultiplier tube compared to the wide intensity range often encountered with intact tissue and compartmentalized cells. Solutions include nonlinear remapping of pixel intensities after image collection and nonlinear collection. A more dramatic improvement in this area is achieved by the slit scanning confocal design, because the image can be viewed directly and the human eye has superior dynamic range. Possible solutions to some of these problems are discussed in more detail in the next section.


## C. Future Prospects

The large size of antibodies limits their penetration into Vibratome sections. Use of the smaller F(ab')$_2$ fragments ($m_r$ 100,000), produced by enzymatic digestion, should allow increased penetration. The extent of avidin penetration supports this possibility. This 66-kDa protein can penetrate at least 50 $\mu$m into Vibratome sections permeabilized with 0.1% Triton X-100. Of course, for indirect immunolabeling it will be necessary to use F(ab')$_2$ fragments of both primary and secondary antibodies.

Changes in lens design that will allow high-numerical aperture lenses to be used at depths below 15–20 $\mu$m from the surface of thick specimens may be forthcoming. High-numerical aperture glycerol immersion objectives would reduce the need to use oil immersion lenses, and thereby eliminate the problem caused by the difference in refractive index between the mounting medium and the coverglass/immersion medium currently encountered with oil immersion lenses. High-numerical water immersion lenses would provide the same solution for live tissue work. As suggested by Inoué (1990), high-numerical aperture oil immersion lenses with a motorized correction collar would allow automated correction as the depth of the focal plane is changed.

There are many fluorescent probes available for live cell work (Haugland, 1992). Because Vibratome sections can be cultured (Mack and Fernald, 1991), LSCM with time-lapse or real-time capability opens up the exciting potential for studying dynamic processes at the subcellular level in living cells within intact tissue (see [2], this volume for a discussion of rapid scanning confocal microscopy). Sections can then be fixed and labeled with antibodies or other probes. An example is the study by O'Rourke et al. (1992), who labeled the plasma membrane with 1,1'-dioctadecyl-3,3,3',3'-tetramethylindocarbocyanine perchlorate (diI) to follow the migration of immature neurons in slices of developing cortex. Branching and directional changes of the neuronal cell leading process and its filopodia could be observed by confocal microscopy. After fixation, radial glia were labeled with anti-vimentin to visualize the spatial relationship between migrating neurons and these cellular substrates. It should be possible to label cells in Vibratome sections of live tissue with organelle-specific probes, voltage-sensitive dyes, or ion concentration indicators, although some of these dyes must be microinjected. It also should be possible to observe binding and uptake of, for example, hormones and drugs. Of course, practical issues, such as those discussed by Cornell-Bell et al. [8], Loew [6], Kurtz and Emmons [5], Terasaki and Jaffe [7], and Art and Goodman [2] (this volume), coupled with the loss of spherical aberration correction with depth into the specimen that occurs with currently available high-numerical aperture lenses, will need to be addressed.

The slit scanning confocal systems introduced by Meridian Instruments, Inc. (Okemos, MI) and Bio-Rad Microsciences Division (Cambridge, MA) promise to facilitate confocal imaging. The fluorescence image can be viewed directly by eye with these microscopes, and recorded by using a 35-mm camera with high-speed film or a sensitive video camera. Direct viewing provides three advantages. First, the time required to view specimens by confocal microscopy is dramatically reduced. The entire section can be scanned and three-dimensional information can be gathered quickly, just as it can in conventional epifluorescence microscopy, simply by observing through the eyepieces while moving the stage and focusing up and down through the tissue. The researcher does not have to wait for several scans to be averaged before a sharp image can be obtained for examination or documentation. Second, the human eye is still the best detector in terms of dynamic range and, although not as good as the human eye, photographic film is better than video cameras or photomultiplier tubes. Thus detail can be seen in bright and dim areas of the tissue at the same time. Third, for double-label work, simultaneous viewing of, for example, green and red fluorescence is possible without splitting the emitted light for detection by separate detectors. Maintaining the full intensity aids double-label work with weak signals. Another benefit is that with the eye or a sensitive color video camera, the wavelength (i.e., color) information can be utilized more effectively to ascertain true colocalization, for instance, structures stained with both fluorescein and rhodamine appear yellow. With separate monochromatic detectors, the inefficiency of barrier filters can make it difficult to distinguish double-fluorescence emission from bleed-through of a single strong emission.

## V. Appendix: Procedures for Immunohistochemical Preparation

### A. Fixing Tissue

We do not perform an initial fixation by vascular perfusion, but this step is desirable for tissues that cannot be rapidly dissected. Cacodylate is preferable to a phosphate buffer for fixation, because its greater buffering capacity can maintain a stable pH. We do not use cacodylate buffer with sodium borohydride, because the combination gives off an unpleasant odor. (See Gard [9], this volume, for phosphate-buffered saline formulation.) Glutaraldehyde fixative should be made with an 8% stock solution (EM grade; Polysciences). We have found that solutions of higher concentration can cause intense autofluorescence, possibly because of lower purity. After formaldehyde fixation, tissues should be stored in fixative for the best preservation, as formaldehyde fixation/stabilization partially reverses in buffer (see Section II,A). Step-by-step instructions are given in Table III.

**Table III**
**Procedure for Fixing Tissue**

**Formaldehyde**

1. Fix small pieces of tissue (1 mm thick—frog retinal thickness is about 300 $\mu$m) by immersion in 4% formaldehyde (granular paraformaldehyde; Electron Microscopy Sciences) in 0.1 $M$ sodium cacodylate, pH 7.3, at 4°C for at least 8 hr. Store tissue in this solution at 4°C
2. Rinse tissue in two changes, 10 min each, of 0.1 $M$ sodium cacodylate. Transfer to phosphate-buffered saline (PBS), pH 7.3, for 10 min. Rinsing will continue during sectioning. Tissue can be rinsed overnight

**Glutaraldehyde–Formaldehyde**

1. Fix in 0.1% glutaraldehyde–4% formaldehyde in 0.1 $M$ sodium cacodylate, pH 7.3, on ice for 30–35 min before transferring them to 4% formaldehyde at 4°C for an additional 4 hr or more
2. Rinse tissue in two changes, 10 min each, of 0.1 $M$ sodium cacodylate. Transfer to PBS, pH 7.3, for 10 min
3. Incubate tissues in three changes, 10 min each, of 0.1% sodium borohydride (Fisher Scientific), a reducing agent, in PBS, pH 8.0, at room temperature (Bacallao *et al.*, 1990). (Add the sodium borohydride to PBS, pH 8.0, just before use.) *Note:* The tissue will float, because bubbles collect on its surface
4. Rinse tissues in three changes, 10 min each, of PBS, pH 7.3. If tissue is still floating, hold at 4°C until it sinks. Tissue can be rinsed overnight

**Table IV**
**Procedure for Agarose Embedding and Vibratome Sectioning**

1. Transfer the tissue to a mold filled with buffer. Remove as much liquid as possible with a pasteur pipette without letting the tissue become dry. Cover the tissue with a 5% solution of low gelling temperature agarose (type XI; Sigma) in PBS, pH 7.3, cooled to just below 40°C. Position tissue as desired. The agarose will gel quickly
2. Once the agarose gels, transfer to 4°C until firm
3. Cut the agarose with a scalpel or razor blade into a small cube around each piece of tissue. Orientation of the tissue in the agarose block determines the sectioning plane, because the orientation of the block and the blade in the Vibratome is fixed
4. Blot the surface of the agarose to be glued and glue the cubes onto supports with cyanoacrylate (Krazy Glue)
5. Fill the boat of the Vibratome with chilled PBS
6. Break a double-edge razor blade in half and clean with ethanol to remove the protective oil coating. Mount the blade and specimen support
7. Set speed and amplitude, and section at desired thickness
8. Collect sections with a small spatula or camel's hair brush. Store sections in PBS at 4°C. As in Section V,A,1, for storage of formaldehyde-fixed tissue longer than a few days, transfer to formaldehyde fixative solution

## B. Agarose Embedding and Vibratome Sectioning

The agarose solution should be cooled to below 40°C, just above the gelling temperature (37°C), before use. An elevated agarose temperature is a major contributor to tissue autofluorescence. Small weighing boats can be used as molds. Be careful not to let tissue embedded in agarose dry out; always keep in a humid chamber. We use a Technical Products International Vibratome 1000 (Polysciences). We have found that low speed, intermediate amplitude settings, and a blade angle of 20–25° perform best for the retina with the sclera removed;

**Table V**
**Procedure for Labeling with Fluorochrome-Conjugated Probes**

**Antibodies**[a]
1. Incubate in normal goat serum (Sigma) diluted 1/50 for 1–2 hr, to block nonspecific staining seen with some antibodies
2. Rinse twice, 10 min each
3. Incubate in primary antibody solution for 18–24 hr (overnight). Dilutions must be determined empirically for each antibody; concentrations previously used for sections of embedded or frozen tissue are useful as a starting point
4. Rinse three times, 15 min each
5. Incubate in secondary antibody solution for 12–18 hr. We have not seen nonspecific labeling with these long incubation times. In our experience, fluorescein (FITC)- and rhodamine (RITC)-conjugated, affinity-purified goat anti-mouse or anti-rabbit antibodies (Cappel Research Products, Organon Teknika Corporation, Durham, NC) work well at a concentration of 50 $\mu$g/ml. Because the signal with Cy3-conjugated secondary antibodies (Jackson ImmunoResearch) is more intense, we suggest a concentration of 7.5 $\mu$g/ml or less
6. Rinse for at least 2–3 hr in several changes of buffer containing detergent before viewing; unbound fluorescent antibody produces an undesirable level of background fluorescence in thick sections
7. Store in plain PBS after the final rinse to minimize the length of time sections are exposed to detergent
8. Store in 4% formaldehyde if sections of formaldehyde-fixed tissue wil be kept for more than a few days

**Phalloidin**
1. Incubate sections in fluorochrome-conjugated phalloidin (Molecular Probes) at a concentration of 10 units/ml in PBS, pH 7.3, containing 0.1% Triton X-100 for 2 hr
2. Rinse for at least 1 hr with several changes of buffer before viewing
3. Store sections as described for indirect immunofluorescence

**Lectins**
1. Incubate sections in fluorochrome-conjugated lectin in standard antibody buffer with 0.1% Triton X-100 and any additional cations recommended by the supplier for 12–18 hr. We have used fluorescent WGA and concanavalin A (Vector Laboratories, Burlingame, CA) at 5 and 10 $\mu$g/ml, respectively
2. Rinse for at least 2–3 hr in several changes of buffer
3. Store sections as described for indirect immunofluorescence

[a] A standard incubation and rinse buffer consisting of 0.5% bovine serum albumin (BSA), detergent of choice (see Section II,C,1), and 0.01% sodium azide (preservative) in PBS, pH 7.3, can be used throughout.

**Table VI**
**Procedure for Mounting Sections**

1. Transfer one or two sections with a spatula to a drop of PBS on an 18 × 18 mm No. 1 coverglass. Remove buffer by blotting with a Kimwipe. For viewing without a coverglass, transfer a section to a small drop of melted agarose (<40°C) on a slide coated with a thin layer of dried-on agarose. Be careful not to let agarose cover the upper surface
2. Add a small drop of 100% glycerol containing 5% *n*-propyl gallate to the section(s)
3. Invert the coverglass onto a glass slide slowly to avoid forming bubbles
4. Affix the coverglass to the slide with nail polish, otherwise it may move when immersion lenses are used. It should be noted that nail polish is highly autofluorescent. *Caution:* Allow the nail polish to dry completely before viewing to avoid getting it on the objective lens

other tissues may require different settings. See Section II,B for a discussion of section thickness. Step-by-step instructions are given in Table IV.

## C. Labeling with Fluorochrome–Conjugated Probes

Sections are incubated free floating. Solutions need to be stirred to achieve even penetration of probes into tissue sections, as well as adequate rinsing. It is also desirable to use small volumes in order to conserve probes. We have found that sections can be immersed and adequately, yet gently, stirred on a rotator (50 rpm) in 400 $\mu$l of solution, using disposable microbeakers (10-ml size; Fisher Scientific), or in 200 $\mu$l or less, using 1.5-ml microcentrifuge tubes or small glass vials laying on their sides. We have found that penetration is better when microbeakers are used, even if microcentrifuge tubes are filled with 400 $\mu$l. All incubations and rinses should be performed at 4°C. In addition, sections should be kept in the dark during incubations in fluorescent probes and subsequent storage. We recommend centrifuging diluted antibody and lectin solutions at 14,000 rpm in a Beckman (Fullerton, CA) microfuge for 5 min to remove large aggregates. The purity and age of the detergent stock used can be critical to good penetration and labeling intensity. Detergents that have been purified for biological applications are recommended. We have found that Triton X-100 loses effectiveness and may become somewhat autofluorescent with time, and suggest storing at 4°C and replacing after several months. Step-by-step instructions are given in Table V.

## D. Mounting Sections

We mount sections no more than a few hours prior to viewing, as background fluorescence can increase after a prolonged period in mountant. Large coverglasses should not be used, because they flex when immersion objectives are used, interfering with *z*-series collection. Thick tissue slices do not appear to be deformed by mounting under a coverglass, probably because the surrounding agarose prevents compression. When oil immersion lenses are used, sections should be mounted directly on the coverglass (see Section III,B). Step-by-step instructions are given in Table VI.

## Acknowledgments

We would like to thank Mr. Robert Gill for expert technical assistance, Dr. Steven Fisher and Mr. Kevin Long for critical reading of the manuscript and valuable suggestions, Dr. William Stegeman at Jackson ImmunoResearch for generously providing CY3-conjugated secondary antibodies before they were commercially available, Dr. Jack Saari for the gift of the CRALBP antibody, Drs. Vijay Sarthy and Robert Molday for the gift of the rhodopsin antibodies, Dr. Michael Klymkowsky for the gift of the $\beta$-tubulin antibody, and Meridian Instruments, Inc. and Bio-Rad Microscience Division for demonstrations of their slit scanning confocal microscopes.

This research was supported by National Institutes of Health Grant EY-07191 to B. Matsumoto.

## References

Art, J. (1990). *In* "Handbook of Biological Confocal Microscopy" (J. B. Pawley, ed.), Rev. Ed., pp. 127–139. Plenum, New York.

Bacallao, R., Bomsel, M., Stelzer, E. H. K., and De Mey, J. (1990). *In* "Handbook of Biological Confocal Microscopy" (J. B. Pawley, ed.), Rev. Ed., pp. 197–205. Plenum, New York.

Barak, L. S., Yocum, R. R., Nothnagel, E. A., and Webb, W. W. (1980). *Proc. Natl. Acad. Sci. U.S.A.* **77,** 980–984.

Bok, D. (1985). *Invest. Ophthalmol. Visual Sci.* **26,** 1659–1694.

Brakenhoff, G. J., van Spronsen, E. A., van der Voort, H. T. M., and Nanninga, N. (1989). *Methods Cell Biol.* **30,** 379–398.

Bunt-Milam, A. H., and Saari, J. C. (1983). *J. Cell Biol.* **97,** 703–712.

Chen, H., Sedat, J. W., and Agard, D. A. (1990). *In* "Handbook of Biological Confocal Microscopy" (J. B. Pawley, ed.), Rev. Ed., pp. 141–150. Plenum, New York.

Cheng, P. C., and Summers, R. G. (1990). *In* "Handbook of Biological Confocal Microscopy" (J. B. Pawley, ed.), Rev. Ed., pp. 179–195. Plenum, New York.

Chu, D. T., and Klymkowsky, M. W. (1989). *Dev. Biol.* **136,** 104–117.

Eckert, B. S., and Snyder, J. A. (1978). *Proc. Natl. Acad. Sci. U.S.A.* **75,** 334–338.

Gaur, V. P., Adamus, G., Arendt, A., Eldred, W., Possin, D. E., McDowell, J. H., Hargrave, P. A., and Sarthy, P. V. (1988). *Vision Res.* **28,** 765–776.

Giloh, H., and Sedat, J. W. (1982). *Science* **217,** 1252–1255.

Goldenthal, K. L., Hedman, K., Chen, J. W., August, J. T., and Willingham, M. C. (1985). *J. Histochem. Cytochem.* **33,** 813–820.

Haugland, R. P. (1992). "Handbook of Fluorescent Probes and Research Chemicals." Molecular Probes, Inc., Eugene, Oregon.

Hicks, D., and Barnstable, C. J. (1987). *J. Histochem. Cytochem.* **35,** 1317–1328.

Hicks, D., and Molday, R. S. (1986). *Exp. Eye Res.* **42,** 55–71.

Inoué, S. (1986). "Video Microscopy." Plenum, New York.

Inoué, S. (1990). *In* "Handbook of Biological Confocal Microscopy" (J. B. Pawley, ed.), Rev. Ed., pp. 1–14. Plenum, New York.

Johnson, G. D., Davidson, R. S., McNamee, K. C., Russell, G., Goodwin, D., and Holborrow, E. J. (1982). *J. Immunol. Methods* **55,** 231–242.

Keller, H. E. (1990). *In* "Handbook of Biological Confocal Microscopy" (J. B. Pawley, ed.), Rev. Ed., pp. 77–86. Plenum, New York.

Larsson, L.-I. (1988). "Immunocytochemistry: Theory and Practice." CRC Press, Boca Raton, Florida.

Lis, H., and Sharon, N. (1986). *In* "The Lectins: Properties, Functions, and Applications in Biology and Medicine" (I. E. Liener, N. Sharon, and I. J. Goldstein, eds.), pp. 293–370. Academic Press, Orlando, Florida.

Mack, A. F., and Fernald, R. D. (1991). *J. Neurosci. Methods* **36,** 195–202.

Matsumoto, B., and Hale, I. L. (1993). *In* "Methods in Neuroscience" (P. C. Hargrave, ed.), Vol. 15, pp. 54–71. Academic Press, San Diego.

Matsumoto, B., Defoe, D. M., and Besharse, J. C. (1987). *Proc. R. Soc. London, Ser. B* **230,** 339–354.

Matus, A., Bernhardt, R., and Hugh-Jones, T. (1981). *Proc. Natl. Acad. Sci. U.S.A.* **78,** 3010–3014.

Nagle, B. W., Okamoto, C., Taggart, B., and Burnside, B. (1986). *Invest. Ophthalmol. Visual Sci.* **27,** 689–701.

Novikoff, P. M., Tulsiani, D. R. P., Touster, O., Yam, A., and Novikoff, A. B. (1983). *Proc. Natl. Acad. Sci. U.S.A.* **80,** 4364–4368.

Ohtsuki, I., Manzi, R. M., Palade, G. E., and Jamieson, J. D. (1978). *Biol. Cell.* **31,** 119–126.

O'Rourke, N. A., Dailey, M. E., Smith, S. J., and McConnell, S. K. (1992). *Science* **258,** 299–302.

Osborn, M., and Weber, K. (1982). *Methods Cell Biol.* **24,** 97–132.

Osborn, M., Webster, R. E., and Weber, K. (1978). *J. Cell Biol.* **77,** R27–R34.

Papermaster, D. S., Schneider, B. G., Zorn, M. A., and Kraihenbuhl, J. P. (1978). *J. Cell Biol.* **78,** 415–425.

Papermaster, D. S., Schneider, B. G., and Besharse, J. C. (1985). *Invest. Ophthalmol. Visual Sci.* **26,** 1386–1404.

Pease, D. C. (1962). *Anat. Rec.* **142,** 342.

Pickel, V. M. (1981). *In* "Neuroanatomical Tract Tracing Methods" (L. Heimer and M. J. Robards, eds.), pp. 483–509. Plenum, New York.

Priestley, J. V. (1984). *In* "Immunolabeling for Electron Microscopy" (J. M. Polak and I. M. Varndell, eds.), pp. 37–52. Elsevier, New York.

Priestley, J. V., and Cuello, A. C. (1983). *In* "Immunohistochemistry" (A. C. Cuello, ed.), pp. 273–321. Wiley, Chichester, England.

Priestley, J. V., Alvarez, F. J., and Averill, S. (1992). *In* "Electron Microscopic Immunocytochemistry: Principles and Practice" (J. M. Polak and J. V. Priestley, eds.), pp. 89–121. Oxford Univ. Press, Oxford, England.

Puchtler, H., and Meloan, S. N. (1985). *Histochemistry* **82,** 201–204.

Sabatini, D. D., Bensch, K., and Barnett, R. J. (1963). *J. Cell Biol.* **17,** 19–58.

Sale, W. S., Besharse, J. C., and Piperno, G. (1988). *Cell Motil. Cytoskeleton* **9,** 243–253.

Southwick, P. L., Ernst, L. A., Tauriello, E. W., Parker, S. R., Mujumdar, R. B., Mujumdar, S. R., Clever, H. A., and Waggoner, A. S. (1990). *Cytometry* **11,** 418–430.

Spencer, M., Detwiler, P. B., and Bunt-Milam, A. H. (1988). *Invest. Ophthalmol. Visual Sci.* **29,** 1012–1020.

Sternberger, L. A. (1979). "Immunocytochemistry," 2nd Ed. Wiley, New York.

Tsien, R. Y., and Waggoner, A. (1990). *In* "Handbook of Biological Confocal Microscopy" (J. B. Pawley, ed.), 2nd Ed., pp. 169–177. Plenum, New York.

van der Voort, H. T. M., and Brakenhoff, G. J. (1990). *J. Microsc. (Oxford)* **158,** 43–54.

Vaughan, D. K., and Fisher, S. K. (1987). *Exp. Eye Res.* **44,** 393–406.

Vaughan, D. K., Fisher, S. K., Bernstein, S. A., Hale, I. L., Lindberg, K. A., and Matsumoto, B. (1989). *J. Cell Biol.* **109,** 3053–3062.

Vaughn, J. E., Barber, R. P., Ribak, C. E., and Houser, C. R. (1981). *In* "Current Trends in Morphological Techniques" (J. E. Johnson, ed.), Vol. 3, pp. 33–70. CRC Press, Boca Raton, Florida.

Weber, K., Rathke, P. C., and Osborn, M. (1978). *Proc. Natl. Acad. Sci. U.S.A.* **75,** 1820–1824.

White, J. G., Amos, W. B., Durbin, R., and Fordham, M. (1990). *In* "Optical Microscopy for Biology" (B. Herman and K. Jacobson, eds.), pp. 1–18. Alan R. Liss, New York.

Willingham, M. C., and Yamada, S. S. (1979). *J. Histochem. Cytochem.* **27,** 947–960.

Wood, J. G., and Napier-Marshall, L. (1985). *Histochem. J.* **17,** 585–594.

Yu, H., Ernst, L., Wagner, M., and Waggoner, A. (1992). *Nucleic Acids Res.* **20,** 83–88.

# CHAPTER 12

## Using Confocal Laser Scanning Microscopy to Investigate the Organization and Development of Neuronal Projections Labeled with DiI

**Gary E. Baker★ and Benjamin E. Reese†**

★W. M. Keck Center for Integrative Neuroscience
Department of Physiology
University of California, San Francisco
San Francisco, California 94143

† Neuroscience Research Institute and
Department of Psychology
University of California, Santa Barbara
Santa Barbara, California 93106

Current address: Gary E. Baker, Department of Human Anatomy, University of Oxford, Oxford OX1 3QX, U.K.

## I. Introduction

The aim of this article is to provide a basic technical framework for any investigator pondering the use of carbocyanine dyes for the study of neuronal connectivity. The focus will be largely on using one such dye, 1,1'-dioctadecyl-3,3,3',3'-tetramethylindocarbocyanine perchlorate (DiI), in combination with confocal laser scanning microscopy, but it should become clear that the choice of whether to choose confocal microscopy to visualize the dye, or more conventional fluorescence microscopy, will ultimately be determined by the specific question being addressed. In addition, although the focus is on the use of DiI in conjunction with confocal laser scanning microscopy, there will be no attempt to expand on the relevant optical principles governing viewing conditions, as these are covered amply in Chapter 1 in this volume. The approach will be solely one that emphasizes the practical aspects of labeling and viewing the neural structures and pathways.

## II. Neuronal Tract Tracing Techniques

From an anatomical standpoint, the pioneering investigators of neural structure were primarily dependent for their analyses on natural and synthetic dyes, which vary in their affinity for various tissue constituents. The use of such dyes gives us an overall view of the way the nervous system is structured, but for neuronal tract tracing a significant addition to the technical armory came with the development of a different class of techniques that enable impregnation of various tissue features with heavy metal derivatives. The opaque deposit produced by these techniques creates a visual contrast between the impregnated cell and its background and therefore enhances viewing conditions for following the course of cellular processes. Tracing such stained structures through adjacent sections, however, can present problems when the tract of interest courses close to, or merges with, another tract. In addition, a projection involving relatively few neurons can be easily lost within the surrounding neuropil. It is therefore of enormous advantage to identify the neurons under investigation exclusively, and this has been a driving force for the subsequent development of modern neuroanatomical techniques.

The most commonly used approach relies on using some experimental "marker" of the relevant pathway. Initial studies capitalized on the reactive changes in neural tissue following lesions of the structures of interest, and consequently relied on the visualization of degenerating, rather than normal, neural profiles. The development of techniques that utilize both the normal physiological uptake mechanisms to introduce the tracer from the extracellular space into the nerve cells, and the axoplasmic transport system of those cells to distribute the tracer to and/or from their processes, represented a quantal leap in tracer technology. A review of the topic is not appropriate here but suffice it to say that a plethora of such techniques is available for investigating both the organizational principles of discrete neuronal populations and the morphological properties of the individual components. The method of choice depends on the specific issue to be addressed—some capitalize on the retrograde transport of the tracer to the cell body whereas others utilize the anterograde transport of the tracer distally into the processes of the cell (Heimer and RoBards, 1981; Heimer and Zaborszky, 1989; Mesulam, 1982). Thus, depending on the particular method or combination of methods used, the morphology and distribution of the labeled cells can be examined. The specificity of the labeled population is governed primarily by the extent of spread of the tracer when it is initially introduced, and the nature of the cellular labeling is determined by whether it is introduced into the region of the cell body or into the region of the axon terminals.

At this stage, one might legitimately ask why yet another tract tracing technique is being developed and what particular advantages are provided by the carbocyanine dyes such as DiI? Despite the wide variety of available techniques, there remain situations in which conventional tracing techniques are, in practical terms, difficult to implement. The relative inaccessibility of structures of interest and the need for substantial postoperative survival periods are two factors that can hinder conventional approaches. One specific example of this is the cochlea, which is surrounded by bone. Any attempt to label the primary afferent neurons at the peripheral level may require a degree of surgical intervention that is incompatible with any substantial postoperative survival. Another, more general example comes from developmental studies in placental mammals. Many of the developmental events in question occur *in utero* and again the problems of accessibility and survivability of the preparation arise. Furthermore, these are not the only difficulties to be surmounted. Conventional tracer substances are generally hydrophilic and as such will diffuse significantly within the extracellular space. Consequently, great care is needed in interpreting the results of experiments in which small populations of cells are presumed to be labeled exclusively. Thus this question of the specificity of labeling can be as much of a problem as that of accessibility or survivability of the preparation.

What properties does DiI possess that provide significant advantages in such situations? As there are detailed reviews of these elsewhere (Honig and Hume, 1986, 1989), only a brief summary will be given. First, DiI is essentially hydrophobic. When implanting or injecting it into the structure of interest there is little initial spread of the label. It is therefore possible to be more confident about specifically labeling small regions than is the case for conventional tracers. Second, it is intensely fluorescent under the appropriate illumination. This is critical for detecting extremely thin processes or lightly labeled somata. Third, it is lipophilic, and diffuses readily in membranes of fixed tissue. This property renders DiI suitable for labeling structures that are difficult to access *in vivo* (in particular, studies that would otherwise require intrauterine surgery), and for studying neuronal connections in the human brain in postmortem tissue. Thus, under conditions in which a difficult dissection is necessary to expose the site of labeling, or when great precision is required when introducing the label, or when only postmortem tissue is available, the use of DiI as the label in a fixed preparation offers significant advantages.

Of course, the hydrophobic nature of DiI and its intense fluorescence have made it of great use in conventional terms and there are a number of published reports describing the use of DiI as a tracer *in vivo* (see, e.g., Simon and O'Leary, 1990; Stuermer, 1988). But judging by the numerous investigations using DiI in previously fixed preparations, it is this particular facet of its properties that has paved the way in making possible investigations that were previously technically problematic, and on which the present article focuses.

## III. Investigating Neuronal Pathways in Fixed Specimens

### A. Specimen Fixation

Specimens are typically fixed with 4% paraformaldehyde in 0.1 $M$ sodium phosphate buffer at 20°C and at pH of 7.4 (see Appendix 1). The precise nature of the fixative and its temperature and pH do not appear to be critical determinants of labeling with DiI. However, the addition of glutaraldehyde to the fixative can result in undesirable levels of background fluorescence when ultimately viewing the preparation. The fixation protocol provided above is commonly used and is generally accepted to conserve the integrity of tissue structures.

To fix the tissues as rapidly as possible, transcardial perfusion with the fixative should be the method of choice. However, when studying the earliest developmental events, this approach is not always feasible because of the small size of the specimen. Under these circumstances, immersion fixation is the alternative, as is also the method required when studying valuable postmortem specimens.

Some investigators have developed their own "witches brew" of fixative for their individual purposes. Some, for example, include a low percentage (e.g., 1%) of dimethylsulfoxide (DMSO) in the fixative under the assumption that this assists the lateral diffusion of the implanted DiI. Although such additives may be beneficial, there is currently no empirical study of their effectiveness, and there may be other reasons for being cautious about their use, particularly in developmental studies. Neighboring axons within a developing neuronal projection are often closely apposed or in intimate contact. If the aim of a particular study is to label and trace a specific subpopulation of such a pathway, then it is essential to minimize the possibility that unrelated cells become labeled by axo-axonal transfer of DiI from cells that are initially labeled by a precisely located implant of the dye (see Section III,F). The effect of adding solvents or detergents to the fixative may, in fact, by their effects on the plasma membrane, increase the likelihood of such artifactual labeling.

Theoretically, the specimen can remain in the fixative *ad infinitum* prior to labeling, but generally the dye is implanted after a postfixation period of hours or days. Labeling can nevertheless be obtained from tissue fixed months or years previously.

## B. Dye Implant

Neural connections can be traced with DiI in either the anterograde or the retrograde direction. For instance, if the dye is administered at a point along a fiber, the dye will diffuse in each direction to reveal both the terminal arborization in the target and the soma and dendritic morphology of the cell of origin. Alternatively, the dye can be administered at the cell group of origin or in the target, and the labeled axons can subsequently be traced along their complete course.

DiI, along with other carbocyanine dyes, is obtained from Molecular Probes, Inc. (Eugene, OR). The dye can be administered either as small crystals, or as a solution obtained by dissolving the crystals in DMSO or in dimethylformamide to the desired concentration. Sonication aids the rate at which the dye goes into solution, which can then be applied to the required site by pressure injection from a micropipette (Bovolenta and Dodd, 1990; Simon and O'Leary, 1991). When the aim is to label as many of the cells as possible another approach is to soak a piece of absorbable gelatin (e.g., Gelfoam; Upjohn, Kalamazoo, MI) in a solution of DiI and insert this into a natural or dissected cavity (e.g., into the posterior chamber of the eye (Erzurumlu *et al.*, 1990). Crystals of DiI can be applied from the tip of an insect pin or micropipette with the aid of an operating or dissecting microscope, the goal being to place the crystal adjacent to the severed membranes. Once implanted, the tissue is placed in a bath of the same fixative and stored in the dark at room temperature, although labeling has been obtained when stored at 4°C (Godement *et al.*, 1987).

Figure 1a shows an example of small crystals of DiI implanted in the retina of a fetal ferret. The anterior chamber and lens were first removed, and the crystals were then carefully inserted at the desired location. The implant site is small relative to the total retinal area, and anterogradely labeled axons (Fig. 1a), as well as growth cones (Fig. 1b), can be seen to course across the retinal surface to the optic disk.

In the case of dye application to central structures, gross dissection of the preparation is often necessary. Although this is unavoidable in some cases, one practical disadvantage is that the tissue is prone to mechanical distortions during the process of dissection. This can disrupt the structural integrity of the tissues and especially of developing axons, which at this stage are of fine caliber. An alternative strategy, and one we find particularly useful when dealing with fetal tissue, is to embed the entire specimen in a gelatin–albumen matrix and then to cut through the specimen with a Vibratome (model 1000; Technical Products International, Polysciences, Warrington, PA) until the desired site for applying the dye is exposed. The entire head of the fetus is embedded in the gelatin–

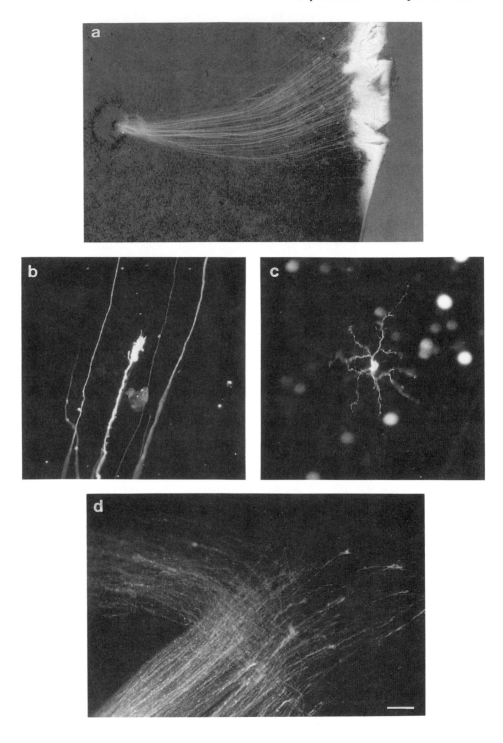

albumen (Appendix 2) and sections are cut through the specimen until the desired level is reached. If necessary, the appropriate location can be monitored each time a section is cut by using a dye such as methylene blue to stain the surface of the section. This provides rapid feedback concerning the gross structure of the exposed surface of the brain. Alternatively, the cut surface of the brain can also be stained with the dye; this allows the desired structure to be identified directly and allows the crystals of dye to be inserted precisely. Figure 2 shows an example of retrograde labeling within the optic chiasm of a fetal ferret in which crystals of DiI had been inserted into the optic tract by this approach. The preparation has retrogradely labeled the ipsilateral and contralateral retinofugal fibers of each optic nerve projecting into the implanted tract, and has additionally labeled the supraoptic fibers of the opposite hemisphere.

This strategy for exposing the desired implant site has several advantages beyond that of avoiding distortion of the tissue in preparation for the dye implant. It ensures accuracy and precision of the implant, and allows for consistency of dye placement. It also frequently enables direct observation of the diffusion "front" of the dye *in situ*. In the instance described above, the process of sectioning the brain horizontally provides a direct view of a portion of the optic chiasm via the third ventricle, through which the dye can be seen, either directly, with a dissecting microscope, or via conventional fluorescence microscopy with a long working distance objective. One can therefore obtain an indication that the pathway of interest is labeled, and avoid premature harvesting of the tissue (see Section III,C).

Cutting sections with a Vibratome is relatively simple at early stages, prior to calcification of the cranium, but at later stages as the skull becomes harder it becomes necessary to remove it with care prior to embedding and cutting. But one must remove only enough to allow sectioning of the appropriate region. Of course, the entire brain can be removed prior to being prepared for dye implant. If, however, the study is focused on a cranial nerve that courses through bone, the problem may be more complicated. In such situations the skull can be decalcified either before or after implanting the dye. Many decalcifying agents are incompatible with the carbocyanine dyes, even if the decalcification is done

---

**Fig. 1** (a) Combined fluorescent–bright-field image of a retinal flat mount from a ferret fetus on day 36 of gestation. DiI-labeled axons course from the site of the implant, along the extreme temporal retinal margin, centrally to exit the eye via the optic disk. (b) Fluorescent image taken from the retina shown in (a). Individual axons, as well as the detailed morphology of growth cones, can readily be observed in such DiI-labeled fetal retinas. (c) The morphology of individual retinal ganglion cells can also be imaged following such retinal implants, particularly with large implants and long postimplantation times, as in this fetal ferret retina on day 39 of gestation, viewed from the vitreal surface. A large temporal retinal implant had been made 4 months prior to harvesting the tissue. (d) Fluorescent image taken from a chiasmal whole mount of the ferret that had received the temporal retinal implant in (a). Growth cones pass through the chiasmatic midline to enter the contralateral optic tract. Bar in (d) = 200 $\mu$m for (a); 20 $\mu$m for (b); 40 $\mu$m for (c); and 80 $\mu$m for (d).

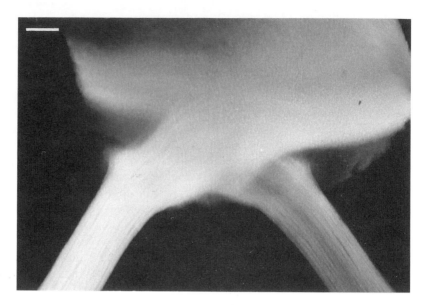

**Fig. 2** Fluorescent image of a chiasmal whole mount from a ferret fetus on day 36 of gestation, viewed from the ventral surface. The DiI was placed in the right optic tract, and has subsequently labeled the contralateral (lower left) and ipsilateral (lower right) optic nerves, and the contralateral supraoptic commissures (upper left). Notice the fascicular nature of the fiber labeling in the optic nerves. Bar = 200 $\mu$m.

in advance (Bartheld *et al.*, 1990), so a careful choice of agent is required. Ethylenediaminetetraacetate disodium salt (EDTA) as such an agent is reported to maintain the label intact, even if the label has been administered in advance (Bartheld *et al.*, 1990).

## C. Tissue Harvesting

Before preparing the implanted specimen for microscopic observation it is important to make as accurate a judgment as possible concerning the complete labeling of the relevant pathway. In some instances, as described above for the retinofugal pathway, the strategy of sectioning and removing much of the overlying tissue allows one to observe portions of the subsequently labeled pathway. Because it is not always possible to directly observe the extent of diffusion along the pathway of interest, the optimum period for adequte postimplant diffusion must be determined empirically. A number of factors need to be considered in making this determination. First, the absolute length of the pathway is of primary importance. The longer the neurons that need to be labeled, the longer the time required for the dye to diffuse sufficiently. Second, rates of diffusion vary with the maturity of the tissue. Six to 7 weeks is sufficient to label a distance of about 1 cm in embryonic neuronal projections (Colello and Guillery, 1990), whereas 6 months may be required to label such distances in fully mature tissue (Mufson *et al.*, 1990). For distances greater than this, substantially longer times may be necessary for adequate diffusion of the DiI (see Godement *et al.*, 1987, for a discussion of the diffusion kinetics of DiI). Third, the time required will also depend on the desired quality of the labeling. If the precise details of the dendritic geometry of retrogradely labled cells are being sought, then it will take longer for the dye to diffuse throughout the dendrites in adequate quantity. A fourth factor may relate to whether the axons are myelinated, because of the lipophilic nature of the dye. Whatever the reason, there are as yet few reports of the use of DiI in adult tissue despite the initial excitement about its potential advantages for such material (Burkhalter and Bernardo, 1989; Friedman *et al.*, 1991; Mufson *et al.*, 1990).

Because of the relatively long periods often necessary to allow for diffusion of DiI, it was inevitable that strategies would be forthcoming that aim to shorten the required delay between dye implant and tissue harvesting. One "informal" protocol to this end has been to store the tissue at 37°C or greater, the higher storage temperature resulting in shorter diffusion times (Bartheld *et al.*, 1990; Snider and Palavali, 1990). Another has been to store the tissue in fixative at an alkaline pH of between 8 and 9. We have not used either of these approaches because the protocol outlined above provides relatively consistent labeling. Engineering of the dyes to increase their fluidity within the plasma membrane may speed up the rate of diffusion, as has been claimed for the molecular modifications of the carbocyanine dyes, Fast DiI and Fast DiO (Molecular Probes Inc., Eugene, OR).

## D. Preparing Tissue for Microscopy

Following the appropriate diffusion period, the tissue is typically cut into sections for microscopic viewing of the labeled components. The tissue should remain moist and is consequently sectioned with a Vibratome, whereby the tissue can be maintained and cut in a bath of the appropriate buffer. Yet there are some preparations in which sectioning of the tissue is not necessary, as in the case of retinal flat mounts (e.g., Fig. 1a–c), or whole mounts of the optic chiasm (e.g., Figs. 1d and 2), or whole mounts of the lateral diencephalon and dorsal midbrain (Erzurumlu *et al.*, 1990; Godement *et al,.* 1987).

Because the ideal fixation for studies using the carbocyanine dyes does not provide the specimen with much rigidity, cutting the brain with a Vibratome can often lead to sections of varying thickness. Embedding the specimen in the gelatin–albumen matrix mentioned above provides sufficient stability for sections of constant thickness, but this is generally true only for sections at least 100 $\mu$m in thickness. The use of confocal laser scanning microscopy overcomes the drawbacks that such thick tissue sections traditionally present to the microscopist (see Section III,E).

If the specimen is initially embedded for the purpose of exposing the site for implanting the dye, the adhesion between the tissue surface and this original embedding medium decreases significantly during the relatively long period in fixative following implantation. It is therefore generally wise to remove the original embedding medium and re-embed in order to restore the necessary rigidity to the tissue block for sectioning. The re-embedding may be additionally useful for providing the appropriate plane of section of the specimen, which may differ from the plane employed to expose the site for implantation.

When the sections are positioned on slides they are coverslipped immediately to avoid any dehydration of the tissue. Organic solvent-based mounting media are not recommended because DiI is soluble in them, but a variety of alternative mountants are available that avoid this problem. We find that mounting the sections in the fixative itself or in phosphate buffer is sufficient. Alternatively, some investigators use glycerol either on its own or with additives such as phenylenediamine (Johnson *et al.*, 1982), which reduce the rate of fading of the fluorescence label in the specimen.

This protocol for mounting sections has the disadvantage that the sections are not adherent to the slide and movement of the sections is possible. This is an unacceptable condition for accurate data collection during confocal microscopy when lengthy viewing times are often the rule and when even the slightest movement will degrade the image. Likewise, it is an equally undesirable situation during conventional fluorescence photomicroscopy when relatively long exposure times are necessary. To minimize such movement of the sections, only enough mounting solution is applied to the slide to coat the area occupied by a coverslip; the coverslip is then secured in place by affixing it to the slide with a rapidly drying substance such as nail varnish.

## E. Microscopy

DiI is viewed with filter sets appropriate for observing rhodamine fluorescence. When preparing to view labeled specimens, using either confocal laser scanning microscopy or conventional epifluorescence, we routinely ensure that the conditions for data storage are available immediately. Our experience, especially when viewing heavily labeled populations of cells or fibers, is that the fluorescent image can deteriorate significantly during irradiation and thus it is advisable to record the data right away.

Because of the high intensity of the fluorescing label, conventional fluorescence microscopic images can suffer from substantial out-of-focus "blur," a particular problem when whole-mount preparations or thick sections are being viewed. The confocal laser scanning microscope, by virtue of its ability to image the fluorescent label in only a single plane of focus, is ideally suited to alleviate this problem.

Figure 3 shows confocal images of DiI-labeled axons in both optic nerves of a fetal ferret in which one optic tract had been implanted with the dye approximately 6 weeks earlier (G. E. Baker and R. J. Colello, unpublished observations). The images obtained from these sections by conventional epi-

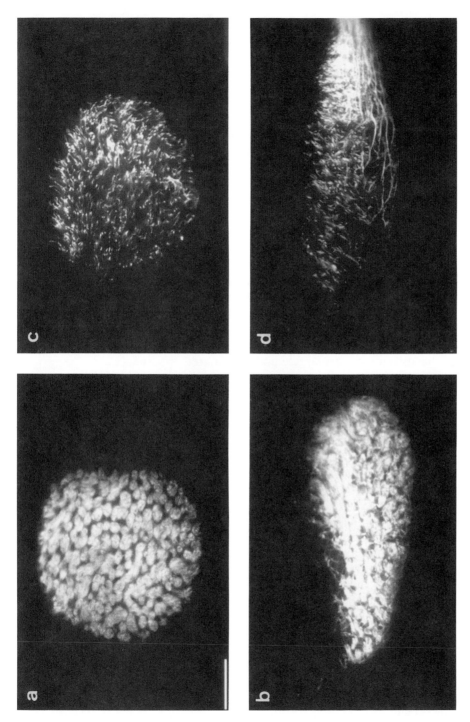

**Fig. 3** Confocal images of sections through the two optic nerves of a fetal ferret on day 28 of gestation. DiI had been implanted into one optic tract, as in Fig. 2, labeling the populations of the crossed and uncrossed optic axons. The optic nerves were sectioned at 100 μm, and the sections were subsequently "optodigitally microtomized," using the laser-scanning microscope. Despite the thickness of the histological preparations and the resultant out-of-focus blur produced by signal in other focal planes, the confocal laser-scanning microscope yields a clear image of a single focal plane, much as if a thin section had been cut and analyzed. (a and b) The optic nerve contralateral to the implanted optic tract. (c and d) The optic nerve ipsilateral to the implanted tract. (a) and (c) come from distal segments of the optic nerves, whereas (b) and (d) come from prechiasmatic segments of the optic nerves. Bar = 50 μm.

fluorescence optics were uninterpretable. As discussed above, because of the thickness of the Vibratomed sections and because of the high fluorescence intensity of the labeled axons, a great deal of out-of-focus blurring is present, prohibiting the detection of individual, punctate fibers cut transversely. As is evident from the clarity of the images in Fig. 3 (see also Fig. 5), the "optodigital microtomy" of the thick sections, using confocal laser scanning microscopy, results in a much clearer demonstration of the organization of the axons at different levels of the developing optic nerve.

Figures 3c and d shows the distribution of the uncrossed optic axons in the nerve at this early developmental age. Even though there are a great number of axons labeled, many individual profiles can be identified, some of which can be observed coursing in the plane of the section (Fig. 3d). Particularly when other fluorescent profiles are in the field of view, the details of individual axons are better resolved with the confocal microscope (see also Colello and Guillery, 1990). Figures 3a and b demonstrates the organization of the crossed optic axons. As is clear from the micrographs, there is substantially more label in these sections due to the primarily crossed retinofugal projection of ferrets, making resolution of individual profiles more difficult. But the labeled axons are arranged into small bundles or fascicles surrounded by unlabeled interfascicular spaces, and the definition of these fascicles is clear. Without confocal imaging, conventional epifluorescent viewing would not resolve these fascicles so well, giving the appearance of a largely undifferentiated optic nerve.

The optodigital microtomy of such thick sections provided by the confocal microscope can be of enormous benefit, particularly when the issue of fiber order in the pathway is of interest (see also Fig. 5). There are of course other solutions that confer additional advantages, such as the long-term stability of the histological preparation and compatibility with electron microscopy. DiI is photooxidized by ultraviolet irradiation in the presence of diaminobenzidine (DAB; Sigma, St. Louis, MO). As with other fluorescent labels, the resultant stable reaction product can be examined under bright-field illumination (Bartheld et al., 1990; Bhide and Frost, 1991; Catalano et al., 1991; Sandell and Masland, 1988). Unlike the fluorescent label, the photoconverted label is permanent and electron opaque and, provided it is embedded appropriately in resin, can allow one to examine the label in 1-$\mu$m sections when convenient or to determine the fine structural features of the labeled profiles in ultrathin sections with the electron microscope. Figure 4 shows such photoconverted axonal profiles in the optic fiber layer of a postnatal ferret in which the axons had been initially labeled anterogradely with DiI from the retinal periphery, as in Fig. 1a. The DiI-labeled retina was subsequently incubated in 0.2% DAB in Tris buffer (Appendix 3) while the relevant region of fluorescent labeling was illuminated for 2 hr with a ×10 objective. The region containing the reaction product was subsequently osmicated, dehydrated, and embedded in Epon/Araldite resin as described elsewhere (Baker, 1990), and 1-$\mu$m sections were cut with an ultramicrotome and counterstained with methylene blue and Azur II. The punctate nature of the resultant label is readily localized within the bundles of the de-

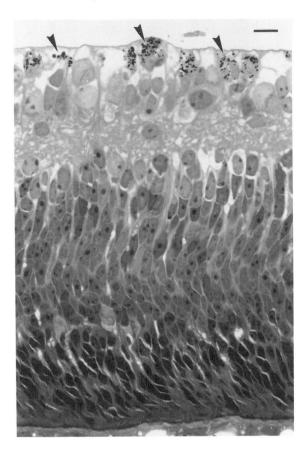

**Fig. 4**  Bright-field image from a 1-$\mu$m thick transverse section through the retina of a ferret on postnatal day 6. In this case, the fixed retina was dissected and flattened first, after which a crystal of DiI was implanted. The consequent labeling was similar to that in Fig. 1a. The fluorescent label in the optic axons was subsequently photoconverted, and a piece of retina containing the photoconverted label was dissected from the whole mount and then osmicated, dehydrated, and embedded in resin. Notice the discrete axonal labeling (some of which is indicated by arrowheads) in the fascicles of the optic nerve fiber layer along the vitreal margin of the retina. Bar = 10 $\mu$m.

veloping fiber layer, and the other tissue components are apparent by virtue of the counterstain. The tissue is also in a condition for examination with electron microscopy, should this be required. This protocol is, however, substantially more time consuming; as fluorescent labels become available for other tissue components, the confocal image may provide a faster route for questions other than those pertaining to ultrastructure. Each approach confers different advantages and, in some instances, both may complement the same study (see, e.g., Finger and Böttger, 1990).

A distinct advantage of the confocal microscope is that $z$-axis reconstructions of labeled profiles are readily produced, as in Fig. 5. Figure 5a is a photomicrograph,

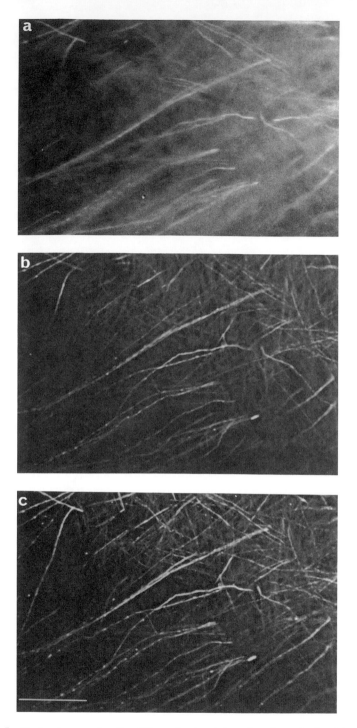

**Fig. 5** Photomicrographs of a 100-μm horizontal section through the chiasmatic region of a 19-day-old cat, showing the course of axons retrogradely labeled by an implant of DiI (beyond the right side of the micrograph). (a) Conventional epifluorescence image. (b) Confocal image of the

using conventional epifluorescence optics, of labeled axons coursing through a 100-$\mu$m thick horizontal section of the optic chiasm of a cat. The specimen had been fixed and a block of tissue containing the chiasmatic region had been dissected out. DiI was implanted in one optic tract (beyond the right border of Fig. 5a) to retrogradely label optic axons coursing from the ipsilateral optic nerve (i.e., from the left of Fig. 5a). Although many of the optic axons are clearly labeled, substantial out-of-focus blur prohibits identification of many profiles and their trajectories, especially near the implant site. By sampling only a single focal plane in the tissue, the optodigital microtomy of the confocal microscope clearly reveals the axonal profiles in Fig. 5b. Furthermore, by combining a series of such confocal images taken at different depths through the tissue, a composite reconstruction of the labeled profiles can be produced, free of the blurring typical of conventional epifluorescence optics. Morphological detail and trajectories of the labeled profiles, especially those of finer caliber, are readily observed in such reconstructions.

## F. Transcellular Labeling: Artifact or Intimacy?

Occasionally, we and others have obtained patterns of labeling with carbocyanine dyes that are clearly transcellular (Godement *et al.*, 1987; Johnson and Casagrande, 1991; Johnson *et al.*, 1990). Several plausible explanations can be advanced for the occurrence of such labeling and the possible reasons deserve mention. As briefly discussed, the ultrastructural appearance of developing axons, particularly growth cones, often indicates close contact with neighboring axons or glia. Neuronal tract tracing with DiI in fixed material relies on the lateral diffusion of the dye along the axonal membranes. Regions of axons that are in close apposition with other axons are therefore potential sites for diffusion of the label from one axon to another. Transcellular labeling has indeed been shown to occur from optic axons to neuroepithelial cells in the chiasmatic region of the embryonic mouse after initial labeling within the retina (Godement *et al.*, 1987; Johnson and Casagrande, 1991).

The likelihood of axoaxonal transfer of DiI would be increased in specimens in which there is poor tissue fixation. The membranes of adjacent axons in poorly fixed developing pathways appear at the electron microscopic level to be "fused" with each other. The problem is undoubtedly exacerbated when extraordinarily long diffusion periods and large implants are employed. For instance, large implants of DiI into fetal retina, coupled with 4-month diffusion periods, can label ganglion cells in both the opposite retina and elsewhere across the same retinal surface (Fig. 1c). Although many of the former cells may reflect

---

same specimen at a similar plane of focus. (c) $z$-axis reconstruction of the same field, from a series of 25 confocal images taken at 3.5-$\mu$m increments through the section. Both (b) and (c) have been contrast enhanced. Bar = 100 $\mu$m.

a true transient retinoretinal pathway (see, e.g., Bunt and Lund, 1981), the latter cells are labeled not by direct transretinal profiles extending to the implant site but rather by their axons from the optic disk. Likewise, a transient uncrossed retinofugal projection from the nasal retina has been observed, during early mammalian development, with DiI (Colello and Guillery, 1990; Godement *et al.*, 1987; Lia, 1991); yet with 4-month diffusion periods and large implants (albeit restricted to one side of the brain), substantially greater numbers of labeled neurons in the retina ipsilateral to the implant can be obtained, presumably via axoaxonal transfer of the dye within the developing optic chiasm. In view of these factors, it may be best to employ only those specimens in which there is good tissue fixation, and to ensure that the time allowed for diffusion of the label is kept to the minimum necessary.

Although the potential for transcellular labeling can be viewed as a feature that limits the interpretability of the data obtained using DiI, it is also a feature that when observed in tissue with good fixation may indicate truly intimate (e.g., tight junctions), and possibly functional, relationships between the cells exhibiting the label (see, e.g., Vaney, 1991). If such transcellular labeling occurs along only discrete portions of the pathway, as with the transcellular labeling of profiles in the developing chiasm, it may be indicative of interactions between growing axons and cells that guide or direct that growth, particularly in regions where directional decisions are made (Godement *et al.*, 1987).

A further example comes from intriguing studies of the innervation of barbel taste buds in the catfish, *Ictalurus punctatus* (Finger and Böttger, 1990). DiI was applied, in fixed preparations, to the peripheral nerve innervating taste bud receptors. In addition to labeling the innervating fibers, DiI was subsequently found to label cells within the taste buds themselves; most of these labeled cells were presumed to be receptor cells, but in a few cases basal cells within the taste bud complex were also labeled. These cells do not possess processes that extend to the site of the implant; thus this strongly supports the view that the labeled cells received the label by transcellular transfer, suggestive of a special relationship between these cells and the primary afferents (Finger and Böttger, 1990).

## G. Other Applications

Although most reports of the use of DiI for neuronal tract tracing in previously fixed tissue have been restricted to studies of developing pathways, its application to the mature nervous system will undoubtedly prove useful. One reason for the relative lack of its use to date may be that other tracers using axoplasmic transport as their basis require such short intervals despite the length of mature pathways. However, some success has been reported. The study of the innervation of the barbel taste bud in catfish cited above is one example. In addition, it has been used to label retinal ganglion cells after implants at the optic disk in mice (Godement *et al.*, 1987); it has been used to demonstrate the topography of spiral ganglion cell projections in hamsters (Collinge and Schweitzer, 1991); and it has been used to label the retinohypothalamic pathway and to reveal the intrinsic circuitry of hippocampal and cerebral cortices of postmortem tissue from humans (Burkhalter and Bernardo, 1989; Friedman *et al.*, 1991; Mufson *et al.*, 1990). It would seem that the prospects for successful labeling in mature tissue are promising, at least for studies of intrinsic circuitry if not for demonstrating long neuronal pathways.

There are increasing numbers of reports of the use of the carbocyanine dyes, and especially DiI, for *in vivo* preparations. Used in this manner, the nature of the staining and the time required for labeling pathways are consistent with active axonal transport mechanisms (Godement *et al.*, 1987). One advantage of using DiI in such situations is that its lipophilic/hydrophobic properties are ideal for precise restriction of the tracer when initially applied. For example, this feature has been applied to the study of the topography of developing retinal ganglion cell projections, in which precisely restricted injections of the dye are placed at various retinal loci, a requirement that has previously been difficult to achieve (Simon and O'Leary, 1990, 1991). When used as a conventional tracer (i.e., transported by the physiological mechanisms of the cell), it is also of use for labeling neuronal pathways in adult animals (Vidal-Sanz *et al.*, 1988).

Another advantage of DiI when used *in vivo* is that the fluorescent properties persist over long postinjection survival periods. This finding, initially observed in cell culture (Honig and Hume, 1986), has also been demonstrated in retrogradely labeled neurons (Vidal-Sanz *et al.*, 1988). This aspect of the label has presented the exciting opportunity for directly observing the development of neuronal systems *in vivo*. The initial study in this vein used time-lapse video microscopy to observe the behavior of labeled growing optic axons as they course along the optic tract of *Xenopus* and enter the optic tectum (Harris *et al.*, 1987), and others have since followed this approach in studies of various systems (Godement and Mason, 1990; Halloran and Kalil, 1991; Myers and Bastiani, 1991; Sretavan, 1990). This strategy has also been extended by incorporating confocal laser scanning microscopy to definitively resolve the three-dimensional structure of the labeled processes. In an elegant study of the developing retinotectal projection of *Xenopus laevis*, DiI-labeled retinotectal arbors were repeatedly observed *in vivo* over a period of days in order to record their changing branching patterns (O'Rourke and Fraser, 1990). Migrating neuroblasts in developing cortical explants have similarly been followed by using this combination of DiI, confocal microscopy, and time-lapse video imaging (O'Rourke *et al.*, 1991).

## H. Future Developments

The various examples of the application of DiI that we have described should provide some sense of how the dye can be used and its potential for examining neuronal morphology and for tract tracing in the future. Like all methodological innovations, many features of a technique that are initially regarded as dogma may eventually be replaced or at least improved under certain circumstances. Further, as investigators attempt to widen its application, the technique will be found to be, or eventually made to be, compatible with others, such as immuno-cytochemistry (Elberger and Honig, 1990).

The use of the confocal laser scanning microscope in studies employing the carbocyanine dyes is more than a matter of taste. Although all studies using such dyes may not find a need for confocal microscopy, it may confer genuine advantages in others. In some circumstances, the benefit is derived solely from the improved resolution of the fluorescent image (e.g., Figs. 3 and 5b); in others, its utility is due to the rapid reconstruction of images of structures that vary in depth (e.g., Fig. 5c). The examples we have provided in which confocal laser scanning microscopy has been a beneficial tool for investigating neuronal projections are meant to convey the exciting potential of the approach. The ultimate uses to which it will be put is limited only by the ingenuity of the investigator.

# IV. Appendices

## Appendix 1: Fixative

Paraformaldehyde (4%) in 0.1 $M$ sodium phosphate buffer (ph 7.4): 500 ml of distilled water, 500 ml of stock 0.2 $M$ sodium phosphate buffer, 40 g of paraformaldehyde, 1 $N$ sodium hydroxide

Add the paraformaldehyde to the distilled water, and stir while heating to approximately 60°C. After the majority of the paraformaldehyde has dissolved, slowly add the sodium hydroxide drop by drop until the solution becomes transparent. This usually requires about 15 to 20 drops of the sodium hydroxide to clear the otherwise cloudy solution. Add the sodium phosphate buffer and cool the solution to room temperature. Filter the solution, adjust the pH as necessary and store at 4°C.

Stock 0.2 $M$ sodium phosphate buffer (pH 7.4): 6.9 g of $NaH_2PO_4 \cdot H_2O$ (mono-basic, monohydrate), 28.4 g of $Na_2HPO_4$ (dibasic, anhydrous), 1250 ml of distilled water

Dissolve the disodium hydrogen orthophosphate in 1000 ml of distilled water, and the sodium dihydrogen orthophosphate in 250 ml of distilled water. Add together and filter.

## Appendix 2: Embedding Medium

Gelatin–albumen solution: 45 g of egg albumen, 0.75 g of gelatin powder, 150 ml of 0.1 $M$ sodium phosphate buffer (pH 7.4)

Slowly stir the egg albumen into 100 ml of the buffer and continue stirring the solution for approximately 1 hr to ensure that the albumen dissolves. Stir the gelatin powder into the remaining 50 ml of buffer and heat until the gelatin dissolves. Allow this solution to cool to room temperature and then stir it into the albumen solution. Continue stirring for a further 10 min to ensure thorough mixing of the two solutions. Store at 4°C.

To use, place the embedding container (e.g., a plastic weighing dish) on a bed of ice. Add 0.6 ml of 25% glutaraldehyde to 15 ml of the gelatin–albumen solution in the embedding boat and mix thoroughly for approximately 5 sec. Position the specimen in the solution in the appropriate orientation and allow the block to harden for at least 1 hr on ice, or at 4°C. Remove the hardened block from the embedding boat, trim to the appropriate size with a razor blade, and the block is ready for sectioning.

## Appendix 3: Photoconversion Solution

Diaminobenzidine (0.2%) in 0.1 $M$ Tris buffer (pH 8.2): 20 mg of 3,3′-diaminobenzidine tetrahydrochloride (DAB), 10 ml 0.1 $M$ stock Tris buffer

Dissolve the DAB in Tris buffer. Immerse the tissue in the DAB solution on a recessed slide, or place a few drops of the solution directly on the tissue section. Irradiate with rhodamine filter block for approximately 2 hr, until the fluorescent label has been photooxidized into a dark brown reaction product, changing the DAB solution every 10–20 min. Rinse in buffer and then mount, dehydrate, clear, and coverslip, or embed in resin for subsequent ultramicrotomy.

Stock 0.1 $M$ Tris buffer (pH 8.2): 9.69 g of Tris base (Sigma), 3.15 g of Tris hydrochloride (Sigma), 1000 ml of distilled water

Dissolve the Tris base in 800 ml of distilled water, and the Tris hydrochloride in 200 ml of distilled water. Add together and filter.

## Acknowledgments

The authors' research has been supported by grants from the Wellcome Trust and from the National Institutes of Health. G.E.B. was a Kleberg Foundation Fellow. The authors gratefully acknowledge the contributions of R. J. Colello in developing some of the technical strategies described herein, and the assistance of Bob Fariss and Brian Matsumoto.

## References

Baker, G. E. (1990). *Eur. J. Neurosci.* **2**, 24–33.
Bartheld, C. S. V., Cunningham, D. E., and Rubel, E. W. (1990). *J. Histochem. Cytochem.* **38**, 725–733.
Bhide, P. G., and Frost, D. O. (1991). *J. Neurosci.* **11**, 485–504.

Bovolenta, P., and Dodd, J. (1990). *Development* **109,** 435–447.

Bunt, S. M., and Lund, R. D. (1981). *Brain Res.* **211,** 399–404.

Burkhalter, A., and Bernardo, K. L. (1989). *Proc. Natl. Acad. Sci. U.S.A.* **86,** 1071–1075.

Catalano, S. M., Robertson, R. T., and Killackey, H. P. (1991). *Proc. Natl. Acad. Sci. U.S.A.* **88,** 2999–3003.

Colello, R. J., and Guillery, R. W. (1990). *Development* **108,** 515–523.

Collinge, C., and Schweitzer, L. (1991). *Hearing Res.* **53,** 159–172.

Elberger, A. J., and Honig, M. G. (1990). *J. Histochem. Cytochem.* **38,** 735–739.

Erzurumlu, R., Jhaveri, S., and Schneider, G. E. (1990). *J. Neurosci. Methods* **33,** 81–89.

Finger, T. E., and Böttger, B. (1990). *J. Comp. Neurol.* **302,** 884–892.

Friedman, D. I., Johnson, J. K., Chorsky, R. L., and Stopa, E. G. (1991). *Brain Res.* **560,** 297–302.

Godement, P., and Mason, C. A. (1990). *Soc. Neurosci. Abstr.* **16,** 1125.

Godement, P., Vanselow, J., Thanos, S., and Bonhoeffer, F. (1987). *Development* **101,** 697–713.

Halloran, M. C., and Kalil, K. (1991). *Soc. Neurosci. Abstr.* **17,** 532.

Harris, W. A., Holt, C. E., and Bonhoeffer, F. (1987). *Development* **101,** 123–133.

Heimer, L., and RoBards, M. T. (1981). "Neuroanatomical Tract-Tracing Methods." Plenum, New York.

Heimer, L., and Zaborszky, L. (1989). "Neuroanatomical Tract-Tracing Methods 2: Recent Progress." Plenum, New York.

Honig, M. G., and Hume, R. I. (1986). *J. Cell Biol.* **103,** 171–187.

Honig, M. G., and Hume, R. I. (1989). *TINS* **12,** 333–341.

Johnson, G. D., Davidson, R. S., McNamee, K. C., Russell, G., Goodwin, D., and Holborrow, E. J. (1982). *J. Immunol. Methods* **55,** 231–242.

Johnson, J. K., and Casagrande, V. A. (1991). *Soc. Neurosci. Abstr.* **17,** 1133.

Johnson, J. K., Jinks, R. N., and Chamberlain, S. C. (1990). *Soc. Neurosci. Abstr.* **16,** 53.

Lia, B. (1991). *Soc. Neurosci. Abstr.* **17,** 1133.

Mesulam, M.-M. (1982). "Tracing Neural Connections with Horseradish Peroxidase," IBRO Handbook Series: Methods in the Neurosciences. Wiley, Chichester, England.

Mufson, E. J., Brady, D. R., and Kordower, J. H. (1990). *Neurobiol. Aging* **11,** 649–653.

Myers, P. Z., and Bastiani, M. J. (1991). *Soc. Neurosci. Abstr.* **17,** 533.

O'Rourke, N. A., and Fraser, S. E. (1990). *Neuron* **5,** 159–171.

O'Rourke, N. A., Dailey, M. E., Smith, S. J., and McConnell, S. K. (1991). *Soc. Neurosci. Abstr.* **17,** 533.

Sandell, J. H., and Masland, R. H. (1988). *J. Histochem. Cytochem.* **36,** 555–559.

Simon, D. K., and O'Leary, D. D. M. (1990). *Dev. Biol.* **137,** 125–134.

Simon, D. K., and O'Leary, D. D. M. (1991). *J. Comp. Neurol.* **307,** 393–404.

Snider, W. D., and Palavali, V. (1990). *J. Comp. Neurol.* **297,** 227–238.

Sretavan, D. W. (1990). *Soc. Neurosci. Abstr.* **16,** 1126.

Stuermer, C. A. O. (1988). *J. Neurosci.* **8,** 4513–4530.

Vaney, D. I. (1991). *Neurosci. Lett.* **125,** 187–190.

Vidal-Sanz, M., Villegas-Perez, M. P., Bray, G. M., and Aguayo, A. J. (1988). *Exp. Neurol.* **102,** 92–101.

# CHAPTER 13

## Three-Dimensional Confocal Light Microscopy of Neurons: Fluorescent and Reflection Stains

**James N. Turner,\*,† John W. Swann,\*,†**
**Donald H. Szarowski,\* Karen L. Smith,\***
**David O. Carpenter,\*,† and Michael Fejtl\***

\* Wadsworth Center for Laboratories and Research
New York State Department of Health
Albany, New York

† School of Public Health
University at Albany
Albany, New York

## I. Introduction

Neurons exhibit enormous variation in three-dimensional structure at the light microscopic level. Knowledge of this three-dimensional microanatomy is critical to our understanding of neuronal function, especially the relationship between cellular anatomy and neuronal network organization and function. The dendritic and axonal fields of neurons extend over large distances, making it difficult to image the extent of these structures if the specimen is prepared and examined by traditional methods. A major limitation of the standard methods is the sectioning process, which physically cuts the neurons into several sections that are thin in comparison to their lateral dimensions. Images collected from serial sections of this type can be reconstructed into a three-dimensional rendition of the object, but this procedure is often difficult. The confocal microscope is a conceptual and practical advance that makes feasible anatomical studies that are either not approachable or not practical by other means.

Confocal microscopy has two advantages over conventional microscopic image modes: first, under the right circumstances, it provides improved resolution by approximately 1.4 times, that is, structures 1.4 times smaller than the Rayleigh limit can be resolved (Brakenhoff *et al.,* 1979; Wilson and Sheppard, 1984). The second is the ability to form high signal-to-noise in-focus images by rejecting out-of-focus light from above and below the region of focus (White *et al.,* 1987). It is the second feature that is exploited in current three-dimensional studies of neurons. These confocal images are optical sections through the specimen that are "thin" by comparison to the lateral dimensions. These sections are formed nondestructively, that is, without physically cutting the specimen. A set of optical sections collected in sequence through the depth of the specimen composes a *z* series, because the *z* direction corresponds to depth in the specimen and to the optical axis of the instrument. Such a series contains three-dimensional information about the object, and can be displayed and manipulated in a number of ways.

A montage of the *z* series is the simplest display, but it is often difficult to integrate this information into a comprehensive three-dimensional image that accurately represents the object. Montages can be useful for studying high-resolution details, which can sometimes be lost in the more complex displays that utilize extensive computer manipulations. The next more sophisticated display is a simple projection of the *z* series or a subset of it. This has the effect of producing a depth of field equal to the *z* dimension of the projected set. Two projections formed with the correct offsets produce a stereo pair that can be fused by the observer into a single three-dimensional image (Boyde, 1985). This is a qualitative image that produces a good perspective of the three-dimensional structure of the object. However, the most generally useful display is a three-dimensional reconstruction, which can be viewed from any perspective with a graphics workstation (Carlsson and Liljeborg, 1989; Turner *et al.,* 1991a).

Confocal imaging, like all other types of microscopy, is highly dependent on contrast enhancement methods to increase the visibility of the details of interest relative to their surroundings. This is particularly important for neurons embedded in thick tissue slices because they are surrounded by large numbers of other cells with identical optical properties. Thus staining and specimen preparation procedures are of critical importance, and it is essential to use selective stains that label only the portion of the specimen that is of interest. This specificity can be achieved by filling a selected space with stain, by exposing the specimen to stains that chemically bind to a particular component(s), or by conjugating the stain to a lectin or antibody that binds specifically to a particular component. There are two general categories of stains used for confocal imaging applied to neurobiology: fluorescent and reflection. When using the former, the illuminating light excites a molecular transition that decays by emitting light at a wavelength longer than the incident light, and the optical system allows only the longer wavelength to be detected. The latter reflects a portion of the incident light back into the objective lens to be subsequently detected to form the image.

## A. Fluorescent Labels

The most commonly used fluorescent labels are space-filling dyes injected into neurons through a microelectrode that can also be used to perform electro-physiological measures (Carlsson and Liljeborg, 1989; Fine *et al.,* 1988; Turner *et al.,* 1991a). Lucifer yellow is most often used for this purpose as it is readily pressure or iontophoretically injected, yields high fluorescent signals, and is relatively photostable, especially in comparison to fluorescein (Stewart, 1978, 1981). For reasons of solubility, the Lucifer yellow solution is usually made from its lithium salt but, at least for some neurons, there are indications that lithium degrades their physiological state (Tseng and Haberly, 1989). We have noted that there are small differences in membrane potential and action potential height and shape. These changes are relatively small and certainly do not affect cell classification based on electrophysiological criteria (J. W. Swann and K. L. Smith, unpublished observations). Other dyes that are not similarly suspect should be investigated for this purpose, and likely candidates include Texas Red, Cascade Blue, Evans Blue, and sulforhodamine. Cascade Blue requires ultraviolet (UV) excitation, which is not available on most laser scanning confocal microscopes, but is available on disk-type instruments, because they utilize arc sources (Boyde *et al.,* 1989). Fluorescein and its various forms are generally too photolabile to be suitable.

Labeling of specific structures can be achieved by chemical partitioning of fluorescent dyes into particular subcellular components. Good examples are lipophilic dyes that are dissolved into the lipids of cell membranes. There are a variety of these dyes and some of them are at least partially selective with respect to the membranes that they label. 1,1'-Dioctadecyl-3,3,3',3'-tetramethylindocarbocyanine perchlorate (DiI) labels the plasma membranes of cells, including neurons, and diffuses over long distances, making it a good retrograde and anterograde tracer. It has been used to delineate the complex multiorgan and tissue-level innervation of the vagus nerve in rats (Berthoud *et al.,* 1990, 1991a,b). DiI can be used as a vital dye providing contrast in living specimens, allowing the growth cones of axons and migrating neurons to be recorded as a function of time (Dailey and Smith, 1991; O'Rourke *et al.*, 1991). Cultured *Aplysia* neurons have been labeled with DiI and observed to change shape as a function of the osmolarity of the medium. As many as 400 optical sections were recorded from individual neurons, which were observed by intracellular recordings to have the same membrane physiology after the imaging session as before (Turner *et al.*, 1991b; Fejtl *et al.*, 1991; Carpenter *et al.*, 1992).

Increased specificity can be achieved by tagging antibodies or lectins with fluorescent molecules and reacting them against particular molecules in the specimen. We have used concanavalin A tagged with rhodamine to contrast the membranes of cultured *Aplysia* neurons, but have found that the background of material on the substrate is much higher than for DiI (Turner *et al.*, 1991b; Carpenter *et al.*, 1992). Cytoskeletal elements can be labeled by the antibody method and monitored as a function of physiological and pharmacological parameters. Changes in glial cell shape were demonstrated to be microtubule mediated and independent of intracellular calcium (Shain *et al.*, 1992).

## B. Reflection Stains

Golgi and peroxidase are traditional neurobiology stains for selectively labeling either portions of the neuronal population or a single selected neuron. Although these stains are imaged by absorption of transmitted light by conventional microscopy, they can be used as reflection stains for confocal microscopy. Golgi-stained rat spinal cord neurons and Golgi–Cox-stained mouse cerebellum Purkinje cells have been imaged by a tandem disk scanning instrument (Boyde, 1985, 1987). Blood vessels in the cortex were imaged 100 $\mu$m below the surface of the specimen by these methods (Boyde, 1988). Freire and Boyde (1990) imaged cerebral pyramidal cells from hamster cortex with sufficient resolution to distinguish dendritic spines, and demonstrated their relationship to blood vessels.

We have imaged Golgi preparations and peroxidase-contrasted neurons from the CA3 region of the hippocampus, using a laser scanning confocal microscope. The peroxidase specimens were prepared either by injection of biocytin, which was detected with streptavidin–horseradish peroxidase (HRP) (Horikawa and Armstrong, 1988; Deitch *et al.*, 1990a), or by direct injection of HRP (Deitch *et al.*, 1990b, 1991). A distinct advantage in each case is that the axonal arborization was well filled and contrasted, and could be readily followed for long distances in all three dimensions. This is not always the case for Lucifer yellow.

The resolution and contrast of the axonal reflection images allowed single varicosities to be imaged under different preparation methods, including embedment for electron microscopy. For the latter, it was possible to locate varicosities with sufficient accuracy to section the block efficiently for transmission electron microscopy (TEM). Varicosities were readily found within a few ultrathin sections for conventional TEM or within thick (0.25 $\mu$m or greater) sections for high-voltage electron microscopy (HVEM) (Deitch *et al.*, 1991). Synapses were identified and correlated with the confocal light microscope images of axonal varicosities and dendritic expansions (Deitch *et al.*, 1991).

Several physical parameters of the specimen and microscope must be optimized to produce high-quality reflection mode images. An instrumental problem is the generation of artifactual high-intensity regions that "swamp" the image signal (Deitch *et al.*, 1990b). This artifact is produced by internal reflection from optical components, usually in the illumination path where the light intensity is high. Because the artifact is essentially constant for given illumination conditions, its effect is particularly prominent when the image signal is low. The detrimental effect of this artifact increases with depth in the specimen because the image signal decreases. However, it can be minimized or eliminated by the addition of polarization components. A quarter-wave plate is placed in both the illumination and image path, and an analyzer is positioned before the detector. This procedure has been implemented in scanning disk-type instruments (Xiao and Kino, 1987) and in laser scanning microscopes (Draaijer and Houpt, 1987; Turner *et al.*, 1990; Szarowski *et al.*, 1992). In the latter, it was shown that both the quarter-wave plate and the analyzer must be rotated to optimize the image.

When peroxidase is contrasted with diaminobenzidine (DAB) or similar molecules, a metal is often used to intensify the stain. This has the effect of increasing the reflectivity and, thereby, the image signal. Nickel is a metal commonly used for this purpose (Deitch *et al.*, 1990a,b; Szarowski *et al.*, 1992), as is osmium (Robinson and Batton, 1989, 1990).

In addition to being reflected, light is absorbed by the specimen both in the stained and unstained portions, and this can have an impact on the image. The pathlength for absorption is twice the imaging depth because the system operates in the epiillumination mode. This can result in significant signal loss, decreasing the signal-to-noise ratio and limiting the depth into the specimen at which images can be recorded. High absorption in stained structures produces shadows that can interfere with the images of structures deeper in the specimen (Deitch *et al.*, 1990b). The solutions in which the specimen is processed can deposit light-absorbing atoms or molecules in the unstained portions of the specimen. Both the illuminating beam and image signal suffer absorption as they traverse the specimen, decreasing both image signal and signal to noise. The effect of light absorption on image quality can be minimized by selecting a wavelength that has low absorption and high reflectivity from the selective stain (Deitch *et al.*, 1990b; Turner *et al.*, 1990; Szarowski *et al.*, 1992). The metals added to intensify the peroxidase–DAB reaction product shift the absorption spectra and alter the choice of wavelengths that should be used (Deitch *et al.*, 1990b).

## II. Thick Tissue Slices

Imaging neurons in the intact brain can be extremely difficult, and is limited to a thin layer at the surface. Even with the confocal microscope the detailed morphology of neurons cannot be observed beyond such superficial layers. Therefore methods to maintain thick slices of brain tissue in essentially physiological conditions have been developed. The slice can be taken from most brain regions and maintained in chambers that provide controlled temperature, nutrients, and oxygen. Individual neurons, particularly those distant from the cut surface of the slice, can be studied intact and in an environment that closely mimics their natural state (Schwartzkroin, 1975; Dingldine, 1984). Because the slices are typically 400–500 $\mu$m thick, many of the neuronal connections are preserved, and the electrophysiological activity of the cells can be monitored as a function of electrical stimuli or drugs that are applied to the perfusate (Swann and Brady, 1984).

### A. Acute Slices

In our studies, the portion of the brain anterior to the cerebellum was gently removed from the skull of 10- to 70-day-old Wistar rats, and rinsed in preoxygenated artificial cerebrospinal fluid. One hippocampus was dissected out, trimmed of adhering tissue, and cut into 500-$\mu$m thick slices, using a mechanical tissue chopper. Four to eight such slices were taken transverse to the longitudinal axis, usually from the ventral half. Slices were placed in a beaker of oxygenated cerebrospinal fluid and transferred to a nylon mesh platform in a perfusion chamber with circulating oxygenated cerebrospinal fluid at the level of the top of the slice (Schwartzkroin, 1975; Swann and Brady, 1984). The slice was allowed to equilibrate for at least 1 hr before being impaled with a 70- to 150-M$\Omega$ microelectrode containing 4 $M$ potassium acetate and 5–10% Lucifer yellow according to the procedures developed by Stewart (1978, 1981). Only cells with physiologically acceptable membrane potential ($-50$ to $-70$ mV), action potentials (50–90 mV), and input resistance (20–45 M$\Omega$) were selected for this study. Lucifer yellow was injected into the neuron by the application of hyperpolarizing current steps (0.1–0.5 nA, 100–250 msec, 1–2 Hz). The injection of the dye was monitored through a dissecting microscope equipped with an epifluorescence illuminator. When electrode placement was important a video camera was used to observe the specimen and the microelectrode. The slices were then removed from the chamber, fixed in 10% neutral buffered Formalin, dehydrated through graded ethanols, and mounted in methylsalicylate in a well slide. Confocal images were collected with a Bio-Rad (Cambridge, MA) MRC-500 or -600 mounted on an Olympus (Lake Success, NY) BH-2 microscope, using the 488-nm line of an argon ion laser.

## B. Explant Cultures

Slices of brain tissue have been maintained in culture for several weeks by the roller tube method, and neurons in these preparations demonstrate the expected electrophysiology while maintaining organotypic tissue-level anatomy (Gähwiler, 1988). However, this method is technically difficult. It requires specialized culture equipment, and is not applicable to repeated long observations requiring manipulation of the specimen outside the tube. Thus we have used the membrane method developed by Stoppini *et al.* (1991). Slices are prepared as above, but are mounted on Millicell Millipore (Bedford, MA) filters and placed in culture dishes with the culture medium level reaching but not covering the top surface of the slice. The medium used was that specified by Stoppini *et al.* (1991). Cultures were incubated at 37°C, in a $CO_2$ incubator. Crystal(s) of DiI were applied to the surface of the slice with the tip of a microelectrode and left in position for the duration of the experiment. DiI diffused into the membranes and through the axons, labeling neurons at long distances from the crystal.

The membrane method can also be used to coculture slices, and we have abutted two slices such that the CA3 region of one was in contact with the entorhinal cortex of the second. A large number of axons grew between the two slices, and DiI applied to one slice diffused to all regions of the second.

## C. Reflection Stains

The use of reflection stains based on peroxidase–DAB required modification of the above procedures. This was due to both preparation and instrumental factors. The penetration of large molecules such as avidin–HRP is slow, requiring that a detergent be added to the incubation solutions and that the slice be sectioned on a Vibratome (model 1000; Technical Products International, Polysciences, Warrington, PA). Thinner tissue slices were also required because of signal-to-noise problems encountered in the reflection imaging mode (Deitch *et al.*, 1990a,b; Szarowski *et al.*, 1992).

Thick slices of hippocampus were prepared and observed electrophysiologically as above, but were injected with either biocytin or peroxidase (Deitch *et al.*, 1990a,b, 1991). Biocytin was injected as a 5% solution in 0.5 m$M$ KCl by passing hyperpolarizing current pulses (0.1–1.0 nA for 100–500 msec at 1 Hz) for 10–20 min (Horikawa and Armstrong, 1988). Slices were allowed to equilibrate for 30–60 min before overnight fixation in 4% paraformaldehyde and 5% sucrose in 0.1 $M$ phosphate buffer, pH 7.4. Most slices were cut into serial 75- to 150-$\mu$m sections, using a Vibratome. The sections were rinsed in 0.1 $M$ phosphate-buffered saline, and the biocytin detected by incubation in avidin–HRP (diluted 1 : 200; Vector Laboratories, Burlingame, CA) for 2 hr at room temperature. Sections were then washed five times in buffer for 20 min each, followed by 15 min in DAB (0.5 mg/ml; Polysciences) with 0.01% $H_2O_2$. The latter was often intensified with 0.04% nickel ammonium sulfate. Triton X-100 (0.5%; Sigma, St. Louis, MO) was added to all the above reaction steps to increase penetration. Whole slices were also processed, but the avidin–HRP incubation was increased to 24 hr.

Because HRP is also an excellent electron microscopic stain, the fixation, dehydration, and mounting procedures were altered to optimize both confocal light microscopy and electron microscopy (Deitch *et al.*, 1990a,b, 1991). Horseradish peroxidase was pressure injected as a 5% solution in 0.5% KCl. The slices were allowed to equilibrate in the experimental chamber for 1–2 hr to allow diffusion and transport of the HRP, and were fixed in 4% paraformaldehyde and 2.5% glutaraldehyde in artificial cerebrospinal fluid at 4°C for 4 hr. Fixing the tissue in its physiological fluid was critical for the preservation of structures at the electron microscopic level (Deitch *et al.*, 1991). The slices were cut into 50- to 100-$\mu$m thick Vibratome sections, and the sections were reacted with DAB (0.5 mg/ml) in 0.13 $M$ phosphate buffer, pH 7.4, with 0.01% $H_2O_2$. Postfixation was carried out in 0.1–1% $OsO_4$ for 30–45 min, and the sections were stained *en bloc* in 2% uranyl acetate for 45 min, dehydrated in methanol series and acetone, and flat embedded in Maraglass between two glass microscope slides coated with dimethyldichlorosilane (Sigma). After curing, one slide was removed, and the specimen examined by confocal light microscopy. The entire neuron could be imaged, and areas identified, cut out, mounted on plastic stubs, and sectioned on an ultramicrotome for electron microscopic observation.

If only light microscopy is to be performed, the $OsO_4$ and uranyl acetate are omitted, and the slice is dehydrated and mounted in the same way as for the Lucifer yellow-injected slices above. Confocal imaging was performed on a Bio-Rad MRC-500 or -600 [with the modifications described in Szarowski *et al.* (1992) and Turner *et al.* (1990)] mounted on an Olympus BH-2 microscope. These include the use of polarization components and a helium–neon laser to optimize image signal to noise, and digital subtraction methods for enhancing the images.

## D. Cellular and Local Neuronal Network Microanatomy

Neurons with the same or similar electrophysiology often have different three-dimensional shapes and interrelationships with other neurons (Turner *et al.*, 1991). The neuron in Fig. 1 is a simple pyramidal cell from the CA3 region of the rat hippocampus. The soma is nearly spherical with a large and long primary apical dendrite. The higher order apical dendrites are simple, forming only two branching structures. Several primary basilar dendrites originate independently from the basilar surface of the soma. Again, they have a simple distribution projecting into a roughly conical volume with few branches. The initial segment of the axon, indicated by the arrow in the basilar dendrites, is seen projecting through these dendrites before branching. One branch projects back through the

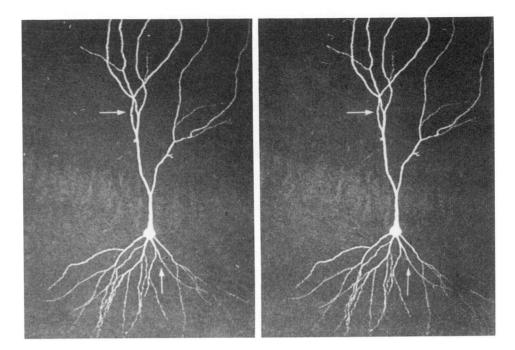

**Fig. 1** A simple pyramidal neuron in a 500-$\mu$m slice that was injected with Lucifer yellow. The pyramidal cell layer runs roughly left to right in line with the cell soma. Apical dendrites project toward the top of the figure and basilar dendrites toward the bottom. The arrow in the apical dendrites indicates the region of Fig. 6a, and the one in the basilar dendrites denotes the initial segment of the axon. The image was collected with a $\times 20$ NA 0.8 oil objective lens, is 115 $\mu$m in the $z$ direction, and is projected with Bio-Rad software run on a PC. The field width is 316 $\mu$m. [Reproduced with permission from Turner *et al.* (1991a). *J. Electron Microsc. Tech.* **18**, 11–23.]

dendrites in the apical direction but on the opposite side of the soma from the initial branching point.

Figure 2 is also a pyramidal neuron from the CA3 region of the rat hippocampus and illustrates the variability in the three-dimensional shape of this cell. This cell is more complex than that in Fig. 1, with a larger soma, but is in the same position relative to the pyramidal cell layer. The primary apical dendrite is shorter, with multiple branchings close to the cell soma, but the apical dendrites are still made up of a few large projections with only a small number of branches. The basilar dendritic field is fairly complex, with a large number of fine dendrites originating from the basilar portion of the double soma as opposed to the widely separated and distinct origin of the basilar dendrites of the neuron in Fig. 1. The initial segment of the axon arises from the most basilar point of the soma, projecting toward the lower left. It branches at a point about one-third the way

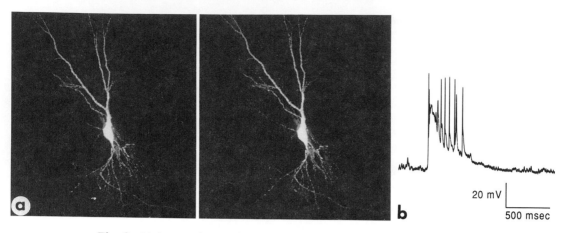

**Fig. 2** (a) A stereo image of a Lucifer yellow-injected pyramidal neuron in a 500-$\mu$m thick slice. The apical dendrites are toward the top and the basilar toward the bottom. The pyramidal cell layer runs horizontally at the level of the soma. The initial segment of the axon and several apical and basilar branches are clearly seen. The reconstruction was volume rendered with the Analyze software system from the Mayo Clinic, running on an IBM RISC 6000 graphics workstation. The image was collected with a $\times$20 NA 0.8 oil objective lens. The image is 86 $\mu$m in the $z$ direction, and the width of field is 316 $\mu$m. (b) An intracellular recording from the cell soma.

through the dendritic field, sending projections in the apical and basilar directions. Both segments branch with projections leaving the field of the image.

We have injected over 200 neurons in thick hippocampal slices with Lucifer yellow, and found at least 35% are dye coupled to one or as many as five other neurons, that is, dye injected into one cell appears to be transported selectively to other neurons. The dye-coupled neurons are usually pyramidal cells, but we have also observed the phenomenon in interneurons (Turner *et al.*, 1991; Deitch *et al.*, 1990a). Other workers have reported similar dye coupling with fluorescent dyes (Andrew *et al.*, 1982; MacVicar and Dudek, 1980), and we have observed it for biocytin injections (Deitch *et al.*, 1990a). Whether dye coupling is a reflection of electrotonic coupling or not is somewhat controversial. Some workers attribute the phenomenon to dye leakage from the microelectrode that is taken up by cut ends of dendrites or axons. Although this is a possibility, in our experience it does not appear to be the case. In every instance in which we observed dye coupling, the coupled cells had dendrites that were in contact, at least within the resolution limits of our confocal microscope. We never observed a secondarily filled cell that did not have such a relationship to the impaled neuron. Finally, some dye-coupled cells were known to be in regions never penetrated by the microelectrode and they had no visible projections into the region of the electrode track. These are of course circumstantial arguments, but they have the weight of a large number of observations behind them.

The only way to verify or refute this phenomenon is to observe the potential contact points by electron microscopy. Correlative techniques using the confocal microscope to localize small structures that are subsequently observed by electron microscopy have been reported (Deitch *et al.*, 1991), providing the methodology to approach the question.

A group of three dye-coupled pyramidal neurons is shown in Fig. 3a. The neuron on the right has a triangular soma with the basilar dendrites projecting mainly from the two lower corners, and with simple apical dendrites branching from the primary. The neuron on the left has a small soma and small dendritic fields. The apical field is composed of a long primary dendrite with few branches projecting between the two second-order apical dendrites of the center neuron. The center and left neurons have a hillock-like area from which the basilar dendrites project, and each has what appears to be dendrites projecting from the center of the soma. The left cell has a fine projection from the center of the left side of the soma and the center cell has two originating near each other from the center right of its soma. There are two potential contact sites between the left and center neurons in the apical dendrites and these are shown in the optical sections (Fig. 3b and c, indicated by arrows). These areas are seen in three dimensions in Fig. 3a, as are a number of potential sites in the basilar dendrites, marked by arrowheads. The latter sites are more difficult to display as they each involve fine processes. Similarly, there are several potential sites in the apical and basilar dendrites of the center and right neurons. Individual optical sections are a powerful way to study detailed regions within the three-dimensional shape that is displayed in a more general format in the stereo image. Any questions of interpretation should always be confirmed with the optical sections as they form the basic data set and have the highest image resolution and contrast, especially in the $z$ direction.

Explant slices are an excellent way to study alterations in neuronal function and three-dimensional structure, especially over a long period of time. Figure 4a is a montage of DiI-labeled regions of two cocultured explants. The two slices were maintained in culture for 2 weeks such that the CA1 region of the top slice was in contact with the entorhinal cortex of the bottom slice. The DiI was applied to the bottom slice in the CA1 subfield 2 days before observation in the confocal microscope. A large number of axons projected between the slices during the culture period and can be observed as individual projections or as large tracts. The dye labeled a number of neurons at large distances from the application site (as far as 2 mm). The nonpyramidal neuron of Fig. 4b was such a cell located in the CA3 region near the arrow in Fig. 4a. This neuron, although located in the pyramidal cell layer, does not display typical pyramidal cell morphology, and is probably best classified as a basket cell. Its dendritic fields are different from those of the neurons in Figs. 1–3. This cell is not as highly polarized, as the dendrites are more distributed in space with little difference between what might be considered the apical and basilar projections. A large

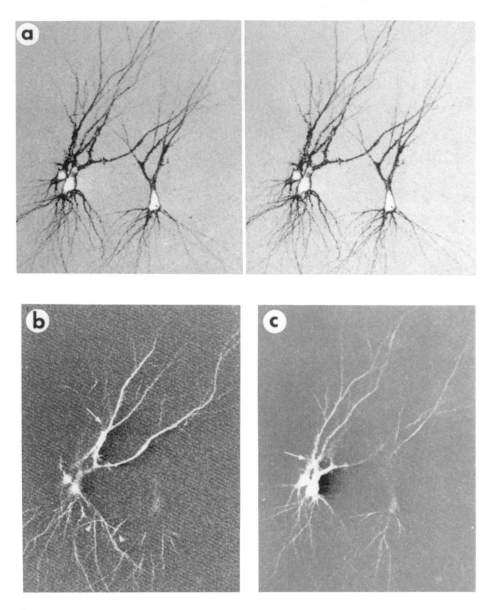

**Fig. 3** (a) A stereo image of a group of dye-coupled Lucifer yellow-injected pyramidal neurons. All the soma lie in the pyramidal cell layer with apical dendrites projecting to the top and basilar dendrites to the bottom. The image is 84 $\mu$m in the $z$ direction. (b) and (c) Optical sections showing potential contact points, indicated by arrows, between the dendrites of the center and left neurons in (a). The arrowheads indicate potential contact points between the basilar dendrites of the right and center neurons. They are, respectively, 36 and 44 $\mu$m below the surface of the slice. All images were collected with a $\times$20 NA 0.8 oil objective lens, and the field width is 316 $\mu$m. The image in (a) was reconstructed with Analyze from the Mayo clinic, and (b) and (c) were projected with VoxelView from Vital Images. Both were run on an IBM RISC 6000 graphics workstation.

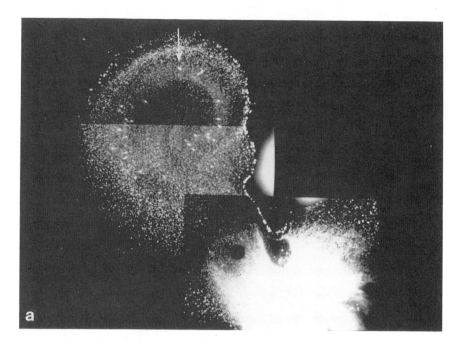

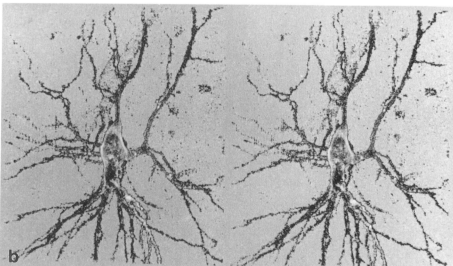

**Fig. 4** (a) A montage of projection images of two explants labeled with DiI. The bright area (*bottom* right) is the site of application of the DiI and a tract of axons is seen projecting from the top center of this area into the upper slice. The "larger dots" of intensity in the top slice are neurons that have been labeled with DiI. The three images forming the montage were recorded at different gain settings because of the large differences in signal level from the various regions. The images were recorded with a ×4 NA 0.13 objective lens. These were collected with the pinhole wide open and no change in $z$. (b) The neuron indicated by the arrow in (a), imaged at higher magnification and reconstructed with the Analyze software package from the Mayo Clinic, running on an IBM RISC 6000 graphics workstation. The optical sections were collected with a ×40 NA 1.0 objective lens over a distance of 52 $\mu$m in the $z$ direction.

primary dendrite arises from the lateral surface and others arise from the center of the somal surface away from the observer in Fig. 4b.

The images of neurons stained with DiI are different from those stained with Lucifer yellow. DiI images are primarily formed from information arising from the surface membrane, and therefore appear as images of the cell surface with nearly equal signal levels throughout the image. This effect is strengthened by the fact that the dye is sequestered in structures having thicknesses much smaller than the depth of field of any objective lens. On the other hand, images formed from space-filling dyes arise from volumes that often are equal to the depth of field for a given pixel. Thus the images appear as volumes that have a wide range of signal levels. The signal can vary from the noise level to the saturation level of the system, and this effect can be enhanced by the uneven distribution of the dye. The signal range can be unmanageable, especially for projection images of the cell soma and large dendrites, because they nearly always saturate the system.

Interneurons are frequently found near the pyramidal cell layer in the hippocampus. They are smaller and have a simpler morphology than the pyramidal neurons. An example of an interneuron filled with biocytin and contrasted with peroxidase–DAB is shown in Fig. 5. It was imaged as described above for reflection stains. The soma is triangular shaped, with a primary dendrite projecting from each apex. The fine projection arising from the soma near the origin of the lower dendrite is probably also a dendrite. Another projection arises from the center of the soma and is directed toward the observer in the stereo pair. This is interpreted to be the initial segment of the axon, but because it leaves the section before branching it cannot definitively be distinguished from a dendrite. This projection arises from the surface directly over the nucleus, which appears as a hole in the soma because the dye does not penetrate it. The other fine projections in this image are from a pyramidal cell with which the interneuron is dye coupled. Biocytin is sufficiently small to pass between cells (Deitch *et al.*, 1990a, 1991).

## E. Axonal and Dendritic Microanatomy

Confocal microscopy is an excellent method to study the three-dimensional distribution and interrelationship of dendrites and axons. A qualitative impression of the density and extent of the projections is easily obtained, as is their interrelationship to each other and to those of other stained neurons in the field (Berthoud *et al.*, 1990, 1991a,b; Deitch *et al.*, 1990a; Turner *et al.*, 1991a). Computer tracing methods can be used to enhance low signal-to-noise images and display dendritic and axonal fields with high contrast and, if desired, in pseudocolor. These techniques allow the reconstructed images to be rotated for viewing from any perspective and to be processed to selectively display either the dendrites or the axon (Turner *et al.*, 1991a).

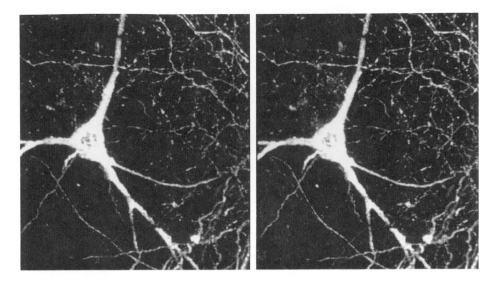

**Fig. 5** A stereo image of an interneuron filled with biocytin and contrasted with HRP–diaminobenzidine. The three primary dendrites arise from the apices of the triangular shaped soma, while a small fourth one projects upward from the center of the soma. The thin, smooth projection originating near the root of the lower primary dendrite and curving away toward the center right of the field is probably the axon. The image was collected with a ×40 NA 1.3 oil objective lens and reconstructed with the Analyze software package running on an IBM RISC 6000 graphics workstation. The $z$ excursion of the image is 19 $\mu$m, and the field width is 150 $\mu$m.

A critical area of application of the confocal microscope is the field of dendritic physiology. Previous electrophysiological studies have impaled dendrites by monitoring recordings in regions of brain tissue known to be rich in dendrites and having few cells. However, these blind impalements cannot be correlated with morphology. The confocal microscope provides the means to make this correlation with sufficient accuracy to determine not only whether a dendrite or small neuron is impaled but also to determine the order of impaled dendrites (Smith *et al.*, 1990; Turner *et al.*, 1991a). A high-magnification image of a portion of the apical dendrites of the pyramidal neuron in Fig. 1 is shown in Fig. 6a. The trace in Fig. 6b was recorded from the third-order dendrite at the site indicated by the arrow. The seizure-like physiological activity demonstrated by the repeating pattern of bursts (afterdischarges) is the result of orthodromic stimulation and bath application of 50 $\mu M$ picrotoxin. The ability of the confocal microscope to accurately locate the site of impalement of the microelectrode allows direct and detailed correlation of dendritic physiology and morphology (Smith *et al.*, 1990; Turner *et al.*, 1991a). Previous studies of dendritic physiology were limited because it was not possible to tell with certainty the location of the recording site. Imaging in three dimensions at high spatial resolution and contrasts has removed these limitations.

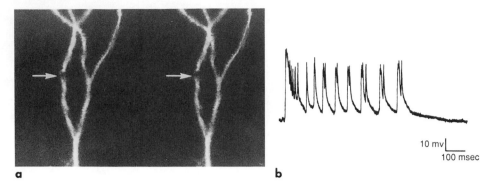

a                                                      b

**Fig. 6** A stereo image of a portion of the apical dendrites indicated by the arrow in Fig. 1. The arrows in Fig. 1 and here indicate the site of impalement of the microelectrode that recorded the trace in (b), showing seizure-like physiological activity in this third-order dendrite. Dendritic spines are seen on the shaft segment in the upper left and on the shaft furthest to the right above the second branch point. The image was recorded with a ×60 NA 1.4 oil objective lens and a ×2 electronic zoom. The $z$ excursion of the image is 15 $\mu$m and the field width is 53 $\mu$m. [Reproduced with permission from Turner *et al.* (1991a). *J. Electron Microsc. Tech.* **18**, 11–23.]

The apical dendrites from three dye-coupled pyramidal neurons are shown in Fig. 7. The three cells were close to each other and their dendrites are intertwined. Three primary dendrites are seen to enter the field at the bottom. Each arises from a different cell, all of which are dye coupled, and each branches multiple times within the volume represented by this stereo pair. The higher-order dendrites form such a complex and intertwined distribution that it is difficult or impossible to determine by stereo viewing which dendrites belong to which neuron. A three-dimensional reconstruction or computer tracing analysis could be used to separate the three populations of dendritic branches (Turner *et al.*, 1991a). Most of the dendrites take a smooth path through the tissue, but some have a sharply corrugated course. It is our opinion that this corrugated structure is an artifact (Turner *et al.*, 1991a). In our experience, such structures increase in severity and frequency when the fixation is questionable. The comparison of images from the same fields in living and fixed slices is expected to help clarify this interpretation.

A stereo image of the basilar dendrites and initial axonal segment from a pyramidal neuron is shown in Fig. 8. The axon is easily distinguished as the smooth projection that is initially thicker than the dendrites shown. It curves first to the right edge of the field and then back toward the center, where it branches to the left and right in a Y shape, and the branches are a smaller caliber than the initial segment. The dendrites have a coarse, irregular structure that undoubtedly represents the spines.

A careful inspection of the fields in Figs. 7 and 8 shows that accurate quantitation of dendritic structure at the level of the number, order, and density of

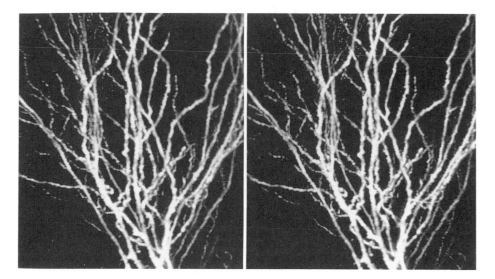

**Fig. 7** A stereo image of the apical dendrites from three dye-coupled pyramidal neurons. The primary dendrites start at the bottom of the field; the somas are below the image. The shaft furthest to the right is a small primary arising from a neuron with a small soma. The two central (and thicker) shafts are the primaries from two other neurons. The image was collected with a ×40 NA 1.0 oil objective lens. The image is 100 $\mu$m along the $z$ direction and the field width is 150 $\mu$m.

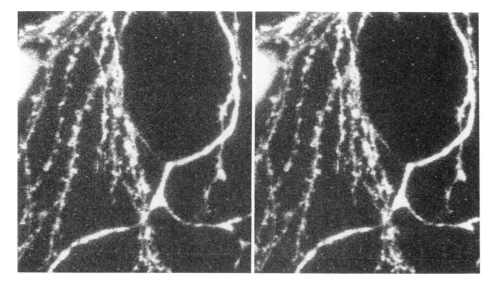

**Fig. 8** A stereo image of the basilar dendrites and axon of a pyramidal neuron. The cell soma is above the field of image. The image was collected with a ×60 NA 1.4 oil objective lens and an electronic zoom of ×3. The $z$ excursion of this image is 50 $\mu$m, and the field width is 33 $\mu$m.

branches is relatively easy, especially with the aid of the appropriate computer support. However, quantitation of fine structure such as dendritic surface area or the number and density of spines is of questionable accuracy. A complication, readily seen in both Figs. 7 and 8, is the uneven distribution of dye. It appears that the dye either is not transported uniformly or, more likely, is excluded by internal structures. In either case, the result is an uneven image of what we have every reason to believe is an even structure. The interpretation of boutons, varicosities, and dendritic thickenings should be approached with caution if their size is near the resolution limit of the light microscope.

## III. Cultured Neurons

It is sometimes an advantage to observe cells in culture rather than in tissue. Individual cells can be easily identified and studied as a function of any number of physiological parameters and time. We are using cultured neurons from *Aplysia* to study physiological and neurotoxic phenomena and to correlate electrophysiology and three-dimensional shape.

Neurons were isolated from all major ganglia of juvenile *Aplysia californica* (10–15 g). After dissection, the ganglia were treated with artificial seawater (ASW) containing 20% sucrose and 0.05% collagenase (Sigma type I) for 30 min, and pinned down to a Sylard 184 (Dow Corning, Midland, MI)-coated culture dish. Connective tissue was removed and the ganglia desheathed with a fine razor blade in the presence of 0.05% DNase (Sigma type 1A). Neurons were mechanically dissociated by trituration with a fire-polished Pasteur pipette, plated in 3.5-cm Falcon culture dishes on poly-L-lysine-coated coverslips, and fed with modified L-15 medium (3 ml/dish) containing 20% *Aplysia* hemolymph. The medium was adjusted to an osmolarity of 1100 mOsm and one-third of the medium was replaced every second day. Cultures were maintained at 22°C.

The health of the cells was gauged by the outgrowth of neurites and the presence of growth cones, which appeared within 2 hr and reached a peak at days 3–4. The cells remained viable for at least 1 week when checked electrophysiologically. Cells typically had resting membrane potentials between $-35$ and $-40$ mV for the smaller neurons and between $-50$ and $-65$ mV for neurons $>100\ \mu m$, and elicited action potentials spontaneously or on a depolarizing test pulse (150 pA for 150 msec). They also showed rebound excitation after similar hyperpolarizing pulses due to the removal of $Na^+$ inactivation (Fejtl *et al.*, 1991; Turner *et al.*, 1991b; Carpenter *et al.*, 1992).

Neurons were stained with either DiI or rhodamine-conjugated lectins. The lectins appeared to stain large amounts of extraneous material, producing some unrepresentative staining patterns and high background areas. DiI appeared to stain the cell surface membrane uniformly and produced a clean outline of the neuron, including its processes. Stock solutions of DiI (1 m$M$) and Pluronic F-127 (20%; Molecular Probes, Eugene, OR) were prepared in dimethylsulfoxide (DMSO). Ten microliters of the stock solution and 10 $\mu$l of Pluronic F-127 were premixed in 3 ml of ASW, resulting in a final concentration of about 0.7% DMSO. This staining solution was applied to the cultures for 1 hr. Stained neurons were observed on an Olympus BH-2 microscope with a modified stage and a Bio-Rad MRC-600 confocal imaging system, using an argon ion laser. The standard Bio-Rad filter set for rhodamine was used.

Neuronal input resistance was measured according to two protocols. The first applied discrete current steps at various membrane potentials measuring the input resistance at each (Fejtl *et al.*, 1991; Carpenter *et al.*, 1992). The second held the membrane potential at its resting level throughout the experiment and hyperpolarizing current pulses (100 pA–1 nA; 150 msec–2 sec) were applied every 5 sec. Care was taken to apply the proper stimulus strength according to the capacitative and resistive properties of the cell membrane.

Neurons swelled or shrank appropriately after exposure to hypo- or hyperosmotic medium, with a larger change associated with the hypoosmotic conditions. In both cases, the neurons returned to their original size and shape on reintroducing the control medium. The cells were never observed to autoregulate, that is, their size remained changed independent of the length of time they were observed at the altered osmotic conditions. Neurons were observed electrophysiologically before and after confocal imaging, which was carried out while the cells were subjected to changes in osmolarity. After recording as many as 450 optical sections, the cells had the same membrane potential, displayed action potentials, and had similar electrophysiological properties in response to hyper- and depolarizing current pulses (Turner *et al.*, 1991b). Thus the membrane physiology was not altered by the dye or the confocal imaging.

Figure 9 shows the effect of a 10% and a 30% hypertonic shock (normal ASW to which sucrose was added). The neuron shrank, reducing its projected diameter by only a small amount in the 10% hyperosmotic medium, with the expected decrease in membrane conductance. However, when 30% hyperosmotic medium was applied, the projected diameter decreased by 10% and the membrane conductance increased. This is a reproducible but unexpected and unexplained result. Figure 10 shows electrophysiological recordings from a cultured *Aplysia* neuron. The neuron is electrically excitable on switching off a hyperpolarizing current pulse (Fig. 10a), and shows reasonable resistive and capacitative properties (Fig. 10b). On changing the perfusion solution from normal ASW to 30% hypertonic ASW (Fig. 10c) the cell depolarized slightly, and resistance fell to about 50% of control. With the return to control ASW there was a slight hyperpolarization, and an increase in resistance (Fig. 10d). Although the cause of the resistance changes is unclear, the resting potential of about $-40$ mV and the presence of action potentials demonstrate a normally functioning neuron.

The electrophysiological response of the neurons could not be confirmed directly during observation, but was verified by performing electrophysiological measures before and after imaging. Resting potentials and action potentials were documented as above and the neurons transferred to the confocal microscope,

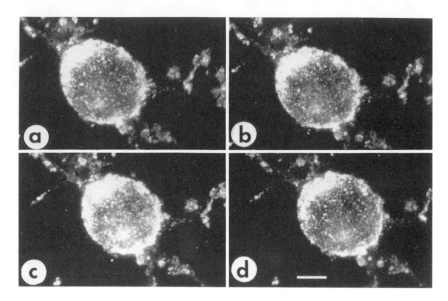

**Fig. 9** Projection images of a cultured *Aplysia* neuron under different osmotic conditions. (a) The control, that is, the cell is in ASW. (b) The change after equilibration in 10% hyperosmotic medium. The reduction in size is reproducible but minimal. (c) The change after equilibration in 30% hyperosmotic medium. The reduction in projected diameter is 10%. (d) The cell after its return to control medium. Images were collected with a ×40 NA 0.5 objective lens. Each image is a projection of 25 optical sections recorded at 2-$\mu$m intervals in the $z$ direction. Bar = 25 $\mu$m. Image projections were formed with Bio-Rad software running on a PC.

where as many as 400 optical sections were recorded. After the imaging session, the neurons were returned to the electrophysiology set-up and the same parameters measured. The observations before and after were identical within experimental error. Neurons also changed shape reversibly and demonstrated the same physiology as a function of osmotic changes in the medium (Turner *et al.*, 1991b; Fejtl *et al.*, 1991; Carpenter *et al.*, 1992).

We have demonstrated that it is possible to form three-dimensional images of living neurons in culture without perturbing the electrical properties of their plasma membrane. The ability to correlate the electrophysiological measures and the three-dimensional shape, including accurate determination of the volume of living cells, has been indirectly demonstrated. Further work in this area will concentrate on performing the three-dimensional imaging and electrophysiology on an integrated microscopy and physiology workstation that has been constructed.

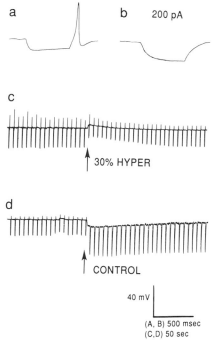

**Fig. 10** Electrophysiological recordings from the neuron illustrated in Fig. 9. (a) The neuron is electrically excitable on switching off of a hyperpolarizing pulse. (b) The effect of applying a hyperpolarizing pulse of 200 pA for 500 msec; the resistive and capacitative properties of the neuron are demonstrated. (c and d) The effects of changing the perfusing solution from normal ASW to 30% hypertonic ASW (added sucrose) at slower speed (50 sec), and return to control. The negative deflections are pulses like those in (b) recorded at slower sweep, in order to monitor membrane resistance. The arrow indicates when the 30% hyperosmotic medium was applied or replaced by normal ASW. Note the reversible increase in membrane conductance.

## Acknowledgments

This work was partially supported by U.S. Public Health Service Grants RR02984, RR06904, and RR01219 awarded by the National Center for Research Resources supporting the Confocal Light Microscope Facility and the Biological Microscopy and Image Reconstruction Resource, and NSF DIR9108492 from the Division of Instrumentation and Instrument Development and Neurobiology. Additional support was derived from PHS Grants NS 18309, AI18997, and ES05203; and from the Austrian Science Foundation, "Erwin Schrödinger Fellowship," Project J-0607.

## References

Andrew, R. D., Taylor, C. P., Snow, R. W., and Dudek, F. E. (1982). *Brain Res. Bull.* **8,** 211–222.
Berthoud, H. R., Jedrzejewska, A., and Powley, T. L. (1990). *J. Comp. Neurol.* **301,** 65–79.
Berthoud, H. R., Carlson, N. R., and Powley, T. L. (1991a). *Am. J. Physiol.* **260,** R200–R207.

Berthoud, H. R., Fox, E. A., and Powley, T. L. (1991b). *Gastroenterology* **100,** 627–637.

Boyde, A. (1985). *Science* **230,** 1270–1272.

Boyde, A. (1987). *J. Microsc. (Oxford)* **146,** 137–142.

Boyde, A. (1988). *Scanning* **11,** 147–152.

Boyde, A., Xiao, G. Q., Corle, T., Watson, T. F., and Kino, G. S. (1989). *Scanning* **12,** 273–279.

Brakenhoff, G. J., Plom, P., and Barends, P. (1979). *J. Microsc. (Oxford)* **117,** 219–232.

Carlsson, K., and Liljeborg, A. (1989). *J. Microsc. (Oxford)* **153,** 171–180.

Carpenter, D. O., Fejtl, M., Ayrapetyan, S. N., Szarowski, D. H., and Turner, J. N. (1992). *Acta Biol. Hung.* **43** (1–4), 39–48.

Dailey, M. E., and Smith, S. J. (1991). *Soc. Neurosci. Abstr.* **17,** 212.6

Deitch, J. S., Smith, K. L., Lee, C. L., Swann, J. W., and Turner, J. N. (1990a). *J. Neurosci. Methods* **33,** 61–76.

Deitch, J. S., Smith, K. L., Swann, J. W., and Turner, J. N. (1990b). *J. Microsc. (Oxford)* **160,** 265–278.

Deitch, J. S., Smith, K. L., Swann, J. W., and Turner, J. N. (1991). *J. Electron Microsc. Tech.* **18,** 82–90.

Dingldine, R., ed. (1984). "Brain Slices." Plenum, New York.

Draaijer, J. S., and Houpt, P. M. (1987). *Proc. Soc. Photo-Opt. Instrum. Eng.* **809,** 85–88.

Fejtl, M., Szarowski, D. H., Ayrapetyan, S. N., Turner, J. N., and Carpenter, D. O. (1991). *Proc. IBRO World Congr. Neurosci. 3rd, Montreal* pp. P5–P15.

Fine, A., Amos, W. B., Durbin, R. M., and McNaughton, P. A. (1988). *Trends Neurosci.* **11,** 346–351.

Freire, M., and Boyde, A. (1990). *J. Microsc. (Oxford)* **158,** 285–290.

Gähwiler, B. H. (1988). *TINS* **11,** 484–490.

Horikawa, K., and Armstrong, W. E. (1988). *J. Neurosci. Methods* **25,** 1–11.

MacVicar, B. A., and Dudek, F. E. (1980). *Brain Res.* **196,** 494–497.

O'Rourke, N. A., Dailey, M. E., Smith, S. J., and McConnell, S. K. (1991). *Soc. Neurosci. Abstr.* **17,** 212.8.

Robinson, J. M., and Batton, B. E. (1989). *J. Histochem. Cytochem.* **37,** 1761–1765.

Robinson, J. M., and Batton, B. E. (1990). *J. Histochem. Cytochem.* **38,** 315–318.

Schwartzkroin, P. A. (1975). *Brain Res.* **85,** 423–426.

Shain, W. G., Bausback, D., Fiero, A., Madelian, V., and Turner, J. N. (1992). *Glia* **5,** 223–238.

Smith, K. L., Turner, J. N., Szarowski, D. H., and Swann, J. W. (1990). *Soc. Neurosci. Abstr.* **16,** 57.

Stewart, W. W. (1978). *Cell* **14,** 741–759.

Stewart, W. W. (1981). *Nature (London)* **292,** 17–21.

Stoppini, L., Buchs, P. A., and Muller, D. (1991). *J. Neurosci. Methods* **37,** 173–182.

Swann, J. W., and Brady, R. J. (1984). *Dev. Brain Res.* **12,** 243–254.

Szarowski, D. H., Smith, K. L., Herchenroder, A., Matuszek, G., Swann, J. W., and Turner, J. N. (1992). *Scanning* **14,** 104–111.

Tseng, G. F., and Haberly, L. B. (1989). *J. Neurophysiol.* **62,** 369–385.

Turner, J. N., Szarowski, D. H., Deitch, J. S., Smith, K. L., and Swann, J. W. (1990). *Proc. Int. Congr. Electron Microsc., 12th* **3,** 152–153.

Turner, J. N., Szarowski, D. H., Smith, K. L., Marko, M., Leith, A., and Swann, J. W. (1991a). *J. Electron Microsc. Tech.* **18,** 11–23.

Turner, J. N., Szarowski, D. H., Fejtl, M., Ayrapetyan, S. N., and Carpenter, D. O. (1991b). *Proc. Annu. Meet. Electron Microsc. Soc. Am., 49th,* pp. 400–401.

White, J. G., Amos, W. B., and Fordham, M. (1987). *J. Cell Biol.* **105,** 41–48.

Wilson, T., and Sheppard, C. J. R. (1984). "Theory and Practice of Scanning Optical Microscopy." Academic Press, Orlando, Florida.

Xiao, G. Q., and Kino, G. S. (1987). *Proc. Soc. Photo-Opt. Instrum. Eng.* **809,** 107–113.

# INDEX

# VOLUMES IN SERIES

**Founding Series Editor**
**DAVID M. PRESCOTT**

**Volume 1 (1964)**
**Methods in Cell Physiology**
*Edited by David M. Prescott*

**Volume 2 (1966)**
**Methods in Cell Physiology**
*Edited by David M. Prescott*

**Volume 3 (1968)**
**Methods in Cell Physiology**
*Edited by David M. Prescott*

**Volume 4 (1970)**
**Methods in Cell Physiology**
*Edited by David M. Prescott*

**Volume 5 (1972)**
**Methods in Cell Physiology**
*Edited by David M. Prescott*

**Volume 6 (1973)**
**Methods in Cell Physiology**
*Edited by David M. Prescott*

**Volume 7 (1973)**
**Methods in Cell Biology**
*Edited by David M. Prescott*

**Volume 8 (1974)**
**Methods in Cell Biology**
*Edited by David M. Prescott*

**Volume 9 (1975)**
**Methods in Cell Biology**
*Edited by David M. Prescott*

**Volume 10 (1975)**
**Methods in Cell Biology**
*Edited by David M. Prescott*

**Volume 11 (1975)**
**Yeast Cells**
*Edited by David M. Prescott*

**Volume 12 (1975)**
**Yeast Cells**
*Edited by David M. Prescott*

**Volume 13 (1976)**
**Methods in Cell Biology**
*Edited by David M. Prescott*

**Volume 14 (1976)**
**Methods in Cell Biology**
*Edited by David M. Prescott*

**Volume 15 (1977)**
**Methods in Cell Biology**
*Edited by David M. Prescott*

**Volume 16 (1977)**
**Chromatin and Chromosomal Protein Research I**
*Edited by Gary Stein, Janet Stein, and Lewis J. Kleinsmith*

**Volume 17 (1978)**
**Chromatin and Chromosomal Protein Research II**
*Edited by Gary Stein, Janet Stein, and Lewis J. Kleinsmith*

**Volume 18 (1978)**
**Chromatin and Chromosomal Protein Research III**
*Edited by Gary Stein, Janet Stein, and Lewis J. Kleinsmith*

**Volume 19 (1978)**
**Chromatin and Chromosomal Protein Research IV**
*Edited by Gary Stein, Janet Stein, and Lewis J. Kleinsmith*

**Volume 20 (1978)**
**Methods in Cell Biology**
*Edited by David M. Prescott*

## Advisory Board Chairman
## KEITH R. PORTER

**Volume 21A (1980)**
**Normal Human Tissue and Cell Culture, Part A: Respiratory, Cardiovascular, and Integumentary Systems**
*Edited by Curtis C. Harris, Benjamin F. Trump, and Gary D. Stoner*

Volume 21B (1980)
**Normal Human Tissue and Cell Culture, Part B: Endocrine, Urogenital, and Gastrointestinal Systems**
*Edited by Curtis C. Harris, Benjamin F. Trump, and Gary D. Stoner*

Volume 22 (1981)
**Three-Dimensional Ultrastructure in Biology**
*Edited by James N. Turner*

Volume 23 (1981)
**Basic Mechanisms of Cellular Secretion**
*Edited by Arthur R. Hand and Constance Oliver*

Volume 24 (1982)
**The Cytoskeleton, Part A: Cytoskeletal Proteins, Isolation and Characterization**
*Edited by Leslie Wilson*

Volume 25 (1982)
**The Cytoskeleton, Part B: Biological Systems and *in Vitro* Models**
*Edited by Leslie Wilson*

Volume 26 (1982)
**Prenatal Diagnosis: Cell Biological Approaches**
*Edited by Samuel A. Latt and Gretchen J. Darlington*

Series Editor
**LESLIE WILSON**

Volume 27 (1986)
**Echinoderm Gametes and Embryos**
*Edited by Thomas E. Schroeder*

Volume 28 (1987)
***Dictyostelium discoideum:* Molecular Approaches to Cell Biology**
*Edited by James A. Spudich*

Volume 29 (1989)
**Fluorescence Microscopy of Living Cells in Culture, Part A: Fluorescent Analogs, Labeling Cells, and Basic Microscopy**
*Edited by Yu-Li Wang and D. Lansing Taylor*

Volume 30 (1989)
**Fluorescence Microscopy of Living Cells in Culture, Part B: Quantitative Fluorescence Microscopy—Imaging and Spectroscopy**
*Edited by D. Lansing Taylor and Yu-Li Wang*